THE ULTIMATE
Women's Guide to
Beating Disease
AND LIVING A HAPPY, ACTIVE LIFE
2017

FROM THE EDITORS OF BOTTOM LINE HEALTH

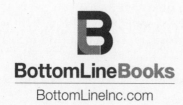

BottomLineBooks

BottomLineInc.com

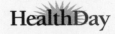

A selection of articles in this book were written by reporters for HealthDay, an award-winning international
daily consumer health news service, headquartered in Norwalk, Connecticut.

Bottom Line Books® publishes the advice of expert authorities in many fields. These opinions
may at times conflict as there are often different approaches to solving problems. The use
of a book is not a substitute for legal, accounting, investment, health or any other professional
services. Consult competent professionals for answers to your specific questions.

Offers, prices, rates, addresses, telephone numbers and websites
listed in this book are accurate at the time of publication,
but they are subject to frequent change.

Bottom Line Books® is a registered trademark of Bottom Line Inc.
3 Landmark Square, Suite 201, Stamford, CT 06901

www.BottomLineInc.com

Bottom Line Books is an imprint of Bottom Line Inc., publisher of print periodicals,
e-letters and books. We are dedicated to bringing you the best information from the most
knowledgeable sources in the world. Our goal is to help you gain greater wealth,
better health, more wisdom, extra time and increased happiness.

Printed in the United States of America

CONTENTS

Contents

3 • STROKE: RISKS, SYMPTOMS, AND SECRETS TO RECOVERY

4 • LUNG HEALTH AND ALLERGIES

Contents

APPENDICES

Appendix 4 • VERY PERSONAL

PREFACE

We are proud to bring to you *The Ultimate Women's Guide to Beating Disease and Living a Happy, Active Life 2017*. This essential volume features trustworthy and actionable life-saving information from the best health experts in the world—information that will help women beat the conditions that are most deadly to them.* In the following chapters, you'll find the latest discoveries, best treatments and scientifically proven remedies to keep you living a long, happy and active life.

Whether it's heart care, the latest on stroke, breast cancer prevention and treatment, breakthrough treatments for hot flashes or cutting-edge nutritional advice, the editors of *Bottom Line Health* talk to the experts—from top women's health doctors to research scientists to leading alternative care practitioners—who are creating the true innovations in health care.

In this 2017 Edition, we've gone beyond diseases and have included two chapters and an appendix of life-enhancing health information on pain, depression, fitness, diet, quality medical care, sexuality and aging...all of which are essential to living a happy, active life. And it's all backed by breaking studies and top health experts.

Over the past four decades, we have built a network of literally thousands of leading physicians in both alternative and conventional medi-cine. They are affiliated with the premier medical and research institutions throughout the world. We read the important medical journals and follow the latest research that is reported at medical conferences. And we regularly talk to our advisors in major teaching hospitals, private practices and government health agencies for their insider perspective.

The Ultimate Women's Guide to Beating Disease and Living a Happy, Active Life 2017 is a result of our ongoing research and connection with these experts, and is a distillation of their latest findings and advice. We trust that you will glean new, helpful and affordable information about the health topics that concern you most...and find vital topics of interest to family and friends as well.

As a reader of a Bottom Line book, please be assured that you are receiving well-researched information from a trusted source. But, please use prudence in health matters. Always speak to your physician before taking vitamins, supplements or over-the-counter medication...stopping a medication...changing your diet...or beginning an exercise program. If you experience side effects from any regimen, contact your doctor immediately.

Be well,
The Editors, *Bottom Line Health*
Stamford, Connecticut

*"Leading Causes of Death in Females," Centers for Disease Control and Prevention (*http://www.cdc.gov/women lcod/2010/index.htm*).

Chapter 1

HEART HELP FOR WOMEN

Shocking Reason Heart Disease May Still Go Undetected in Women

Tests used to confirm heart disease will probably pick up the same symptoms in women and men, according to a recent study out of Duke Clinical Research Institute in Durham, North Carolina.

The two most prominent symptoms for cardiovascular disease—chest pain (angina) and shortness of breath—are common to both sexes, concludes a study of more than 10,000 people in both the United States and Canada.

"In most cases, symptoms of possible blockages in the heart's arteries are the same [for women] as those seen in men," said study lead author Kshipra Hemal, of the Duke Clinical Research Institute in Durham, North Carolina.

However, the study also found that because standard evaluations don't include certain heart disease risk factors more common to women than men, it may still be tougher for women to receive an accurate diagnosis.

The Study

For the research, Hemal's team compared the test results of people with suspected heart disease. She noted that the research included "one of the largest cohorts of women ever evaluated in a heart disease study."

The researchers found that chest pain was the main symptom for about 73% of women and 72% of men, followed by shortness of breath, which occurred in 15% of both women and men.

Women were more likely than men to have back, neck and jaw pain, or palpitations as their main symptom. But, the percentage of both sexes with these symptoms was extremely low: back pain, 1% of women, 0.6% of men; neck or jaw pain, 1.4% of women, 0.7% of men; palpitations, 2.7% of women, 2% of men.

Compared to men, women in the study: tended to be slightly older (62 versus 59); were more likely to be non-white; were less

Kshipra Hemal, Duke Clinical Research Institute, Durham, North Carolina.

Howard Levite, MD, director of cardiology, Staten Island University Hospital, Staten Island, New York.

David A. Friedman, MD, chief, heart failure services, Northwell Health's Franklin Hospital, Valley Stream, New York.

American College of Cardiology, news release.

likely to smoke or be overweight; and were more likely to have high blood pressure, high cholesterol, a history of stroke, an inactive lifestyle, history of depression and a family history of early onset heart disease.

Women also scored lower than men when it came to assessing their risk for heart disease. According to Hemal's team, that could be due to the fact that heart disease risk factors that are more common in women—depression, inactivity, and family history of early onset heart disease—are not included in most risk assessments.

The study was published in the *Journal of the American College of Cardiology: Cardiovascular Imaging*.

Implications

"For health care providers, this study shows the importance of taking into account the differences between women and men throughout the entire diagnostic process for suspected heart disease," Hemal said. "Providers also need to know that, in the vast majority of cases, women and men with suspected heart disease have the same symptoms."

Important Heart Attack Differences

One expert stressed that while symptoms of heart disease may be similar for men and women, that's not always the case for the signs of actual heart attack.

The new findings "run counter" to recent data "on differences between symptom presentation between men and women when it comes to heart attacks," said Howard Levite, MD, director of cardiology at Staten Island University in New York City.

For example, the American Heart Association notes that while men typically feel crushing chest pain when a heart attack hits, symptoms can be more subtle for women.

Women may feel chest pain—it is still the most common symptom for both sexes—but this pain can also be intermittent, the AHA

said. Other symptoms tend to be more common in women than men, such as pain in one or both arms, the back, neck, jaw or stomach; shortness of breath with or without accompanying chest pain; cold sweats, nausea or lightheadedness, the AHA said.

Recommendations for Women: Get the Care You Need

In any case, if a person experiences any or all of these symptoms, they or a loved one should called 911 and receive hospital care as soon as possible, the AHA said.

The key to preventing heart attack is spotting and treating heart disease early. But Dr. Levite believes that current testing protocols may leave women at a disadvantage.

"Women are fighting an uphill battle when it comes to convincing doctors that they are having heart-related symptoms, because the standard scoring tests assign them to a lower risk category," he said.

"Factors more commonly found in women, such as anxiety and depression, are not in the current risk scores," Dr. Levite added.

David A. Friedman, MD, is chief of heart failure services at Northwell Health's Franklin Hospital in Valley Stream, New York. He agreed that a thorough patient examination is key to good cardiac care.

"A high-quality clinical history of present illness—taking into account a good review of all patient complaints including symptom type, onset, duration, intensity, worsening and improving associated problems—can help us get a 'back-to-basics' approach, which can help further define patients' potential cardiac risk profile," Dr. Friedman said.

For more on women and heart disease, head to the American Heart Association website, *goredforwomen.org*, and search "heart disease in women."

Heart Health Is Not a Big Concern for Women...But It Should Be

C. Noel Bairey-Merz, MD, medical director, Women's Heart Center, Cedars-Sinai Medical Center, Los Angeles. American Heart Association, news release.

Heart disease is the leading cause of death among American women, but few feel a personal link with the disease, new research shows.

Survey Results

A nationwide survey of more than 1,000 women between the ages of 25 and 60 found that only 27% could name a woman in their lives with heart disease and only 11% could name a woman who died from it.

Age made a difference. Among those between 50 and 60 years of age, 37% knew a woman with heart disease, compared with 23% of the younger group.

Respondents who knew a woman with heart disease were 25% more likely to be concerned about it for themselves and 19% more likely to bring up heart health with their doctors, the Women's Heart Alliance survey found.

The study was presented at the American Heart Association's annual meeting in Orlando, Florida.

Implications

"Since women who report knowing another woman with heart disease are more apt to express concern and, importantly, bring up this issue with their doctor, awareness of heart disease is crucial," said study author C. Noel Bairey-Merz, MD, medical director of the Women's Heart Center at Cedars-Sinai Medical Center in Los Angeles.

The survey also found that doctors tend to focus more on women's weight than other heart disease risk factors, while men are more likely to be told their cholesterol or blood pressure levels are too high.

"We are stalled on women's awareness of heart disease, partly because women say they put off going to the doctor until they've lost a few pounds. This is clearly a gendered issue," Dr. Bairey-Merz said.

Advice

"Women should be screened for heart disease, including finding out their atherosclerotic cardiovascular disease (ASCVD) score —also called the 'A-risk score.' This figure uses your age, sex, race, blood pressure, cholesterol levels, blood pressure medication use, diabetes status and smoking status to get a 10-year cardiovascular disease risk and a lifetime risk score," Dr. Bairey Merz said.

She said every woman aged 40 and older needs to get her A-risk score, and those under 40 need to know their blood pressure and cholesterol.

The U.S. Office on Women's Health has more information about heart disease at *womenshealth.gov*. Search "heart disease."

Heart Attack or Anxiety? What Every Woman Must Know

Kim Lavoie, PhD, professor, psychology, University of Quebec at Montreal, and director, Chronic Disease Research Division, Hopital du Sacre-Coeur de Montreal, Canada.

Karla Kurrelmeyer, MD, cardiologist, Houston Methodist DeBakey Heart and Vascular Center, Houston, Texas.

Circulation: Cardiovascular Quality and Outcomes.

In women who had never been diagnosed with heart disease, researchers found that those with anxiety were 75% more likely than women without anxiety to have reduced blood flow to the heart during activity.

And researchers suggest doctors may sometimes miss signs of heart disease in these women. Anxiety and depression are possible risk factors for heart disease.

Background

Heart disease kills about the same number of women as men in the United States every year and is the leading cause of death in American women, causing one in every four female deaths, according to the U.S. Centers for Disease Control and Prevention (CDC).

Women can experience different symptoms from men during a heart attack. For example, women are more likely to describe chest pain that is sharp or burning and more frequently have pain in the neck, jaw, throat, abdomen or back, the CDC says.

When a mood or anxiety disorder is added into the mix, a woman's true health status can be misinterpreted, the new study suggested.

The Study

For the study, the researchers looked at more than 2,300 patients, including 760 women, who underwent an exercise stress test and a psychiatric interview.

The exercise stress test looked for reduced blood flow (ischemia), which can cause a shortage of oxygen to the heart, and the effects of gender and mood/anxiety on this condition.

Kim Lavoie, PhD, a professor of psychology at University of Quebec at Montreal, and her team found that women with anxiety were far more likely to show ischemia than women without anxiety. They found no similar effects in men.

The study was published in the journal *Circulation: Cardiovascular Quality and Outcomes*.

Implications

Dr. Lavoie says the findings may indicate that anxiety symptoms such as chest discomfort or palpitations—which can overlap those of heart disease—may mask heart disease in women. This could lead to misdiagnosis, she said.

"If you're a woman and you say you're tired, short of breath, and really anxious about it, and you have no preexisting heart disease, it's possible that doctors are con-

founding the two problems," said Dr. Lavoie, also the director of the Chronic Disease Research Division at Hopital du Sacre-Coeur de Montreal in Canada.

"Doctors may be more likely to attribute those symptoms to anxiety than heart disease," she added. "So, in other words, a diagnostic bias may occur."

Expert Commentary

Karla Kurrelmeyer, MD, a cardiologist at Houston Methodist DeBakey Heart and Vascular Center in Texas, said physicians have been working for years to decipher the link between anxiety and heart disease, "because we realize there's a connection between being distraught or anxious and it affecting the nervous system."

Dr. Kurrelmeyer agreed with Dr. Lavoie that the women with anxiety who exhibited reduced blood flow to the heart might actually have had heart disease that previously went undiagnosed.

"Women with anxiety should be treated seriously because frequently they have ischemia…and doctors need to do more diagnostic testing to make sure symptoms are due to anxiety instead of obstructive coronary artery disease," said Dr. Kurrelmeyer, who wasn't involved in the new research.

Advice

Dr. Lavoie said women with anxiety or depression who are concerned about heart disease can ask their doctor to order tests to check their heart health.

"Clinicians need to recognize that anxiety presents with the same symptoms as heart disease and can mask the symptoms of heart disease if you don't rule that out with objective tests," she said.

The American Heart Association offers more information about heart attack symptoms in women. Go to *heart.org* and search "heart attack in women."

14 Little Things You Can Do for a Healthier Heart

Joel K. Kahn, MD, clinical professor of medicine at Wayne State University School of Medicine, Detroit, and founder of The Kahn Center for Cardiac Longevity. He is author of *The Whole Heart Solution: Halt Heart Disease Now with the Best Alternative and Traditional Medicine.* DrJoelKahn.com

Heart disease is America's number-one killer. But just because it's a major health risk does not necessarily mean that you must make major lifestyle changes to avoid it. *Here are 14 simple and inexpensive ways to have a healthier heart...*

Doable Diet Tips

1. Don't eat in the evening. Research suggests that the heart (and digestive system) benefits greatly from taking an 11-to-12-hour break from food every night. One study found that men who indulge in midnight snacks are 55% more likely to suffer from heart disease than men who don't. So if you plan to eat breakfast at 7 am, consider your kitchen closed after 7 or 8 pm.

Warning: You cannot produce the same health benefits by snacking at night and then skipping breakfast. This might create an 11-to-12-hour break from eating, but skipping breakfast actually increases the risk for heart attack and/or death—by 27%, according to one study. Our bodies and minds often are under considerable stress in the morning—that's when heart attack risk is greatest. Skipping the morning meal only adds to this stress.

2. Use apple pie spice as a topping on oatmeal and fruit. Some people enjoy it in coffee, too. This spice combo, which contains cinnamon, cloves, nutmeg and allspice, has been shown to reduce blood pressure, improve cholesterol levels and lower the risk for heart disease.

3. Take your time with your tea. Tea contains compounds called flavonoids that have

been shown to significantly reduce the risk for heart disease—green tea is best of all. But you get the full benefits only if you have the patience to let the tea leaves steep—that is, soak in hot water—for at least three to five minutes before drinking.

4. Fill up on salad. It's no secret that being overweight is bad for the heart. But most people don't realize that they can lose weight without going hungry. Salad can make the stomach feel full without a lot of calories. But don't add nonvegetable ingredients such as cheese, meat and egg to salads...and opt for balsamic or red wine vinegar dressing—they are rich in nutrients, including artery-healing resveratrol.

As a bonus, vegetables...and fruits...contain nutrients that are great for the heart regardless of your weight—so great that eating a plant-rich diet could improve your blood pressure just as much as taking blood pressure medication. In fact, one study found that increasing consumption of fruits and vegetables from 1.5 to eight servings per day decreases the risk for heart attack or stroke by 30%.

One strategy: Become a vegetarian for breakfast and lunch. That way you still can enjoy meat at dinner, but your overall vegetable consumption will be increased.

5. Marinate meat before grilling it. Grilling meat triggers a dramatic increase in its "advanced glycation end products" (AGEs), which stiffen blood vessels and raise blood pressure, among other health drawbacks. If you're not willing to give up your grill, marinate meat for at least 30 minutes before cooking it. Marinating helps keep meat moist, which can slash AGE levels in half. An effective marinade for this purpose is beer, though lemon juice or vinegar works well, too. You can add herbs and oil if you wish.

6. Sprinkle Italian seasoning mix onto salads, potatoes and soups. This zesty mix contains antioxidant-rich herbs such as oregano, sage, rosemary and thyme, which studies suggest reduce the risk for heart disease and cancer.

7. Avoid foods that contain dangerous additives. There are so many food additives

5

that it's virtually impossible to keep track of them all. Focus on avoiding foods that list any of the following seven among their ingredients—each carries heart-related health risks. The seven are aspartame…BHA (butylated hydroxyanisole)…BHT (butylated hydroxytoluene)…saccharin…sodium nitrate…sodium sulfate…and monosodium glutamate (MSG).

8. Savor the first three bites of everything you eat. When people eat too fast, they also tend to eat too much. One way to slow down your eating is to force yourself to pay close attention to what you are eating. If you cannot do this for an entire meal or snack, at least do it for the first three mouthfuls of each food you consume. Chew these initial bites slowly and thoroughly. Give the food and its flavor your undivided attention, and you will end up eating less.

9. Prepare your lunch the night before if you won't be home for your midday meal. People who intend to make their lunch in the morning often are in too much of a rush to do so…then wind up resorting to fast food.

10. Buy organic when it counts. Higher pesticide levels in the blood predict higher cholesterol levels as well as cardiovascular disease. Organic food is free of pesticide—but it can be expensive. The smart compromise is to buy organic when it counts most—when traditionally grown produce is most likely to contain pesticide residue. According to the Environmental Working Group, the foods most likely to contain pesticide residue are apples, celery, cherry tomatoes, collard greens, cucumbers, grapes, hot peppers, kale, nectarines, peaches, potatoes, spinach, strawberries, summer squash and sweet bell peppers.

Important: If your options are eating conventionally farmed fruits and vegetables or not eating fruits and vegetables at all, definitely consume the conventionally grown produce. The health risks from small amounts of pesticide residue are much lower than the health risks from not eating produce.

Easy Lifestyle Habits

11. Stand two to five minutes each hour. Recent research suggests that sitting for extended periods is horrible for your heart. Sitting slows your metabolism and reduces your ability to process glucose and cholesterol. But standing for as little as two to five minutes each hour seems to significantly reduce these health consequences (more standing is even better). Stand while making phone calls or during commercials. Buy a "standing desk," then stand when you use your computer.

12. Take walks after meals. Walking is good anytime, but walks after meals have special health benefits, particularly after rich desserts. A 20-minute postmeal stroll significantly improves the body's ability to manage blood sugar. Maintaining healthful blood sugar levels reduces risk for coronary artery blockage.

13. Exercise in brief but intense bursts. Research suggests that exercising as intensely as possible for 20 seconds…resting for 10 seconds…then repeating this seven more times provides nearly the same benefits for the heart as a far longer but less intense workout. Try this with an exercise bike, rowing machine, elliptical machine or any other form of exercise. Do an Internet search for "Tabata training" to learn more. There are free apps that can help you time these intervals. Download Tabata Stopwatch in the iTunes store if you use an Apple device…or Tabata Timer for HIIT from Google Play if you use an Android device.

Caution: Talk to your doctor. High-intensity training could be dangerous if you have a preexisting health condition.

14. Get sufficient sleep. One study found that the rates of heart disease for people who get seven to eight hours of sleep a night are nearly half those of people who get too little or too much sleep.

Cut Your Risk of Dying from Heart Disease in Half with One Simple Workout

Barry A. Franklin, PhD, director of preventive cardiology/cardiac rehabilitation at William Beaumont Hospital in Royal Oak, Michigan. He is a past president of the American Association of Cardiovascular and Pulmonary Rehabilitation and the American College of Sports Medicine and coauthor of *One Heart, Two Feet*. CreativeWalking.com

What if there were a piece of exercise equipment that could cut your risk of dying from heart disease by nearly half?

This is actually possible by simply using a treadmill—in a strategic way. The approach is not complicated or even that difficult, but few people take advantage of it.

The "MET" Secret

We all know that walking is an excellent form of exercise. What makes a treadmill so efficient is that you can control your pace and/or incline so that you maintain your desired intensity and get the maximum benefit from your exercise routine.

The treadmill's winning secret is that it gives you the ability to monitor energy expenditure, also called a MET, which stands for metabolic equivalent. Every one MET increase in your fitness level cuts your risk for death from heart disease by 15%, so increasing METs by three, for example, will cut risk by 45%. Many treadmills display METs readings. You can also estimate METs with an app for your smartphone or tablet. The Exercise Calculator for the iPhone or iPad displays METs when you enter your weight, type of activity and length of time exercising.

Simply put, METs allow you to track the intensity of your workout by estimating the amount of oxygen your muscles are burning to fuel you through various activities. For example, sitting requires one MET…and normal walking requires two to three METs—that is, two to three times as much oxygen and calories as you'd burn while relaxing in a chair. Light jogging requires eight METs…and running at a 6 mph pace, 10 METs.

With immediate feedback from your METs reading, you can effectively gauge how hard you're working out…and receive the motivation to push yourself at the safest and most effective intensity levels.

Important: If you've been sedentary, start your treadmill walking at 2 mph to 3 mph with no incline. Gradually increase your speed over the next eight to 10 weeks, then progress to graded treadmill walking or slow jogging. If symptoms such as shortness of breath, dizziness and/or chest pain develop, stop and tell your doctor.

Here's how to most effectively use a treadmill for specific exercise goals…

• **Quick but effective workout.**

What to use: Incline and speed. When it comes to getting the most out of exercise, intensity and duration are inversely related. By combining higher treadmill inclines with increased speeds, you'll bolster your MET level and reach your target heart rate sooner. Working at your target heart rate helps improve fitness. With fast, graded treadmill walking, you can get a great workout in just 20 to 30 minutes.

Example: Increase speed slightly (0.1 mph to 0.2 mph) every minute for five minutes. Then increase the incline setting, which is measured as a percentage, by 0.5% (for example, going from 1% to 1.5% incline) and walk for five minutes. Alternate this sequence once or twice (increasing speed and incline each time) until you feel you're working hard, but can still carry on a conversation.

• **Weight loss.**

What to use: Incline. With incline walking, more muscle mass—especially in the quadriceps and glutes—is activated with each stride. And the more treadmill incline you use, the more calories you'll burn.

A mere increase of just 1% on the incline setting (for example, going from 1% to 2%)

at a comfortable walking speed (such as 1.5 mph to 2.5 mph) will boost your energy expenditure by about 10%, and you shouldn't feel a difference. If you walk faster, you'll burn even more calories because you'll be working at a higher MET level.

Research shows that regular brisk walks of at least 30 minutes five or more days a week is the best approach to weight loss. Walking on level ground at 2 mph or 3 mph equates to about two or three METs. To help protect your knees, slow your pace as you gradually work up to higher levels of inclines.

Good news: At high inclines, walking may burn as many calories as jogging or running.

Don't Forget Strength Training

To get the most from your treadmill walking—or any cardio activity—be sure to add some resistance or strength training to further build your muscle strength. Strength training complements aerobic exercise, reducing your risk for heart disease. You'll also improve your insulin sensitivity (to help fight diabetes) and boost your bone mass (to guard against osteoporosis).

Best: Target various upper and lower body muscle groups, including the chest, back, shoulders, abdomen, quadriceps and hamstrings, using hand weights and/or weight machines. Some yoga poses can also increase muscle strength and endurance.

Aim for eight to 10 exercises…and do at least one set of 10 to 15 reps per set, at least twice a week.

Bonus Tools

You've probably seen people at the gym wearing ankle weights while walking on the treadmill. That's not a good idea. They can strain the lower extremities, increasing your risk for orthopedic or musculoskeletal problems.

Better approach: Try walking with a backpack carrying a comfortable amount of weight. You'll burn more calories than you would if you were walking without one. A snug fit will keep the weight close to your spine and hips—

which may help you avoid balance problems and improve your bone density.

And don't forget your headphones. Music (whatever genre you like) can reduce perceived exertion and may make your workout seem easier. It can be more motivating than watching TV.

Treadmill Safety

Treadmills are generally a safe way to exercise, but accidental falls can happen. *To stay safe…*

• **Always straddle the treadmill before turning it on,** and don't assume it will always start at a slow, comfortable speed.

• **Lightly hold the handrail for support while walking.**

• **Always warm up and cool down before and after the aerobic phase of your workout.** Never suddenly stop the treadmill.

The Best Walking Speed for Your Heart

Study titled "Usual Walking Pace Is More Strongly Associated with Lower Risk of Heart Failure Than Total Physical Activity in the Women's Health Study," Brigham and Women's Hospital and Harvard Medical School, both in Boston, presented at the American Heart Association's Epidemiology and Prevention and Lifestyle and Cardiometabolic Health 2016 Scientific Sessions.

Like to walk? Try picking up the pace—just a little. Your heart will thank you.

In an analysis of 40,000 women (average age 55), among those who walked in their leisure time, about 80% of them—the brisk walkers—were 23% less likely to develop heart failure over the next 17 years than women who simply strolled. The researchers believe that similar benefits would happen in men of the same age.

The pace difference? At least one extra mile per hour. The slowest walkers in the study averaged two or fewer miles per hour—a stroll.

The fastest ones? A brisker three or more miles an hour—which is a good pace to aim for.

If you walk on a treadmill, it's easy to pick the best pace for an optimal heart-healthy workout. If you like to walk outside—walking your dog, heading out for errands, a hike before breakfast—you might be able to use your smartphone to check how long it takes to you to walk one mile so you can figure out your walking speed. If your regular pace is just a leisurely stroll, practice picking up the pace.

Divorce Increases Heart Attack Risk

Divorce increases heart attack risk, especially for women. Compared with people who remained married, women who had been divorced once were 24% more likely to have a heart attack, while those who had multiple divorces faced a 77% higher risk. There is no evidence that a second marriage reduced heart attack risk. Women who remarried were 35% more likely to suffer a heart attack than those who stayed married to their first husbands. Men who had been divorced two or more times were 30% more likely to have a heart attack than men who remained married or remarried once.

Study of nearly 16,000 US adults over two decades by researchers at Duke University, Durham, North Carolina, published in *Circulation: Cardiovascular Quality and Outcomes*.

More Problems with PPIs

Popular antacids are associated with heart attack. Analysis of the medical records of more than three million people found that taking proton pump inhibitors (PPIs), such as Prilosec, Protonix and Nexium, had a modest association (20%) with heart attack risk. The analysis showed no increased heart attack risk among patients taking acid-suppressing histamine blockers, such as Tagamet, Pepcid and Zantac.

Nigam H. Shah, MBBS, PhD, is assistant professor of medicine, Biomedical Informatics Research at Stanford University School of Medicine, California, and leader of a data analysis published in *PLOS ONE*.

Hot Flashes Linked to Heart Disease

Rebecca Thurston, PhD, associate professor of psychiatry, psychology, epidemiology and clinical and translational science at University of Pittsburgh and director of the Women's Biobehavioral Health Laboratory there. She has led several studies on the link between hot flashes and cardiovascular disease.

More than 70% of women experience hot flashes around the time of menopause. Not only are hot flashes bothersome (to say the least)—but research has also connected them with increased cardiovascular disease risk in certain women. In a recent ultrasound study, we found that "super flashers"—women who report at least five or six flashes daily—had significantly thicker carotid artery walls than other women. Other research has shown that the thicker the arterial walls, the greater the risk for heart disease and stroke. Having hot flashes infrequently (an average of four or fewer daily) does not seem to be linked to greater carotid thickness.

"Early-onset flashers"—women who have hot flashes at a relatively early age—also may be at higher risk. In another ultrasound study, we measured how well patients' blood vessels dilated after a cuff was released. Women who first experienced hot flashes at age 42 or younger had significantly worse responses than those whose flashes began later in life. Poor blood vessel responses are associated with the development of cardiovascular disease.

Self-defense: Consult your physician about whether you are up-to-date on cholesterol testing and other cardiovascular screenings. If you smoke, stop. Eat a healthful diet.

Exercise regularly. If overweight, commit to a weight-loss plan.

Stop a Heart Attack Before It Happens

John A. Elefteriades, MD, the William W.L. Glenn Professor of Surgery and director of the Aortic Institute at Yale University and Yale–New Haven Hospital. He is the author of several books, including *Your Heart: An Owner's Guide.* HeartAuthorMD.com

---

Chest pain…shortness of breath…feeling faint…and/or discomfort in the arm—or even the neck, jaw or back. If you are overcome by such symptoms and perhaps even have an intense and sudden "sense of doom," you're likely to suspect a heart attack and rush to a hospital.

But wouldn't it be better to get a heads-up beforehand that a heart attack is on the way?

What most people don't realize: For about 60% of heart attack victims, warning symptoms do occur days or even weeks before the actual heart attack. But all too often, these signs are missed or shrugged off as something trivial.

What's behind this early-warning system? The blockage that creates a heart attack often develops over time and its symptoms, though they may be mild and elusive, should not be ignored.

Knowing the early red flags—including those you might not immediately connect to a heart problem—can allow you to see a doctor before a life-threatening heart attack occurs. Women, especially, can have symptoms that do not immediately bring heart disease to mind.

Important: If these symptoms are extreme and last for more than a few minutes—especially if they are accompanied by any of the more typical symptoms such as those described above—call 911. You could be having an actual heart attack. Even if these symptoms are mild to moderate but seem unexplained, call your doctor. If he/she

cannot be reached but you're still concerned, go to the emergency room.

The following are examples of the subtle symptoms that can precede a heart attack—sometimes by days or weeks…

• **Fatigue.** If you feel more tired than usual, it's easy to tell yourself you're just growing older or getting out of shape. But pay attention! It could be the early-warning sign of heart trouble.

If your usual daily activities, whether it's walking the dog or cleaning the house, leave you feeling more tired than normal, talk to your doctor.

• **Flulike symptoms.** If you get hit with extreme fatigue, as well as weakness and/or feelings of light-headedness, you may think you're coming down with the flu. But people report having these same symptoms prior to a heart attack.

Call your doctor if you experience flulike symptoms but no fever (a telltale flu symptom).

Another clue: The flu generally comes on quickly, while flulike symptoms associated with heart disease may develop gradually.

• **Nausea and/or indigestion.** These are among the most overlooked symptoms of a heart attack—perhaps because they are typically due to gastrointestinal problems.

But if you are feeling sick to your stomach and throwing up, it could be a heart attack rather than food poisoning or some other stomach problem—especially if you're also sweating and your skin has turned an ashen color. If indigestion comes and goes, does not occur after a meal or doesn't improve within a day or so—especially if you're using antacids or antinausea medication—this could also mean heart problems. See a doctor.

• **Excessive perspiration.** If you are sweating more than usual—especially during times when you're not exerting yourself—it could mean that there are blockages. This can cause your heart to work harder, which may lead to excessive sweating. See your doctor. Clammy skin and night sweats also can be warning signs. This is likely to be a cold sweat, instead of the heat experienced in menopausal hot flashes. If sweating occurs with any of the classic heart attack symptoms described above, don't think twice—call 911.

• **Shortness of breath.** If you notice that you are beginning to feel more winded than usual, see your doctor. Shortness of breath can be a precursor to heart attack. If shortness of breath becomes stronger or lasts longer than usual, call 911. Shortness of breath may be your only symptom of a heart attack and may occur while you are resting or doing only minor physical activity.

• **Sexual dysfunction.** Men with heart problems that can lead to heart attack often have trouble achieving and/or keeping an erection. Because poor blood flow to the penis can be a sign of possible blockages elsewhere in the body, including the heart, erectile dysfunction can be an early-warning sign to get checked for cardiovascular disease. Men should absolutely discuss this symptom with their doctors.

Women, Pay Attention!

After a woman goes through menopause— when the body's production of heart-protective estrogen declines—her risk for a heart attack dramatically increases.

Important facts for women: More women die of heart disease each year than men. Nearly two-thirds of women who died from heart attacks had no history of chest pain. The higher death rate for women is likely due to the fact that women don't seek medical attention as promptly as men because they are afraid of being embarrassed if the symptoms turn out to be nothing serious. Don't let this fear stop you from seeking immediate care. If the symptoms turn out to be nothing serious, the emergency medical team will be happy!

What to watch for: While most (but not all) men experience crushing or squeezing chest pain (usually under the breastbone), women are more likely to have no chest pain (or simply a feeling of "fullness" in the chest). Also, women are more likely than men to suffer dizziness, shortness of breath and/or nausea as the main symptoms of heart attack.

Most women (71%) experience sudden onset of extreme weakness that feels like the flu.

Sudden Cardiac Arrest Is Not Always Sudden

About half of cardiac arrest patients had warning signs in the month before the attack, according to recent findings, including symptoms not typically associated with heart problems, such as nausea, back pain and abdominal pain. If you have these symptoms and high blood pressure, high cholesterol, diabetes or a family history of heart disease, or if you have more typical symptoms such as chest pain and pressure, seek medical attention.

Sumeet S. Chugh, MD, is associate director of Cedars-Sinai Heart Institute, Los Angeles, and leader of a study published in *Annals of Internal Medicine.*

Bystanders Less Likely to Help Women Having Heart Attacks

Nicole Karam, MD, MPH, interventional cardiologist, European Hospital Georges Pompidou, Paris. European Society of Cardiology, news release.

Women are less likely than men to be helped by bystanders if they suffer cardiac arrest, a new study finds.

"There is a misconception that women don't have heart problems so they don't get as much help from the public and they are not treated the same by doctors," said study author Nicole Karam, MD, MPH. She is an interventional cardiologist at the European Hospital Georges Pompidou in Paris.

The Study

Researchers reviewed records of more than 11,400 people who had a cardiac arrest in public areas in and around Paris between 2011 and 2014.

Cardiac arrest, the sudden loss of heart function, is often caused by abnormal heart rhythms.

Even though bystanders were more likely to be present when women suffered cardiac arrest, researchers found only 60% of women received basic life support—such as CPR and use of an automated external defibrillator—compared with 70% of men. Eighteen percent of women and 26% of men reached the hospital alive, the investigators found. The study was released by the European Society of Cardiology.

Possible Explanation

"When a man has a cardiac arrest he is less likely to have witnesses, but they perform CPR more frequently. Probably people are more afraid to do CPR in women because we look fragile. They may also not believe that she is really having a cardiac arrest—even though we found that 40% of patients were women," Dr. Karam said.

The frequency of heart disease in women is increasing so it's no longer a "man's problem," she added.

Implications

"When it does happen, doctors need to manage women just as they would manage men. We can only improve women's survival from cardiac arrest when doctors, emergency medical services, the public, and women themselves accept that it can happen to anyone regardless of gender," Dr. Karam concluded.

The American Heart Association has more information about cardiac arrest at *heart.org*. Enter "cardiac arrest" in the search line.

Why Women's Heart Attacks Are Deadlier Than Men's

Laxmi Mehta, MD, chair, American Heart Association writing group, and director, Women's Cardiovascular Health Program, Ohio State University, Columbus.

Gregg Fonarow, MD, professor, cardiology, University of California, Los Angeles.

Suzanne Steinbaum, DO, director, Women's Heart Health, Lenox Hill Hospital, New York City.

Circulation, online.

Heart attacks in women often have different causes and symptoms than those in men, and they're deadlier, too.

That's the premise of a scientific statement from the American Heart Association (AHA) that hopes to raise awareness about key differences in heart attack indicators and treatment in women.

Women who don't recognize their heart attack symptoms won't seek needed medical care, said Gregg Fonarow, MD, professor of cardiology at the University of California, Los Angeles.

"These delays in care contribute to higher mortality rates experienced by women, particularly younger women," he said.

Background

Worldwide, cardiovascular disease is the leading cause of death for women. Since 1984 in the United States, heart attack survival has improved for women. But the heart death rates among women still outpace heart deaths in men, according to the AHA statement.

New Statement

The new statement reviews current scientific evidence, points out gaps in knowledge and discusses the need for more research in women, said Laxmi Mehta, MD. She is chair of the statement writing group and director of the Women's Cardiovascular Health Program at Ohio State University.

Dr. Mehta knows firsthand the dangers that heart disease pose to women. "I was inspired to write this [statement] as both my grandmothers died from heart attacks at age 60 and had presented with atypical [not typical] symptoms," she said.

The statement is published in the American Heart Association journal *Circulation*. *Among the highlights…*

• **Plaque buildup in the arteries**—a frequent cause of heart attack—can differ between the sexes. Women are less likely to need stenting to open a blocked artery, but they still suffer blood vessel damage that reduces blood flow to the heart, causing a heart attack.

• **High blood pressure is a stronger risk factor for women than for men.** And diabetes raises a young woman's heart disease risk up to five times higher compared to young men.

• **Guideline-recommended medications are underused in women,** compared to men, and women are referred less often for cardiac rehabilitation. When they are re-ferred, they are less likely than men to go or to finish it.

• **For men and women, chest pain or discomfort is the most common heart attack symptom,** but women are more likely to report shortness of breath, back or jaw pain, and nausea and vomiting.

• **Black women of any age have a higher incidence of heart attacks than white women.** And black and Hispanic women have more risk factors such as obesity, diabetes and high blood pressure at the time of heart attack compared to white women.

Expert Reaction

The new statement "provides a comprehensive review of current knowledge and key directions needed to further reduce death and disability," said Dr. Fonarow.

This new AHA statement was needed, agreed Dr. Suzanne Steinbaum, DO, director of Women's Heart Health at Lenox Hill Hospital in New York City. "It is time that both the medical community and women address these issues and understand that open communication and awareness are critical to changing these statistics," she said.

What to Do

Dr. Mehta stressed that women need to "know their numbers"—including blood pressure, cholesterol, blood glucose, body mass index (BMI, a ratio of weight to height) and waist circumference. "Take action to keep these numbers in the normal ranges," she advised.

"Lead an active, healthy lifestyle and be accountable for your decisions," she added. "This includes exercising on a regular basis, following a healthy diet and not smoking."

To learn more about heart attack symptoms in women, visit the American Heart Association website, *americanheart.org*, and search "heart attack symptoms in women."

Gender and the Heart

In men, the muscle that wraps around the left ventricle gets thicker with age…in women, it stays the same or gets smaller. Implication: Women with heart failure might get less benefit from drugs that reduce heart-muscle thickness.

Radiology.

This Supplement May Save Your Life (And Your Heart)

Study titled "Effect of Purified Omega-3 Fatty Acids on Reducing Left Ventricular Remodeling After Acute Myocardial Infarction...," Harvard Medical School, and Brigham and Women's Hospital, both in Boston, presented at the American College of Cardiology's 64th Annual Scientific Session in San Diego.

You've survived a heart attack. But you're worried—could another one be waiting to happen? After all, it's a vulnerable time. As your surviving heart muscle works harder to compensate for damaged tissue, you can experience further scarring and inflammation that can weaken your heart even more. But there's a simple, safe, natural, food-based supplement that cardiologists now recommend that can greatly improve your odds of keeping your heart healthy. And while it's no surprise that omega-3s are linked with heart health, this is different—a particular kind and dose of omega-3 could literally keep you alive. *Here's how to save your heart in three seconds a day...*

Omega-3 for a Broken Heart

Omega-3 fatty acids, the kind primarily found in cold-water fish such as salmon, have had a heart-healthy reputation for a long time. It's good for your heart to eat fish twice a week or, if you don't eat fish, to add other omega-3-rich–foods to your diet. And omega-3 supplements have been shown to reduce the risk for irregular heartbeat (arrhythmia) and prevent related fatalities, as well as reduce high triglycerides and high blood pressure, although there isn't enough evidence to determine whether taking them helps healthy people prevent heart disease, according to NIH's National Center for Complementary and Integrative Health.

The latest research makes it clear that there is at least one group of people for whom the benefits of high doses of omega-3s are extraordinarily powerful—people who've had a heart attack.

Eight Ounces of Salmon In a Pill

In this study, 358 patients who had had heart attacks were randomly assigned to take four grams of purified prescription-only omega-3 fatty acids (about the amount found in eight ounces of salmon) or a placebo (a capsule of corn oil) each day for six months. They started within one month of the heart attack. *The researchers wanted to know how omega-3 fatty acids affected...*

• **The left ventricle of the heart,** which usually deteriorates after a heart attack

• **The size of the area damaged by their heart attacks,** which can enlarge after a heart attack

• **Signs of inflammation.**

Results: Compared with placebo, the omega-3 fatty acids were a powerhouse of heart help. Patients taking omega-3 fatty acids were 39% less likely to show deterioration in heart function than those taking placebo. Their hearts also showed much less scarring—very important because the more scarred the heart tissue is, the less well it functions. The omega-3 fatty acids also had a powerful anti-inflammatory effect, with inflammatory enzymes being way down in patients in the omega-3 group compared with patients in the placebo group.

Take These Results to Heart

Four grams of omega-3 fatty acids is a high dose—for Americans. The study researchers noted that most Americans do not get the amount of omega-3 they need, in large part because we don't eat oily fish such as sardines, tuna, trout and salmon twice a week as recommended by the American College of Cardiology and the American Heart Association. In fact, in the study of heart attack survivors, omega-3 blood levels in patients in the high-dose omega-3 group increased quite a bit, but only up to the same levels generally seen among some populations in

14

Japan whose diet is rich in fish—and who have lower risks for heart disease and sudden death from heart attack than Americans.

Nor did the researchers report any side effects, such as interference with blood clotting, which is a concern since omega-3s are natural anticoagulants. Still, check with your doctor before taking high-dose omega-3s, especially if you are on a blood thinner. These researchers used a prescription-only form of omega-3 supplement, Lovaza, which is FDA-approved for reducing high triglyceride levels. There are many good omega-3 supplements on the market, but you'll want to see what your insurance will cover.

All of us can safely benefit from improving our blood levels of omega-3s by eating fatty fish twice a week or by getting omega-3s from other foods. But if you've had a heart attack or know someone who has, a discussion with the cardiologist about taking four grams of omega-3s in a supplement might be a lifesaving conversation.

Women Still Aren't Getting the Heart Treatments They Need

Deepak Bhatt, MD, MPH, executive director, interventional cardiovascular programs, Brigham and Women's Hospital Heart & Vascular Center, Boston.

Stacey Rosen, MD, vice president, women's health, Katz Institute for Women's Health, North Shore-LIJ Health System, New Hyde Park, New York.

American Heart Association annual meeting, Orlando, Florida.

Women are less likely than men to get the recommended treatments for heart attack survivors, and that could explain much of the gender gap in long-term survival, a new study finds.

Looking at records for nearly 50,000 older Americans hospitalized for a heart attack, researchers found that women were 8% less likely to be on "optimal care" when discharged.

Optimal care means that patients are sent home with prescriptions for all of the standard therapies that are appropriate for them. According to guidelines after a heart attack, that can include counseling on smoking cessation, referral to a cardiac rehab program, and prescriptions for a low-dose daily aspirin, a cholesterol-lowering statin or blood pressure drugs such as beta blockers and ACE inhibitors.

Study Details

The findings are based on Medicare records from more than 49,300 Americans who were hospitalized for a heart attack at one of 366 US hospitals between 2003 and 2009. Overall, more than 16,000 people died within three years of their hospital discharge, with the risk higher among women whose care was suboptimal.

Implications

The finding that men are more likely to get recommended heart attack therapies is nothing new, said Deepak Bhatt, MD, MPH, executive director of interventional cardiovascular programs at Brigham and Women's Hospital in Boston, and co-author of the new study.

Past studies have found the same pattern, he noted.

But what's key here, Dr. Bhatt said, is that "suboptimal" care accounted for the gender gap in heart attack patients' long-term survival. When women received optimal treatment, they were just as likely as men to be alive three years later.

When treatment was subpar, women faced a 23% higher risk of dying in the next three years versus men, the study found.

"I think you can look at this as 'good news,'" Dr. Bhatt said, "because that is an actionable finding. If we just give women these simple, guideline-recommended therapies, we can close the mortality gap."

Dr. Bhatt presented the findings at the American Heart Association's annual meeting, in Orlando, Florida.

Expert Commentary

Stacey Rosen, MD, a heart association spokesperson who was not involved in the study, agreed that the results are actually positive in that women's higher mortality can be changed.

"This should empower patients to make sure they work with their doctor to optimize their health," said Dr. Rosen, who is also vice president of women's health at the Katz Institute for Women's Health, North Shore—LIJ Health System in New Hyde Park, New York.

Conclusions

When women see their doctor for follow-up appointments after a hospital discharge, Dr. Rosen said, they should not be shy about asking questions—including whether they've been prescribed all of the therapies that are right for them.

Drugs such as aspirin, statins and beta blockers are not appropriate for everyone, Dr. Bhatt said. But, he added, that did not explain why women in this study were less likely to receive optimal therapy.

It's not clear why women were less likely than men to receive all of the appropriate post-heart attack treatments, Dr. Bhatt said. But whatever the reason, he added, the pattern needs to shift.

"We're not even talking about fancy, expensive interventions," Dr. Bhatt said. "Simple, low-cost treatments, like a daily aspirin, could close the gender gap in heart attack mortality."

Dr. Rosen agreed. "The disparity disappeared when women in this study received optimal therapy. That's a pretty irrefutable finding," she said.

For answers to your questions on recovering from a heart attack, visit the website of the American Heart Association, *heart.org*, and search "heart attack recovery."

Have Heart Disease? Get Your Eyes Checked Now

Study titled "Severity of Coronary Artery Disease Is Independently Associated with the Frequency of Early Age-Related Macular Degeneration" by researchers in the department of ophthalmology, Centre for Vision Research, Westmead Millennium Institute, University of Sydney, and Westmead Hospital, Australia, published in *British Journal of Ophthalmology*.

Macular degeneration is one of the most common causes of vision loss in adults age 50 and older, yet there often are no symptoms in its earliest stages. But now there is strong evidence that if you have another common disease of aging that it's time to get your eyes checked—immediately. The new research also provides a more clear-eyed view of the path to preventing this vision thief.

What Your Heart Has to Say About Your Eyes

Researchers have long suspected that there's a link between heart disease and age-related macular degeneration (AMD). The two diseases share many risk factors beyond simply age—smoking, high blood pressure, high blood cholesterol levels, diabetes and obesity. But research attempting to connect the dots between these risk factors and the two diseases has been inconsistent. One study found an association with stroke but not coronary heart disease, while another found an association with coronary heart disease but not stroke.

A new study from "down under" used a more powerful measure than risk factors—clinical evidence of the extent and severity of coronary heart disease. The Australian researchers carefully studied the eyes of men and women with suspected heart disease who were already scheduled to have an angiogram. The results have implications both for early diagnosis and prevention of AMD.

Early Signs of a Leading Cause of Blindness

While the more than 1,600 subjects ranged in age from 23 to 92, the average age of those who had coronary heart disease was just over 60. By contrast, the late stage of macular degeneration that actually causes vision symptoms (problems with ability to see fine detail, reading and driving and eventually even seeing faces) often doesn't occur until people reach their late 70s or early 80s. Early macular degeneration, and often the intermediate stage, has no symptoms, although it can be detected by a comprehensive eye exam. By the time that vision is impaired, it's harder to treat.

The men and women in the study all had coronary angiography, a procedure in which dye injected into a catheter shows how blood flows through the arteries to the heart. The angiograms allowed cardiologists to take precise measurements to grade the severity of blockage in the coronary arteries. Severity was quantified two ways—first by the number of vessels with significant obstruction, and then by using a Gensini score, a more sophisticated calculation that places emphasis on the more important artery segments. The participants also had their eyes checked out very carefully for signs of AMD.

Results: About 6% of the men and women had early AMD and 1.4% had late AMD. Those who had serious artery blockage were much more likely to have early AMD. After adjusting for age, gender, body mass index, smoking, diabetes and other risk factors, the participants with a narrowing of more than 50% in any one artery segment were nearly twice as likely to have early AMD compared with participants without artery narrowing. Those with narrowing in all three main coronary arteries were 2.7 times more likely to have early AMD. The Gensini score was also highly associated with early AMD—participants with the highest Gensini scores were more than twice as likely as those with the lowest scores to have early AMD.

There were some differences between men and women, too, another indication that heart disease affects the genders differently. For women, there was no link between artery blockage and early AMD, but those with the highest Gensini score were five times more likely to have early AMD. More research is needed to understand how coronary artery disease affects the genders differently and how this relates to early AMD risk, the researchers conclude. But clearly there was risk for both genders.

A Clear and Present Danger

The take-away messages from this study couldn't be clearer…

• **If you or someone you know has coronary heart disease,** don't wait to get your eyes checked. According to the Agency for Healthcare Research and Quality, all adults with no risk factors should have a comprehensive eye exam (which includes AMD testing) every five to 10 years. Those aged 40 to 54 may need to have it repeated only every two to four years…aged 55 to 64, every one to three years…those 65 and over, every one to two years. That's fine for the general population, but this study suggests that people with heart disease should be checked immediately—and ask their doctor how often they should get rechecked.

• **Go to your optometrist, ophthalmologist or retina specialist for a comprehensive eye exam.** While many (not all) optometrists do screen for signs of AMD, opthamologists, (including those who are retina specialists) generally have much more sophisticated equipment. So you may be referred to one if an eye exam finds something suspicious. Opticians generally don't screen for AMD.

• **There's no cure for this sight-robbing disease,** but the process can be slowed down with a heart-healthy lifestyle and supplements, and it needs to be monitored so that when it does need treatment in the late stage, that starts right away.

• **If you have both conditions, make sure your cardiologist and your eye specialist both know all of the medications and**

supplements you are taking. Blood thinners—prescription medications as well as aspirin and fish oil, for example—may cause bleeding problems, including in your eyes, that could make vision problems worse.

The recent research also reinforces that a healthy lifestyle is important for the prevention of a wide variety of age-related diseases. Preventing macular degeneration is about more than just taking the right vitamins. According to the American Academy of Ophthamology, other eye diseases that are related to cardiovascular health include cataracts and retinopathy, often found in people with diabetes. Take care of your heart and you may be taking care of your eyes, too.

Cholesterol Drugs May Cause Cataracts

G.B. John Mancini, MD, professor of medicine, University of British Columbia, Vancouver, Canada. His study was published in *Canadian Journal of Cardiology*.

Doctors are telling us that they expect the incidence of cataracts to continue to increase as the population ages. But a question persists about whether some other reason, in addition to aging—a lifestyle habit or medication perhaps—is a contributing factor. It turns out that widely used cholesterol-lowering drugs might have something to do with cataracts, too.

A Problem of Aging Or Something More?

Cataracts are a condition whereby the lens of the eye slowly clouds over. Your vision becomes increasingly blurry, and people looking at you see an eerie gray disk where your pupil and iris are supposed to be. With loss of vision comes loss of independence. People with untreated cataracts lose their ability to read, drive and otherwise get around on their own, and they can no longer see the faces of their loved ones. For some, cataracts are a casualty of aging. With age, the lenses in your eyes can thicken and become less transparent as eye tissue breaks down and clumps together, causing cloudiness within the lens.

But while this may be a natural but unfortunate aspect of aging in some people, research is also linking statins to cataract formation. Previous research has been inconclusive, but two new studies at the University of British Columbia show important results. They analyzed data from of two very large databases—one from Canada and the other from the US.

The Canadian database included women and men who had visited an ophthalmologist, and the US database included men who had seen any type of doctor. The studies compared people who had had cataract surgery with a large group of people of the same age who never had cataracts. In all, the study included more than 200,000 people with cataracts and 1.1 million without and their prescription records to look for patterns of statin use. Researchers also controlled for age and other risk factors for cataracts, such as diabetes and high blood pressure.

The Statin–Cataract Link

The association was clear. Among Canadian patients, the risk for cataracts was 27% higher among those who used statins for at least one year compared with people who didn't take statins at all. Risk for the US male-only group was 7% higher than men who didn't use statins—not as big an increase but still significant (more men than women use statins, but this is changing). The increased cataract risk shown in this study is but one more of the side effects of statin use.

For reasons unknown, the association between statin use and cataracts was 20 percentage points higher among the Canadian study group than the American group. One important risk factor—cigarette smoking—could not be controlled for because the databases didn't provide any information about it. So it is possible that cigarette smoking—not statin use—was behind cataract development in some of these folks.

You May Not Need Those Statins You're Taking

Study titled "Implications of Coronary Artery Calcium Testing Among Statin Candidates According to American College of Cardiology/American Heart Association Cholesterol Management Guidelines" by researchers at Baptist Health South Florida, Miami, The Johns Hopkins Ciccarone Center for the Prevention of Heart Disease, Baltimore, et al. published in *The Journal of the American College of Cardiology*.

Khurram Nasir, MD, MPH, director, Center for Healthcare Advancement & Outcomes, Baptist Health South Florida, Miami, and director, High Risk Cardiovascular Clinic, Baptist Health South Florida, Miami.

I t's sobering—your doctor tells you that you have an elevated chance of having a heart attack or stroke over the next 10 years. So he recommends that you start taking a statin drug right away—and stay on it for the rest of your life.

But what if your doctor is wrong? What if your cardiovascular risk actually is much lower? The online risk calculator that is being used by the medical community to figure out who needs statins, it turns out, is seriously flawed.

Nearly half the time, a patient's actual risk is so much lower that he/she doesn't even qualify for statins, according to recent research.

The good news is that there is a simple, standard, relatively inexpensive test that your primary care doctor can order that can dramatically improve the accuracy of cardiovascular risk assessment—so that you can make the best decision.

The Statin Net Is Too Wide

In 2013, new guidelines by the American College of Cardiology and the American Heart Association swept an estimated 13 million more Americans into the "you're a good candidate for statins" group. In all, about 45 million Americans now are candidates for statins.

But Americans need to be more cautious before they blindly agree to start taking statins, which can come with some serious side effects. These include muscle and joint pain (the most common complaint, which is sometimes severe and can include nighttime leg cramps), digestive problems such as nausea, diarrhea or constipation, memory loss, rhabdomyolysis (a rare but severe form of muscle injury that can cause kidney failure) and a slightly increased risk of developing diabetes.

Statins offer the most benefit to people with existing cardiovascular disease, and those who have high LDL ("bad") cholesterol in combination with other risk factors, such as a genetic predisposition toward heart disease. If you don't already have cardiovascular disease, taking statins won't reduce your chances of dying, studies show.

The 2013 guidelines were designed to identify people who are at such high risk of having a heart attack or stroke that they would benefit from statins.

The primary tool—an online risk calculator. You or your doctor enters information about age, gender, total and HDL cholesterol, systolic blood pressure (top number) and smoking status into the web-based tool to estimate your chance of having a heart attack or stroke within 10 years. *Here's what you're supposed to do…*

•**If your 10-year risk is 5% to 7.5%, you should "consider" taking a statin.**

•**If your 10-year risk is higher than 7.5%, statins are "recommended."**

Danger: The calculator widely overestimates risks, according to a recent study in *Journal of the American College of Cardiology.*

To the Rescue: Calcium Scans

Lead study author Khurram Nasir, MD, MPH, a cardiologist at Baptist Health South Florida in Miami, and his team studied 4,758 women and men ages 50 to 68 who were already enrolled in a long-term heart study and were followed for 10 years. Applying the 2013 guidelines, the researchers calculated that two-thirds of the participants were either recommended or considered for moderate-to-high-intensity statins.

But the researchers shed light on a better way to determine risk in these people. Each had undergone a coronary artery calcium scan, a computed tomography (CT) scan that can detect calcium deposits in arterial plaque, a primary driver of heart disease. A high calcium score (CAC) can predict heart disease well before symptoms arise. A low score means your risk is likely low as well. *The findings…*

• **Of those patients "recommended" for statins,** 41% had calcium scores of zero, meaning that they showed no buildup of plaque in their coronary arteries. The zero-calcium score lowered their 10-year risk for these patients to 4.9%.

• **Of those "considered" for statins because their 10-year heart attack risk fell between a 5% and 7.5% threshold,** 57% had coronary calcium scores of zero. That lowered their 10-year risk to 1.5%.

"When you combine these two groups, about 45% have a calcium score of zero, and their average 10-year risk is 4.5%, which is much below the threshold where the guidelines suggest you should be on statins," said Dr. Nasir.

Should You Get a Calcium Scan?

A calcium scan is a good option to discuss with your physician if your 10-year cardiovascular risk is in the broad middle range of risk score between 5% and 20%. For people in this group, a low calcium number can tip the balance in helping you to decide whether

Statins and Aggression

The popular cholesterol-lowering statins *simvastatin* (Zocor) and *pravastatin* (Pravachol) were found to increase aggressive acts (such as slapping someone or self-harm) in postmenopausal women but reduced aggression in men in a recent six-month study of 1,000 adults.

Theory: Statins not only reduce cholesterol but may also influence testosterone levels and sleep patterns, which affect men and women differently.

Beatrice Golomb, MD, PhD, professor of medicine, University of California, San Diego.

to embark on a lifetime of statin pills or focus on a nondrug approach.

If your risk score is lower than 5%, it's likely you'd have a calcium score of zero, and you're not even a candidate for statins…and if it's higher than 20%, it's unlikely that the scan results would change your doctor's recommendation to take a statin.

Like all tests, a calcium scan has risks. It delivers less radiation than many CT scans but more than a digital mammogram. The test is highly accurate in predicting risk for coronary artery disease, the most common form of heart disease, but if your score is high, you may need additional tests to confirm the finding.

While the test is noninvasive and widely available, at an average cost of about $100 to $400, it's not usually covered by insurance.

Dr. Nasir encourages patients to feel empowered to ask for the calcium scan test to help them decide whether to take this medication—and then decide what's right for themselves. "If you have a much lower risk than anticipated," said Dr. Nasir, "you have the option of forgoing a lifelong commitment to pills and just focusing on lifestyle—exercising, sleeping and eating well, maintaining your weight and not smoking."

Statins Can Cause Memory Loss

Statins can cause memory loss in some patients, despite a new study that found they don't have cognitive side effects. The study was a generalized statistical study—not a personalized look at vulnerable patients. Some people who are susceptible do have "statin brain." Symptoms stop when the drug is stopped. These patients should talk to their doctors. Anyone considering starting a statin should ask about every-other-day rather than daily dosing.

Linda L. Restifo, MD, PhD, professor in the department of neurology at University of Arizona, Tucson.

What You Need to Know Before Starting Aspirin Therapy

Randall S. Stafford, MD, PhD, a professor of medicine at the Stanford Prevention Research Center and the director of the Program on Prevention Outcomes and Practices, both at the Stanford School of Medicine in Palo Alto, California.

It seems harmless enough…popping an aspirin from that familiar little bottle tucked away in your medicine cabinet.

In fact, millions of Americans take an aspirin daily as a blood thinner to help prevent the artery-clogging blood clots that cause most heart attacks and strokes. But for many of these people, aspirin is doing more harm than good.

Recent finding: In a study of 68,800 adults taking daily aspirin therapy for heart attack and/or stroke prevention, nearly 12% were doing so unnecessarily based on their limited chances of actually suffering from one of these conditions over the next decade. In doing so, these individuals were found to be increasing their risk for potentially dan-

gerous side effects, such as internal bleeding, for no good reason.

A tragic toll: Among the more than 16,000 deaths each year linked to bleeding associated with use of nonsteroidal anti-inflammatory drugs (NSAIDs), about one-third of these deaths occur in those who take low-dose (81-mg) aspirin.

Is Aspirin Right for You?

You may assume from these frightening statistics that aspirin is never worth the risk, but that would be a mistake. Whether you're trying to prevent a heart attack, stroke or cancer, to make the best decision about using aspirin, you and your doctor need to weigh your potential benefits against your potential harms and then make a choice based on your preferences. *When aspirin use may help…*

Heart Attack or Stroke

If you've already had coronary bypass surgery, a heart attack or ischemic stroke (caused by a blood clot), taking aspirin and/or another blood-thinning drug, such as *clopidogrel* (Plavix) or *warfarin* (Coumadin), is wise. That's because study after study shows that aspirin significantly reduces the risk for a second heart attack or stroke. (A person whose risk for bleeding is extremely high may be an exception.)

If your goal is to prevent a first heart attack or stroke, the decision is a bit more complicated. Guidelines from the American Heart Association (AHA) and the US Preventive Services Task Force recommend aspirin for primary prevention in people at high risk for cardiovascular disease. In 2014, the FDA weighed in, releasing a statement that warned against widespread use in people of average risk.

My advice: I advise some—but not all—of my male patients who are over age 45 to take aspirin for primary prevention. For women, I advise aspirin for most who are age 65 and older. There are exceptions, especially for those who are at high risk for bleeding. Meanwhile, men and women younger than these ages sometimes have enough risk factors for heart attack and stroke that they will benefit from aspirin.

Scientific Evidence: An analysis of multiple studies published in *The Journal of the American Medical Association,* involving nearly 100,000 people, showed that in women, the greatest benefit of daily aspirin—for reduction in ischemic stroke and heart attack—occurs for those age 65 and older.

What's my criteria for recommending aspirin? If the patient's chance of having a heart attack or stroke in the next 10 years is higher than 5% to 10%.

To determine your heart attack and stroke risk: Use the cardiovascular disease (CVD) "risk calculator" created by the American College of Cardiology and the AHA. To download the calculator onto your computer or an app onto your smartphone, go to *My.AmericanHeart.org* (click on "Statements & Guidelines," then on "Prevention Guidelines").

If your risk is above 5% to 10%, talk to your doctor about whether you should be taking aspirin.

Important: Once you have your result from the risk calculator, you must balance your potential benefit from taking aspirin to prevent a heart attack or stroke against possible harm. Have you had gastrointestinal (GI) bleeding in the past? Are you regularly taking another anti-inflammatory medicine such as ibuprofen (Motrin), which also increases your risk for GI bleeding?

Are you age 80 or over? Aspirin might help you, but there's no solid evidence to guide your decision. Nonetheless, older adults have the most to gain from aspirin, but need to be particularly careful to avoid bleeding problems.

Could PMS Raise Women's Risk for High Blood Pressure?

Elizabeth Bertone-Johnson, associate professor of epidemiology, University of Massachusetts, Amherst.

Stacey Rosen, MD, vice president of women's health, The Katz Institute for Women's Health, New Hyde Park, New York.

Deena Adimoolam, MD, assistant professor, medicine, endocrinology, diabetes and bone disease, Icahn School of Medicine at Mount Sinai, New York City.

University of Massachusetts, Amherst, news release.

Millions of women suffer through premenstrual syndrome (PMS), and now new research suggests that those with moderate-to-severe PMS may be at heightened risk for high blood pressure later in life.

Study Details

The investigators tracked nearly 1,260 women who developed clinically significant PMS between 1991 and 2005, as well as more than 2,400 women with mild PMS. Both groups were followed until 2011.

Women with moderate-to-severe PMS were 40% more likely to develop high blood pressure than those with mild or no PMS symptoms, the researchers found.

This higher risk remained after the researchers adjusted for high blood pressure risk factors such as being overweight or obese, smoking, drinking, inactivity, use of birth control pills, postmenopausal hormone use, and family history of high blood pressure.

The link between moderate-to-severe PMS and high blood pressure was strongest among women younger than 40, said study leader Elizabeth Bertone-Johnson, ScD, an epidemiologist at the University of Massachusetts, Amherst. In this age group, those with clinically significant PMS were three times more likely to develop high blood pressure.

"To my knowledge, this is the first large long-term study to suggest that PMS may be related to risk of chronic health conditions in later life," said Dr. Bertone.

The study was published in the *American Journal of Epidemiology*.

B Vitamin May Protect Against Hypertension

Dr. Bertone and her colleagues did find that moderate-to-severe PMS did not increase the risk of high blood pressure in women with high intakes of the B vitamins thiamine and riboflavin. Recently, the researchers found that women who consumed high levels of those vitamins were 25% to 35% less likely to develop PMS.

Clinically significant PMS affects as many as 8% to 15% of women, the researchers said. However, they believe that it may be possible to reduce the risk of high blood pressure in these women by increasing their intake of B vitamins.

Expert Commentary

Two experts said the new findings could be important, but questions remain.

"The study is important in identifying an important condition that should lead to closer observation for the onset of high blood pressure," said Stacey Rosen, MD, vice president of women's health at The Katz Institute for Women's Health in New Hyde Park, New York.

She added, however, "one important limitation is that the average age of these patients was 27 years—it would be helpful to see if this association persisted in younger women as well."

Deena Adimoolam, MD is assistant professor of medicine at the Icahn School of Medicine at Mount Sinai in New York City. She said that, right now, "many physicians don't consider PMS as a risk factor for hypertension."

And while the study findings are "interesting," she added, "I don't think women should be overly concerned about this association for a few reasons."

First, the study didn't identify and exclude women with conditions that can look like PMS—chronic fatigue syndrome, anxiety dis-

orders and irritable bowel syndrome, for example—so, "PMS might have been wrongly diagnosed in some patients," Dr. Adimoolam said.

"Also, high blood pressure was self-reported by study participants and not diagnosed by a physician, which makes me question if certain participants truly developed hypertension," she added.

Conclusion

While the study couldn't prove cause-and-effect, the finding may mean that "women with PMS should be screened for adverse changes in blood pressure and future risk of hypertension," said Dr. Bertone-Johnson and her team.

For more information on premenstrual syndrome, visit the website of the U.S. Office on Women's Health, *womenshealth.gov*, and search "premenstrual syndrome."

Are You at Triple Risk for Heart Disease?

Karen Allesoe, Ph.D. student, University of Southern Denmark, Odense.
European Journal of Preventive Cardiology, news release.

Having a physically demanding job and high blood pressure may triple a woman's risk of heart disease, a new study contends.

The Study

Researchers looked at more than 12,000 female nurses in Denmark, and found that those with high blood pressure and highly active jobs were much more likely to develop heart disease than those with normal blood pressure and moderately active jobs.

"Previous research has shown that men and women with physically demanding jobs have an increased risk of heart disease," said study author Karen Allesoe, a Ph.D. student at the University of Southern Denmark.

Take BP Meds at Night

Take blood pressure medicine at night to control hypertension more effectively and reduce the risk for diabetes. Over nearly a six-year period, people who took their medicine at night had a greater drop in night-time blood pressure and a 57% lower risk for diabetes than people who took it in the morning. Talk to your doctor before changing your medication schedule.

Study of 2,012 people by researchers at University of Vigo, Spain, published in *Diabetologia*.

"The two risk factors appear to work together, resulting in an even greater incidence of heart disease," Allesoe said. "To our knowledge, this has not been shown before among women."

However, the study only showed an association for heart disease risk, not a cause-and-effect relationship.

The study was published in the *European Journal of Preventive Cardiology*.

Possible Explanations

The study defined high-activity jobs as those that included standing and walking with lifting, carrying and other physical exertion. Moderately active jobs involved mainly standing and walking with no physical exertion.

"Lifting and carrying cause a rise in blood pressure, and may put people with hypertension [high blood pressure] at particular risk of a cardiovascular event," Allesoe said.

"For nurses, physically demanding jobs may involve high-force demands during patient handling, or standing and walking all day with no time for breaks," Allesoe said.

"Our results may also apply to other occupations that require lifting or carrying heavy loads and standing or walking for many hours, but this needs to be confirmed in other studies.

"We need more information on which aspects of physically demanding work are harmful. Until then we cannot make specific recommendations on how much lifting, and for how many hours, is safe for women with hypertension," she said.

For more information on how to lower risk for heart disease, visit the website of the U.S. National Institutes of Health, *www.nhlbi.nih. gov*, and search "lower heart disease risk."

Even Borderline High Blood Pressure Can Harm Unborn Baby

Anna-Karin Wikstrom, MD, PhD, associate professor, obstetrics, Uppsala University, Sweden.

James Ducey, MD, director, maternal-fetal medicine of obstetrics and gynecology, Staten Island University Hospital, New York City.

Jennifer Wu, MD, obstetrician and gynecologist, Lenox Hill Hospital, New York City.

Hypertension, online.

Even slightly elevated blood pressure in late pregnancy may increase the risk of having an underweight or stillborn infant, new research suggests.

Women with prehypertension—sometimes called borderline high blood pressure—at 36 weeks of pregnancy had about 70%—greater odds for low birth weight or stillbirth compared to women with normal blood pressure, the new Swedish study found.

But even mothers-to-be whose blood pressure rose in late pregnancy without becoming prehypertensive were more likely to have small babies, researchers said.

The researchers stressed, however, that their study showed only an association, not a cause-and-effect relationship, between blood pressure and fetal outcomes.

Infants with low birth weight are more likely to have health problems than normal-weight babies, according to the U.S. Centers for Disease Control and Prevention.

The study authors said prevention, rather than treatment, is key.

"We do not suggest treating women with medications, since earlier studies have not shown that this is beneficial to the mother or unborn child," said lead researcher Anna-Karin Wikstrom, MD, PhD, an associate professor of obstetrics at Uppsala University in Sweden.

For the study, Wikstrom and colleagues collected data on more than 150,000 women listed in a Swedish obstetric database. Only women who carried their babies for 37 weeks or longer, whose blood pressure never rose above 140/90 millimeters of mercury (mm Hg) during pregnancy, and were having a single baby were included in the study.

Prehypertension is a systolic pressure (the top number) between 120-139 mm Hg or a diastolic pressure (the bottom number) between 80-89 mm Hg, or both.

High blood pressure—140/90 mm Hg or more—has been linked with low birth weight and stillbirth, but it wasn't known if borderline high blood pressure is related to birth complications.

About 11% of the women in the study developed prehypertension. Overall, more than 2,400 babies were born underweight and 194 were stillborn, the researchers found.

Women whose diastolic blood pressure rose 15 points or more and developed prehypertension were more likely to have an underweight baby, Wikstrom said.

A rise in diastolic blood pressure that didn't reach prehypertension still increased the risk of low birth weight, with the likelihood rising 2% for every point, the researchers found.

These findings remained significant even after the researchers took into account the mother's age and weight, smoking history and diabetes.

Wikstrom suspects widespread obesity may be contributing to blood pressure increases. "We are worried about the global epidemic of obesity, since obesity has a strong association with maternal cardiovascular health and risk of prehypertension," she said.

Obese women who plan a pregnancy in the near future should "change their lifestyle in order to lose weight before conception to optimize their own health and the health of their fetus during pregnancy," Wikstrom said.

The report was published online in the journal *Hypertension*.

Expert Commentary

"Women who have a rise in blood pressure should have close surveillance," said Dr. Jennifer Wu, an obstetrician and gynecologist at Lenox Hill Hospital in New York City.

Wu said she would consider inducing delivery early if the baby is in danger of being stillborn.

These women should have frequent ultrasound to look at blood flow and fluid levels and "catch any signs of growth restriction or deterioration of the health of the baby," she said.

Dr. James Ducey, director of maternal-fetal medicine at Staten Island University Hospital in New York City, agreed that these pregnancies need to be watched closely.

The first step is to see how well blood is flowing to the baby, Ducey said. "Once we see this rise in blood pressure, we should try to prevent the stillbirths," he said. "This might involve an earlier delivery."

Drug-Free Help for High BP

Acupuncture can lower blood pressure for up to a month and a half in patients with mild-to-moderate hypertension.

Recent finding: 70% of patients given acupuncture had systolic (top number) pressure reductions averaging 6 mmHg to 8 mmHg and diastolic (bottom number) reductions averaging 4 mmHg. They also had significant declines in blood levels of norepinephrine, which constricts blood vessels and increases blood pressure.

John C. Longhurst, MD, PhD, is a professor of cardiology at Susan Samueli Center for Integrative Medicine, University of California, Irvine, and leader of a study published in *Medical Acupuncture*.

For more on blood pressure during pregnancy, visit the March of Dimes at *http://www.marchofdimes.org/complications/high-blood-pressure-during-pregnancy.aspx*.

Shake It Up, Baby: How to Vibrate Your Way to Lower Blood Pressure

Study titled, "Whole-Body Vibration Exercise Training Reduces Arterial Stiffness in Postmenopausal Women with Prehypertension and Hypertension" by Arturo Figueroa, MD, PhD, associate professor of vascular exercise physiology at Florida State University, Tallahassee, and colleagues, published in *Menopause*.

"Jiggle" machines to lose weight—those belts that vibrate around your middle while you just stand there—go back to the 19th century.

News flash: They don't work too well… for weight loss, that is. The best that can be said is that they may help with weight loss… if you also cut calories. Thanks a lot.

But a new generation of "whole-body vibration" (WBV) machines is showing up in some gyms, in physical therapy clinics and even as home fitness equipment. What gives? It turns out that new research is uncovering other health benefits. They help build muscle, and there is some evidence that they may help build bone, too.

The latest benefit—lowering elevated blood pressure.

Keeping Your Arteries Flexible

Three 30-to-40-minute sessions a week with WBV can bring down blood pressure by an average of 12 mmHg systolic and 6 mmHg diastolic over a three-month period.

That's enough to bring you down an entire blood pressure category. That is, if you are "prehypertensive" (aka "borderline"), with a reading between 120/80 and 139/89, WBV treatment could bring you into the "normal" category—below 120/80. If you are hypertensive, with a reading of 140/90 or higher, you could drop down to prehypertensive—and you might no longer require medication.

How does jiggling work therapeutically? WBV has been shown to make the arteries more flexible—less stiff. Arterial stiffness is a process in which the arteries lose their elasticity. A stiffer artery makes the heart work harder, raising blood pressure and cardiovascular risk. WBV may make arteries—including the peripheral ones that go throughout the body—more flexible by improving the functioning of their lining cells (the endothelium) and by stimulating production of nitric oxide, which helps arteries contract and dilate more efficiently.

Ready to Rumble?

To put this research into perspective, remember that regular exercise also reliably lowers high blood pressure, although not as dramatically. Exercise with WBV is no substitute for aerobic exercise and strength training, which have many more benefits for the body and the mind than can be expected from WBV. Indeed, these machines often are used in physical therapy clinics for people who can't do conventional exercise, such as someone recovering from a stroke or with severe arthritis.

Want to add WBV to your exercise routine? First, if you're being treated for hypertension or other ailments, get an OK from your doctor—and don't stop taking any medications without his or her approval. Next, try out one of these machines at a gym or physical therapy clinic that has one—especially before sinking hundreds or thousands of dollars into buying one for home use.

Be aware of possible side effects. As with any exercise, you can experience fatigue and muscle soreness. You may also experience skin redness and itching during the initial sessions due to the increased blood flow to your legs. These are minor. Swelling (edema) in the legs also can happen, but it is rare—if you experience this, tell your doctor.

The most important advice: Whether you use a WBV machine at a gym or get one for home use, you'll get the most benefit if you first get trained by someone who knows how to work with WBV, such as an exercise physiologist. In fact, gyms that have these machines often stick them in an out-of-the-way room because no one knows how to use them properly. There are many personal trainers who are not prepared to provide advice for WBV training. Physical therapists use them with patients who wear shoes during the vibration exercise. That dampens the beneficial effects, negating some of the benefits. There are other subtleties such as how to bend your knees to get the best benefit, but they're easy to learn from a trained instructor the first time you use one of these machines.

The High-Fat Path to Low Blood Pressure... and a Healthier Heart

Study titled "Comparison of the DASH (Dietary Approaches to Stop Hypertension) Diet and a Higher-Fat DASH Diet on Blood Pressure and Lipids and Lipoproteins: A Randomized Controlled Trial" by researchers at Children's Hospital Oakland Research Institute, Oakland, California, and College of Pharmacy, Touro University California, Vallejo, published in *American Journal of Clinical Nutrition.*

The DASH diet is one of the most healthful diets ever created. But it's not that easy to stick to.

One reason that it's so tough is that it's low in fat, especially the saturated fat found in "real" dairy foods that we love so much. In particular, you're supposed to give up full-fat cheese and yogurt and whole milk in favor of low-fat and fat-free versions.

Not very tasty.

And, according to the latest study, not at all necessary.

More Saturated Fat, Less Sugar

The DASH diet started out as a way to lower blood pressure—hence the name, an acronym for "Dietary Approaches to Stop Hypertension." That it does well. People who follow the diet have also been found to have less risk for heart disease, stroke, diabetes, kidney stones, colon cancer and dementia. Oh, yes, it's also great for weight loss.

The diet emphasizes plenty of fruits and vegetables, whole grains and low-fat dairy, along with lean poultry and fish, nuts, beans and seeds.

But it's also a low-fat diet, with a particular emphasis on keeping saturated fat low.

Here's the problem: Saturated fat, especially the kind found in dairy foods, doesn't appear to be bad for the heart. Meanwhile, sugar is—and the diet allowed sugar-laden fruit juices to be counted toward the fruit servings.

So the researchers wondered: What if we allowed DASH dieters to eat full-fat cheeses, high-fat yogurt and whole milk—while asking them to cut back on fruit juices and other sugar sources?

Bingo.

A Tastier, Healthier Diet

To test out the idea that full-fat dairy could make DASH both more palatable and just as healthy, researchers put 36 men and women on different diets over about two-and-a-half years—a control diet, similar to the standard American diet...a traditional low-fat DASH diet...or a high-fat DASH diet. By letting dieters have whole-fat dairy, the total fat went up from 27% in the traditional DASH to 40%...and saturated fat nearly doubled, from 8% to 14%. By cutting back on sugar, mainly from fruit juice, daily consumption went down from 158 grams a day on the traditional DASH to 93 grams.

No doubt, the high-fat DASH was tastier. But it was also just as effective at lowering blood pressure, both systolic and diastolic, as the low-fat DASH. Plus, it had extra benefits: Compared with the low-fat, higher-sugar traditional DASH diet, it lowered triglycerides—blood fats that raise the risk for heart disease and diabetes. The high-fat DASH also was better at reducing very low density lipoprotein (VLDL), which is particularly associated with heart disease risk.

That makes this already heart-healthy diet even heart-healthier.

And more enjoyable.

A-Fib Causes Bigger Problems for Women Than Men

Connor Emdin, doctoral student, cardiovascular epidemiology, University of Oxford's George Institute for Global Health, England.

Suzanne Steinbaum, DO, director, women's heart health, Heart and Vascular Institute, Lenox Hill Hospital, New York City.

Christopher Granger, MD, cardiologist, Duke University, Durham, North Carolina.

BMJ, online.

The world's most common type of abnormal heart rhythm appears to pose a greater health threat to women than men, a new review suggests.

Atrial fibrillation is a stronger risk factor for stroke, heart disease, heart failure and death in women than it is in men, according to an analysis published in the *BMJ*.

About Atrial Fibrillation

Atrial fibrillation occurs when rapid, disorganized electrical signals cause the heart's two upper chambers—the atria—to contract in a herky-jerky manner, according to the U.S. National Institutes of Health.

The condition is most often associated with an increased risk of stroke, because the irregular rhythm allows blood to pool and clot in the atria. Clots can then enter the circulation and travel to the brain where they may obstruct blow flow to areas of the brain.

Atrial fibrillation is a leading cause of heart disease and stroke worldwide, with an estimated 33.5 million people affected in 2010, the researchers pointed out.

Study Findings

But women with atrial fibrillation are twice as likely to suffer a stroke than men with the condition are, researchers concluded after reviewing evidence from 30 studies involving 4.3 million patients.

Women with atrial fibrillation also are 93% more likely to die from a heart condition, 55% more likely to suffer a heart attack, 16% more likely to develop heart failure and 12% more likely to die from any cause, when compared to men, the investigators found.

"This study adds to a growing body of literature showing that women may experience cardiovascular diseases and risk factors differently than men," said review author Connor Emdin, a doctoral student in cardiovascular epidemiology at the University of Oxford's George Institute for Global Health, in England.

Possible Explanations

Women may do worse with atrial fibrillation because their symptoms aren't as apparent as those in men, said Suzanne Steinbaum, DO, director of women's heart health for the Heart and Vascular Institute at Lenox Hill Hospital in New York City.

"It's reasonable to consider that it's diagnosed later, or it's not as recognized or that the symptoms are not the same," Dr. Steinbaum said.

Women might wave off symptoms like fatigue or shortness of breath, chalking them up to stress or feeling tired rather than seeing them as warning signs for heart disease, she said.

Christopher Granger, MD, a cardiologist at Duke University in Durham, North Carolina, agreed that atrial fibrillation might not be as easy to recognize in women as in men.

However, Dr. Granger added that a worse problem is a lack of proper treatment for both women and men with atrial fibrillation.

"Most of them should be on an anticoagulant [anti-clotting drugs] to prevent stroke, and many of them are not," Dr. Granger said. "That's even more of a concern in women than in men because, as this study shows, they are at higher risk for dangerous and even deadly complications."

Emdin said that another explanation might be that "atrial fibrillation in women may be more severe than atrial fibrillation in men, on average, and thereby cause death and cardiovascular disease at a higher rate."

The association could also be a coincidence, since the studies reviewed were not clinical trials and so couldn't draw a direct cause-and-effect link, Emdin added.

"It may be that the associations we report are not causal, and that women with atrial fibrillation are more likely to have comorbidities [co-existing medical conditions] in addition to atrial fibrillation that cause death and cardiovascular disease," he said.

Advice

In any case, all three experts recommended that women with atrial fibrillation should focus on improving their health by exercising, eating right, managing their stress and controlling their blood pressure and cholesterol levels.

"Recent research has demonstrated that lifestyle modification can reduce the severity of atrial fibrillation," Emdin said. "And if they have not already done so, women should consult with their physician about use of anticoagulant therapy."

For more on atrial fibrillation, visit the National Heart, Lung and Blood Institute website, *nhlbi.nih.gov*, and search "atrial fibrillation."

"Work Out" Your Way to Better A-Fib Treatment

In a recent four-year study of overweight atrial fibrillation (a-fib) patients, 84% of those with a high level of cardiorespiratory fitness (a measure of how well the heart, lungs and muscles supply oxygen during workouts) had no arrhythmias, compared with 17% who had a low level of this type of fitness. How does one improve cardiorespiratory fitness? Work with your doctor to design an exercise program—and stick with it!

Some good options include: Cycling, brisk walking and swimming.

Prashanthan Sanders, MBBS, PhD, director, Centre for Heart Rhythm Disorders, The University of Adelaide, Australia.

Chapter 2

BEST WAYS TO BEAT THE BIG C: BREAST CANCER BREAKTHROUGHS AND MORE

Rethinking Breast Cancer Treatment: Good News But Misunderstandings Abound

One-third of all new cancers diagnosed in women are breast cancers. The American Cancer Society estimates that more than 230,000 cases of invasive breast cancer will be diagnosed in the US in 2015.

But no one should let the fear of breast cancer obscure some very encouraging facts. The overall five-year survival rate from breast cancer now is close to 90%. Less than 7% of breast cancers are diagnosed before the age of 40—those diagnosed later in life tend to be easier to treat. Many women with breast cancer will never need highly aggressive (or disfiguring) treatments.

Despite such good news, misunderstandings about breast cancer are common. *Here's what you need to know now…*

•**Lumpectomy often is the best choice.** Many women assume that a mastectomy is the "safest" way to beat breast cancer. It makes intuitive sense that removing an entire breast would improve long-term survival.

Not true. Survival has nothing to do with the amount of additional healthy tissue that's removed during surgery. About 60% to 75% of breast cancer surgeries are lumpectomies, in which only a small amount of tissue is removed. If your doctor gives you a choice, you can assume that the probability of survival for both procedures will be essentially the same.

The advantages of lumpectomy are obvious. The surgery is less extensive and women need less anesthesia, both of which are associated with shorter recovery time—and the breast probably will look much the same as it did before the surgery.

Downside of lumpectomy: About 25% of women will need a second procedure to remove cancer cells that were left behind during the first surgery if clear "margins" aren't achieved. Most patients will require a five-to-seven-week-long course of radiation. And the risk of the cancer coming back is slightly

Elisa Port, MD, chief of breast surgery at Mount Sinai Medical Center, director of the Dubin Breast Center and an associate professor of surgery at the Icahn School of Medicine at Mount Sinai in New York City. She is author of *The New Generation Breast Cancer Book: How to Navigate Your Diagnosis and Treatment Options—and Remain Optimistic—in an Age of Information Overload.*

higher (usually less than 5%) in women who choose a lumpectomy rather than mastectomy (1% to 2%). Despite the slightly higher risk for local recurrence in the breast, the survival rates between lumpectomy and mastectomy are the same for women who are eligible for both.

A lumpectomy often is the best choice for tumors that are smaller than 4 centimeters (cm) to 5 cm. Some women feel that they'll have peace of mind only when the entire breast is removed. This can be a valid decision as long as you understand that the medical outcomes are roughly the same.

Of course, there is no "one size fits all," and absolutely, there are cases where a mastectomy is the better choice for an individual patient. For example, most women who are genetically predisposed to breast cancer and test positive for the BRCA genes are at much higher risk for recurrence with lumpectomy alone. In these cases, mastectomy—and often removal of both breasts, bilateral mastectomy—is recommended.

• **You may respond well to neoadjuvant chemotherapy.** Chemotherapy usually is considered for women whose cancer has spread to the lymph nodes and for those with large tumors. It's typically given after surgery. For certain types of cancer, however, a different approach is highly effective. In this approach, the chemotherapy is given first.

This therapy, called neoadjuvant chemotherapy, is used to shrink a tumor prior to surgery. In some cases, it will allow women who would otherwise need a more extensive surgery, such as a mastectomy, to have a lumpectomy instead. It's also the only recommended approach for women with inflammatory breast cancer, which involves the whole breast along with the overlying skin. It also can be a good choice for women with "triple negative" cancers, which don't respond to hormonal treatments (see next column), and those with HER2/neu-positive cancers. In some cases, this treatment shrinks a tumor so much that surgeons can find no residual cancer (but surgery still is necessary to ensure that this is the case).

• **Consider drugs that block hormones.** Between 60% and 70% of all newly diagnosed breast cancers are estrogen/progesterone-receptor positive. This means that exposure to these hormones can increase the risk for a recurrence.

Women with these types of cancers are almost always advised to take medication that reduces their risks. *Tamoxifen* (Nolvadex) is recommended for women prior to menopause. Aromatase inhibitors (such as *letrozole*, or Femara) are used after menopause.

The medications kill tumor cells that might have spread beyond the breast...reduce the risk that cancer will come back in a treated breast...and reduce the risk for cancer in the opposite breast. Women who take them can reduce their risk for a cancer recurrence by 40% to 50%. Patients usually take one pill a day and continue the treatment for five to 10 years.

Important: New research has shown that premenopausal women who take tamoxifen for 10 years usually have a greater reduction in cancer recurrences than those who take it for only five years.

The medications can cause unpleasant, menopause-like side effects, such as hot flashes and/or vaginal dryness. Tamoxifen also is associated with some rare but serious side effects such as a slightly higher risk for uterine cancer and blood clots, and aromatase inhibitors can affect bone density, which can be a problem for women with osteoporosis. But the side effects usually are minor, and many women feel the side effects are an acceptable trade-off for the superior protection.

What Else Can You Do?

Studies have shown that surgeons who treat a lot of patients (more than 50 cases a year) have better results. Ask your doctor to recommend a surgeon who specializes in breast cancer. *Also helpful...*

• **Ask your doctor if being in a clinical trial makes sense for you.** Most clinical trials are conducted by top hospitals and doctors. You'll get very sophisticated (and attentive) care. In many cases, even if you're assigned to a control group, you still will get the same treatment that you would have gotten if you hadn't joined the study. Those in the "active" group will get something that's expected to be at least as good—and possibly better.

Even if your doctor isn't personally involved in a clinical trial, he/she can talk you through the issues, including the pros and cons of participating...where to look for studies that involve your type of cancer...and what the studies are likely to involve.

•**Keep your weight down.** There's no evidence that specific dietary changes affect recovery from breast cancer. However, there is good evidence that maintaining a healthy weight is important, particularly for women with estrogen-sensitive cancers. (Much of a postmenopausal woman's estrogen is produced by fatty tissue.) Women who maintain a healthy weight may have up to a 5% survival advantage compared with those who are obese. Normal-weight women are less likely to get postsurgical infections and blood clots—particularly important for those who take tamoxifen, which slightly increases the risk for clots.

There isn't clear evidence that regular exercise helps prevent breast cancer, but I have found that cancer patients who exercise tend to recover more quickly—and of course, they find it easier to maintain a healthy weight.

Put Down That Moisturizer! It Can Increase Breast Cancer Risk

Tracey J. Woodruff, PhD, MPH, director, Program on Reproductive Health and the Environment, University of California, San Francisco.
Health Insider research.

Chances are, you've already put something on your skin today that can promote breast cancer. It could be in your soap, your shampoo, your shaving cream, your makeup, your moisturizer, your sunscreen—or all of the above.

We're talking about parabens, the most widely used class of chemical preservatives in cosmetics and personal-care products. They're hormone disrupters, suspected of increasing breast cancer risk. They mimic estrogen, producing similar effects that can cause human breast tumor cells to multiply.

Until now, though, the risk seemed relatively small, because parabens appeared to act only as very weak hormone disrupters. While avoiding them in your sunscreen and other products might be prudent, there wasn't strong evidence that they could play a significant role in causing breast cancer cells to proliferate.

But a new study finds that, under the right circumstances, these chemicals are 100 times more potent at stimulating breast cancer cell growth in the presence of growth factors.

Find out how to protect yourself...

A New Look at Parabens

Dale Leitman, MD, PhD, a gynecologist and adjunct professor of nutritional sciences and toxicology at University of California, Berkeley, and his research team tested parabens not by themselves, as other studies have done, but in combination with another compound made by the body.

They looked at *heregulin*, a naturally occurring growth factor made by breast tissue. In the lab, they combined breast cancer cells, parabens and heregulin...and compared that with breast cancer cells treated just with parabens.

The result: As other studies have found, parabens triggered estrogen receptors to turn on genes that make the cancer cells proliferate. But here's the really disturbing part—parabens combined with heregulin were 100 times more potent! In other words, in the presence of heregulin, it took just 1/100 of the dose of parabens to get breast cancer cells to grow rapidly. The research is evidence that earlier studies of parabens and other hormone disrupters may have vastly underestimated the cancer risk by focusing on just one chemical at a time.

While more research is clearly needed, that doesn't mean it's too early to act. According to Dr. Leitman, women should minimize or avoid the use of parabens—especially anyone with a family history of breast cancer. In fact, this study also suggests that excessive exposure to parabens and other xenoestrogens (chemical compounds that imitate estrogen) might increase the risk for breast cancer in men—about 1% of breast cancers occur in men, and 90% of those are estrogen positive.

Dr. Leitman believes the same logic applies to other known hormone disrupters, such as phthalates, compounds added to nail polish, hair spray and other cosmetics. He plans to study the phthalate combination in future studies, and he expects a similar cancer-promoting effect in the presence of growth factors. "We expect the same effects as with parabens because phthalates show similar types of biological behavior," he says.

In fact, parabens were never actually shown to be safe, according to Tracey J. Woodruff, PhD, MPH, director of the program on reproductive health and the environment at University of California, San Francisco, who is not affiliated with the study. "I don't think there was enough scientific evidence to show that parabens were 'safe,' only that they were not shown to be harmful. Studies often do not account for the way real bodies work and people live. Thus the quality of the studies and the evaluation are often insufficient to say one way or the other. Proving that something is safe is a pretty high bar."

If you're ready to get hormone disrupters off of your skin and out of your body, read on.

How to Primp Without Parabens (and Other Disruptors)

A segment of the cosmetic and personal-care product industry has caught on to concern over parabens and other potentially toxic chemicals and has been creating "paraben-free" and "phthalate-free" products for several years. But these hormone-disrupting chemicals are still perfectly legal to include in products, and they are still widespread.

While the FDA does not require premarketing safety testing of any chemicals in cosmetics, the federal Fair Packaging and Labeling Act (FPLA) does require manufacturers to list all ingredients so consumers can decide for themselves which products—and ingredients—they want to steer clear of. *Here's how…*

To avoid parabens…

• **Look for products that are labeled "paraben-free."**

• **If you don't see "paraben-free" on the label of your cosmetics and personal-care products,** read the ingredient lists and avoid products that list methylparaben, propylparaben, butylparaben or benzylparaben—the most commonly used parabens—in the ingredients. Also avoid anything that ends in "paraben."

To avoid phthalates…

• **Look for products labeled "phthalate-free."**

• **If you don't see "phthalate-free" on the label,** check the ingredients list for dibutyl phthalate (DBP), dimethyl phthalate (DMP), diethyl phthalate (DEP) and anything that ends in "phthalate."

• **Go fragrance-free.** The FPLA does not require the listing of individual fragrance ingredients, and phthalates are commonly used in fragrances. So avoid products that include "fragrance" in their ingredient list.

• **You can seek out "phthalate-free" fragrances but will have to rely on the manufacturer's word.**

One good bet: Choose products that rely on essential oils or other natural-based, rather than synthetic, fragrances.

The Big Picture: What's Safe on Your Skin?

You could wait until the thousands of chemicals that can be added to skin products are tested, but don't hold your breath. Most have never been tested and will never be tested. Plus, even when a chemical such as a paraben or a phthalate has been removed, the

Skip the Midnight Snack

Longer periods of overnight fasting may reduce risk for breast cancer. According to a recent study, for every three hours women didn't eat at night, glucose decreased by 4%, regardless of how much they ate the rest of the day.

Theory: Since diabetes is a risk factor for breast cancer, keeping normal blood sugar levels is a good way to stave off both conditions. Prolonged overnight fasting may also reduce risk for other types of cancer and heart disease.

Ruth E. Patterson, PhD, program leader, cancer prevention, Moores Cancer Center, University of California, San Diego.

replacement chemical may turn out to have similar effects, says Dr. Leitman. His advice—minimize exposure to products that contain ingredients that may affect hormones. That's why many people choose to protect themselves by minimizing exposure to synthetic chemicals in personal-care products. *Here are some tips…*

• **Limit your products to those with just a few ingredients**—and research them.

• **When in doubt, check your product, or the product's company,** against databases that track safe or unsafe use of chemicals in cosmetics and personal-care products such as the Environmental Working Group Skin Deep Database, Campaign for Safe Cosmetics or the Good Guide.

• **Don't rely solely on a label that claims a product is "100% natural"** or "made with organic ingredients" or some other variation of some healthful-sounding claim. "There is no guarantee that products labeled 'natural' or 'organic' are safe," says Dr. Woodruff.

• **Consider making your own cosmetics or skin creams.**

And lastly, get involved and vote, according to Dr. Woodruff. There are literally thousands of chemicals in cosmetics and personal-care products, and, unlike foods

or drugs, there is no regulatory requirement that they be tested before they go on sale. Says Dr. Woodruff, "The government should require that the burden be on the manufacturers to make sure these chemicals are safe before they go on the marketplace."

Can Coffee Prevent Breast Cancer?

Donald Northfelt, MD, professor of medicine and physician, Mayo Clinic, Scottsdale, Arizona. *Health Insider* Research.

Great health news about coffee is no longer a jolt to the system. So we weren't surprised to read a recent study about coffee and breast cancer that showed protection.

This one looked at more than 1,000 Swedish women who were already being treated for breast cancer. It found that women who drank more than two cups a day tended to have smaller tumors, and a lab component of the study reported that caffeine and caffeic acid (another coffee component) suppressed the growth of breast cancer cells in test tubes.

So should you drink more coffee—or start drinking coffee—to prevent or treat breast cancer? One study alone isn't enough to go on. To get the bigger picture, we went to Donald Northfelt, MD, a professor of medicine and oncologist at the Mayo Clinic in Scottsdale, Arizona, who has extensive experience in breast cancer research.

Coffee, Breast Cancer and a Million Women

While small studies such as the recent one from Sweden are part of the picture, Dr. Northfelt suggested a better approach. Look at a recent meta-analysis that pooled data from 37 studies with nearly one million women—including 59,000 with breast cancer. Such studies can use the power of statistics to suggest conclusions that can't be teased out of any one study.

While there was no overall effect of coffee or caffeine on breast cancer risk, either positive or negative, the larger analysis did find that coffee was protective for postmenopausal women. For them, breast cancer risk declined by about 2% for each two cups of coffee daily.

To put that in perspective, walking briskly for an average of 75 to 150 minutes a week may reduce breast cancer risk by 18%, while drinking two to five alcoholic drinks a day may increase risk by 50%, according to the American Cancer Society. So the risk reduction associated with drinking coffee in postmenopausal women was slight, in comparison.

But still—reducing risk is a good thing, especially when it involves something you may actually enjoy doing. If you like coffee and are concerned about breast cancer, go ahead and pour yourself a few cups—or more. If you've been through menopause, it might protect you—a little. Plus, there are a whole host of other health benefits. Regular coffee drinking reduces the risk for diabetes, cardiovascular disease, cognitive decline, Parkinson's Disease, liver cancer and less life-threatening conditions such as tinnitus

(ringing in the ears) and migraines. A coffee habit may even lead to longer life.

No beverage is perfect, of course—even coffee. If you have fibrocystic breasts, which can be lumpy, tender and sore, caffeine (from any source) may make symptoms worse. "It can induce discomfort and greater lumpiness in the breasts, especially at certain times in the menstrual cycle," says Dr. Northfelt. The good news is that having fibrocystic breasts is entirely benign and doesn't increase the risk for breast cancer.

The New Mammogram

Mary Pronovost, MD, a breast surgeon at Bridgeport Hospital in Connecticut.

About 40% of women have dense breasts, but 95% of them don't know it. Why does this matter? Studies have shown that women with dense breasts are more likely to develop breast cancer. Small tumors that are readily apparent on mammograms of "normal" breasts are harder to spot in dense breast tissue. You can't see or feel breast density…it shows up only on mammograms.

Recent development: In 21 states, the law now requires women to be told when they receive their mammograms whether they have dense breasts. (Legislation is pending elsewhere.) The laws also require doctors to inform women that tumors may be invisible on mammograms…and that additional tests should be considered. Does this added information really help? *Pros and cons…*

It's true that ultrasound or an MRI can detect tumors that mammography misses, but research has not shown that finding these cancers saves more lives. For many women, the cancers are not life-threatening.

Many women also experience tremendous anxiety when they learn from these other tests that a tumor might be present. They're more likely to undergo costly biopsies, many of which will prove to be unnecessary. Of course, some of the tumors will be serious enough to require treatment.

Dense Breast Calculator: Do You Need Additional Screening?

Not all women with dense breasts need additional screening for breast cancer. Women with dense breasts have a higher risk for breast cancers, but only 24% benefit from extra screening. A calculator (*Tools.bcsc-scc. org/BC5yearrisk/intro.htm*) from the National Cancer Institute's Breast Cancer Surveillance Consortium can help women ages 35 to 79 decide whether extra screening is warranted. Discuss the results with your doctor.

Karla Kerlikowske, MD, a professor in the departments of medicine and epidemiology/biostatistics at University of California, San Francisco, and an internationally recognized expert on breast cancer screening.

Best advice for now: After your next mammogram, ask about breast tissue, particularly if you live in a nondisclosure state—and ask your doctor if he/she advises further tests.

MRI vs. Mammogram

Recent research does indicate that for women at high risk for breast cancer, an MRI can significantly improve cancer detection rates by as much as 90%. But there is currently no evidence that MRIs find additional cancers in women at average risk for the disease.

Start by talking to your doctor about such factors as your family history of the disease and any known genetic mutation you might have that predisposes you to breast cancer. Also, there are some excellent online resources, such as the American Cancer Society, that can point you toward your appropriate risk group. If you do fall into a high-risk category, talk to your doctor about whether an MRI is right for you. For patients with an average risk for breast cancer, routine mammography still is the recommended method of screening.

Constance D. Lehman, MD, PhD, FACR, professor and vice-chair of radiology, section head of breast imaging, University of Washington School of Medicine, Seattle, and director of imaging at Seattle Cancer Care Alliance.

Ultrasound and Mammography Equally Effective at Detecting Cancer

Lusi Tumyan, MD, radiologist and assistant clinical professor, City of Hope Cancer Center, Duarte, California.

Wendie Berg, MD, professor, radiology, Magee-Womens Hospital of UPMC, Pittsburgh.

Journal of the National Cancer Institute.

Ultrasound and mammography appear equally likely to detect breast cancer, a recent study says.

The finding is good news, particularly for women who live in developing countries that typically have more access to ultrasound than to mammography, the researchers said.

Background

Ultrasound is generally used as a follow-up test once a potential breast tumor has been discovered through a mammogram or a physical exam, according to the American Cancer Society (ACS). The ACS says that ultrasound is a valuable tool that's widely available and noninvasive.

Study Findings

The new study involved 2,600 women living in the United States, Canada and Argentina who had ultrasound and mammogram annually for three years. They had no symptoms of breast cancer at the study's start, but they did have dense breast tissue—considered a risk factor for breast cancer—plus at least one other risk factor for breast cancer.

Separate radiologists interpreted each of the two scans the women received.

At the end of the study, 110 women were diagnosed with breast cancer. Detection rates were similar between the two tests. Rates of false-positive results (where a scan erroneously suggests a tumor) were higher for ultrasound compared to mammography, the researchers reported.

Overall, the researchers found that 32% of more than 2,500 women without cancer were asked to come back for additional testing at least once after an ultrasound. That compared to 23% of women who'd had mammography, the study said.

The study was published in the *Journal of the National Cancer Institute*.

Implications

While the detection rate with ultrasound was comparable to that of mammography, "it looks like ultrasound does better than mammography for node-negative invasive cancer," said study leader Wendie Berg, MD, professor of radiology at Magee-Womens Hospital of UPMC in Pittsburgh. Node-negative invasive cancer is cancer that hasn't invaded the lymph nodes, but has grown past the initial tumor, according to the U.S. National Cancer Institute.

"The downside [to ultrasound] is, there were more false positives," Dr. Berg said.

The findings suggest that for women who don't have a high risk of breast cancer but have dense breasts, "we find many more cancers if we do ultrasound in addition to mammography," Dr. Berg said.

Dr. Berg said the cost of mammography and ultrasound are comparable in the United States. "The issue is: what are the cancers we most need to find," she said. "The cancers you need to find are the invasive, node-negative ones. More of the cancers found with ultrasound were invasive and node-negative than those found with mammography."

General Guidelines On Screening

Guidelines about breast cancer screening vary among organizations. Current ACS guidelines advise women to consider beginning screening at age 40, depending on individual risk factors. They then recommend that women undergo annual screening with mammography from ages 45 to 54. At age 55, the ACS suggests continuing annual screening or switching to screening every two years, depending on risk factors. Some women, due to family history or other risk factors, should also be screened with MRIs, according to the ACS.

Expert Commentary

At least one expert doesn't expect this study to change current screening practice in the United States.

"For US patients, what [this study] really confirms is, ultrasound should be used as a supplemental screening exam in dense breast patients," said Lusi Tumyan, MD, a radiologist and assistant clinical professor at the City of Hope Cancer Center, in Duarte, California.

She reviewed the findings but was not involved in the study.

"At this time we do not have enough data to support or refute ultrasound as a screening tool for average-risk patients," Dr. Tumyan said.

Insurance coverage for breast ultrasounds also varies, according to Dr. Tumyan.

"Ultrasound coverage varies with different insurance companies and different state laws. California has passed a law that requires radiologists to inform patients if they have dense breasts. But California law does not require insurance companies to pay for supplemental screening. However, in other states, the dense breast law requires insurance companies to pay for supplemental screening," she explained.

Advice

The take-home message for women in the United States, she added, is to discuss their specific risks with their physician and decide together which screening test is best for them.

To learn more about breast ultrasound, visit the American Cancer Society website, *cancer.org*, and search "breast ultrasound."

DCIS Breast Cancer: What You Need to Know Now

Steven A. Narod, MD, professor, Dalla Lana School of Public Health, University of Toronto, Canada. His study was published in *JAMA Oncology*.

One woman in five who learns from a mammogram that she has breast cancer will be told she has ductal carcinoma in situ (DCIS)—abnormal cells found only in the milk ducts. It hasn't spread, even to the breast glands. It's such an early cancer that it's often called "Stage 0." Indeed, many experts don't think it's cancer at all but rather a possibly precancerous condition. Yet some women with DCIS go on to develop breast cancer...and some ultimately die from it.

So it's commonly treated to prevent future breast cancer, most often by removing the lump (lumpectomy) or sometimes by removing the entire breast (mastectomy)...followed by radiation...and then years of anxiety about the cancer recurring.

Now a major study suggests that some treatments are unnecessary. The new finding is bound to change the way medicine treats this common condition...plus it reveals clues to understanding those cases in which DCIS does lead to invasive breast cancer.

Treatment That Doesn't Save Lives

The researchers used data from 108,000 women diagnosed with DCIS. The average age was 54 at the time of diagnosis. Most women had some sort of treatment—lumpectomy with radiation was most common. The researchers compared the risk of dying from breast cancer within 20 years between the women with DCIS and the general population (women without breast cancer). *Key findings...*

• **The overall risk of dying from breast cancer in women with DCIS was about 80% higher** than that of the average American woman but still relatively low—about 1% over the next 10 years and 3.3% over the next 20 years.

• **Age mattered.** Women who were diagnosed before age 35 had a death rate that was 17 times higher than average. (This is a small group...only 5% of women diagnosed with DCIS are under age 40.) The older a woman was when diagnosed with DCIS, the lower were her chances of dying from breast cancer.

• **Race mattered, too.** Black women were at higher risk—with an overall 7% risk of dying over 20 years rather than 3.3%.

But the truly explosive finding was about the outcome of treatment. When the researchers compared lumpectomy alone with lumpectomy plus radiation and/or mastectomy, they found that the simple treatment had the same mortality outcome as the more extensive one. In other words, adding radiation

or mastectomy did not lead to longer lives, on average.

The study will almost certainly lead many women diagnosed with DCIS and their doctors to reconsider what kind of treatment to opt for. But it also raises important questions about whether certain kinds of DCIS may require different treatment.

Some DCIS Really May Be Cancer

The research confirms what some experts have already suspected—DCIS is not a precursor to invasive breast cancer.

How can that be, if women with DCIS had a higher risk of dying from breast cancer?

A small subset of the DCIS tumors acted very differently from the others. More than half of the women who did die of breast cancer after a DCIS diagnosis were never diagnosed with invasive breast cancer—meaning cancer that had spread beyond the milk ducts into breast tissue. While it's possible that some of those cases were misdiagnosed and invasive breast cancer was present but not found, it's more likely that some DCIS tumors actually were cancerous already...and metastasized (spread to other parts of the body). The recent findings open doors to more research aimed at identifying which DCIS tumors are actually dangerous...and which will never turn into cancer at all. DCIS in younger women, for example, may be a very different condition. Researchers are also looking into whether DCIS is best treated with immunological approaches currently being studied rather than with lumpectomy/radiation.

What to Do Now

The recent research certainly puts women... and cancer doctors...in a confusing situation. Getting a DCIS diagnosis means you are at somewhat increased risk of dying from breast cancer...but going for the most radical treatment will not necessarily increase your chances of survival.

Remember, however, that these are averages, and every case is different. If you get a DCIS diagnosis, talk to your doctor, and find out how the specific characteristics of your case affect a treatment decision. That's especially true if you are 35 or younger...or black. Other characteristics, including whether the tumor is affected by hormones, as well as genetic risk factors, may also lead to a conclusion that treatment is warranted. In some cases, the recommended treatment may be hormonal, with medications such as tamoxifen or raloxifene, rather than surgery/radiation, experts suggest. But more research is clearly needed to find out if a hormonal approach actually prevents cancer and cancer deaths.

One thing is clear—the era of routine lumpectomy-followed-by-radiation for women diagnosed with DCIS is coming to an end. In general, your risk of dying from breast cancer is very low and treatment, even aggressive treatment, may not do anything to further reduce that risk.

A diagnosis of DCIS is not an emergency that requires that surgery be scheduled in the next two weeks. You have time to consider your options. You will also want to work with your doctor to make sure that you get regular screenings and double down on your cancer-preventive lifestyle—a proper diet, regular exercise, drinking alcohol in moderation if at all—and avoiding hormone therapy for the treatment of menopausal symptoms.

Family History of Prostate Cancer Raises Breast Cancer Risk

A woman whose father, brother or son has or had prostate cancer may have a 14% higher risk for breast cancer. And women with a family history of both prostate and breast cancer have a 78% elevated risk for breast cancer.

Self-defense: Discuss screening options with your doctor.

Jennifer L. Beebe-Dimmer, MPH, PhD, is associate professor at Barbara Ann Karmanos Cancer Institute and Wayne State University School of Medicine, Detroit. She led a study published in *Cancer*.

When Should You Have a Healthy Breast Removed?

Deborah Axelrod, MD, medical director, clinical breast services and breast programs, Laura and Isaac Perlmutter Cancer Center, NYU Langone Medical Center, New York City.

Call it the Angelina Effect. More women are choosing to have double mastectomies.

Many celebrities have gone that route—Sharon Osbourne, Wanda Sykes, and more recently, Amy Robach and Sandra Lee.

Nor is it only celebrities. Between 1998 and 2011, the rates of women with breast cancer having a double mastectomy for single-breast disease zoomed from less than 2% to more than 11%, according to a recent study published in *JAMA Surgery*.

Here's the catch: Some women are choosing to remove healthy breasts even when doing so isn't likely to help them avoid cancer...or live longer.

What's a good reason to have a healthy breast removed? What's a bad reason? To help women faced with this difficult decision, we spoke with Deborah Axelrod, MD, surgical oncologist at NYU Langone Medical Center and coauthor of *Bosom Buddies*, a guide for women with breast cancer.

Reasons to Remove a Healthy Breast—or Not

"There are indeed many reasons why you may want to remove the 'other' breast...and they're not all purely medical," said Dr. Axelrod. "But you shouldn't be pressured. It's important to understand that most women overestimate their risk for breast cancer returning or getting a cancer in the other breast."

In her practice, when Dr. Axelrod asks patients what they are thinking about their condition and treatment options, she hears a number of reasons for choosing a double mastectomy. *Here are the four reasons she hears most often—and the science that supports or negates them…*

REASON #1: "I Never Want to Have to Worry about Breast Cancer Again."

"This is possibly the worst reason to choose a double mastectomy," said Dr. Axelrod. That's true whether you are newly diagnosed with cancer in one breast…or have already gone through treatment. Why? "Removing the second breast won't have any effect on the cancer that you have been diagnosed and treated for," said Dr. Axelrod. "A bevy of credible research has found no meaningful survival benefit in women who have had cancer in one breast and elect to undergo a double mastectomy. Women who die of breast cancer most likely die of cancer that has spread outside the breast and the lymph nodes. If your breast cancer is going to recur, it will happen locally in the same breast—we can never remove all of the tissue—or systemically, meaning it traveled from the lymph nodes to another part of your body, most typically the bones, liver, lungs and brain. Removing the other, healthy breast is not going to prevent either type of recurrence from happening."

REASON #2: "I've Got the Breast Cancer Gene."

As a carrier of the BRCA1 gene mutation, Angelina Jolie had an 87% lifetime risk of developing breast cancer and a 50% lifetime risk of developing ovarian cancer. Her diagnosis hit close to home, too—her mother died of ovarian cancer at the age of 56. Angelina Jolie eventually had not only both her breasts but also her ovaries removed as a preventive measure. Said Dr. Axelrod, "Carriers of the well-publicized BRCA1 or BRCA2 genes, as well as a number of other genes that have been discovered more recently, including TP53 (Li-Fraumeni syndrome), pTEN (Cowden's disease), CDH1, and PALB2 have

a significantly higher risk. And as in Jolie's case, removing the breasts and ovaries even when there is no cancer present will greatly reduce the odds of both forms of the disease and bring peace of mind.

"Still, you don't have to go to this extreme—with your breasts anyway. Ovarian cancer is harder to diagnose in the early stages, so there is a good argument for having your ovaries removed." With your breasts, however, it's a more complicated decision. You can choose to be closely monitored for very early signs of breast cancer, which is 98% curable if caught in Stage 0 or 1. "However, women who are BRCA1 carriers have a higher rate of small aggressive cancers," she said, "and preventive mastectomy substantially reduces that risk."

REASON #3: "I Have a Family History of Breast Cancer."

"Many women have close relatives—mothers, sisters, grandmothers—who have been diagnosed with breast cancer, yet testing has not revealed any genetic link." That's actually the case most of the time, since only 5% to 10% of women who get breast cancer have known genetic risk factors. "That doesn't rule out a genetic predisposition," she said. "It could well mean that we haven't yet discovered the particular gene mutation that you have. But it's not a good argument for removing a healthy breast. You can avoid unnecessary surgery with close monitoring."

REASON #4: "I Want Both My Breasts to Look the Same."

"While this is not a medical reason, it is a valid personal reason why one may choose to remove a healthy breast along with a diseased one," Dr. Axelrod said. "Breast reconstruction has come a long way, but there is still a big difference between a natural breast and a reconstructed one, and if you're going to have both reconstructed, better symmetry can be achieved if you choose to have them done at the same time. In addition, if you choose to have a TRAM (transverse rectus abdominis) flap (in which some of the abdominal muscle is used to create the new breast) or a DIEP flap (which uses abdominal skin and tissue but no muscle), it can be performed only once, so choosing to have both breasts done makes sense to many women. Bear in mind, however, that the length of time you will spend on the operating table for this procedure is at least double that of traditional reconstruction with implants, and your recovery time will be longer because you're also having abdominal surgery, which also increases the risk for complications. You'll likely be in the hospital for five days as opposed to two or three.

And not every woman is a candidate for this procedure: If you're thin, you likely won't have enough belly tissue. Women who have had multiple cesarean deliveries or other abdominal surgeries also may not be candidates."

All of this adds up to a very personal decision in which you must consider your comfort, convenience, recovery, appearance, family history and fears. "Take your time and consider all the options," said Dr. Axelrod. No doctor should tell you that you need to be on the operating table ASAP, nor should any doctor casually say, 'how about taking off the other breast?' Both kinds of comments are warning signs that you need another opinion."

Why False-Positive Mammograms Increase Your Breast Cancer Risk

Study titled "Increased Risk of Developing Breast Cancer after a False-Positive Screening Mammogram" by researchers at University of North Carolina-Chapel Hill School of Medicine published in *Cancer Epidemiology, Biomarkers & Prevention.*

Half of all women who get mammograms regularly will have a "false positive" within 10 years—a "suspicious" finding that turns out to not be cancer after all. When they find out that their "positives" are false, they're relieved.

But a large new study shows that women who get false positives may be at higher risk for breast cancer after all. Researchers analyzed data from 1.3 million women aged 40 to 74. Compared with women who had only negative mammograms, those who had had false positives were 39% more likely to get breast cancer in the next 10 years—and those who had gotten biopsies because of their potentially positive results were 76% more likely to get breast cancer.

Researchers aren't sure why false positives would be an indicator of greater cancer risk, but it's possible that what medical science currently labels as "false" results could actually indicate changes in breast tissue that are not cancer but that stand a reasonable chance of developing into it.

The increased risk percentages sound scary but the actual level of risk for women who had false positives is much smaller than you might think. That's because the vast majority of women, even those who have had false-positive mammogram results, don't get breast cancer. In the study, women with true negative mammograms had a 10-year risk of developing breast cancer of 0.4%, while those with a false positive had a 0.5% risk, and those who had a false positive and then a biopsy had a 0.7% risk. Even in the highest-risk biopsy group, then, 99.3% will not get breast cancer in the next decade.

It may be that as the science improves, some of today's mammogram results that are simply considered "false positives" and forgotten about will come to be considered actual positives—not for cancer, but for increased risk, albeit small.

Women with a strong family history of breast cancer, especially those with genetic markers for the disease, are already at higher-than-average risk. While this study didn't look at these groups of women in particular, they already have reason to be extra vigilant.

For women who aren't aware of any extra risk, however, this study may be an added incentive—if you've ever had a false-positive mammogram result, you now have even more reason to monitor your breast health.

Better Breast Cancer Treatment

Radiation of lymph nodes is usually not given to women whose early-stage breast cancer has spread to just a few nodes.

New research: Among women with early-stage breast cancer who had surgery, 82% of those who also had radiation to the breast and nearby lymph nodes were cancer free over the following 10 years, compared with 77% who received surgery alone. Side effects included skin rash, chronic swelling of the arm and inflammation of the lungs.

Timothy Whelan, BM, BCh, professor of oncology, McMaster University, Hamilton, Ontario, Canada.

When It Comes to Breast Cancer Treatment, Timing Is Key

Richard J. Bleicher, MD, associate professor, surgical oncology, Fox Chase Cancer Center, Philadelphia.

Mariana Chavez MacGregor, MD, assistant professor, breast medical oncology, University of Texas MD Anderson Cancer Center, Houston.

Lauren Cassell, MD, chief, breast surgery, Lenox Hill Hospital, New York City.

Frank Monteleone, MD, chief, breast services and director, Breast Health Center, Winthrop-University Hospital, Mineola, New York.

Charles L. Shapiro, MD, director, Translational Breast Cancer Research, Mount Sinai Health System, New York City.

Fox Chase Cancer Center, news release.

JAMA Oncology, news release.

The sooner early-stage breast cancer patients have surgery following their diagnosis, and chemotherapy after their surgery, the better their chances of survival, two new studies find.

Study #1

In one study, researchers at Fox Chase Cancer Center in Philadelphia analyzed data from more than 94,500 American women ages 66 and older. All were diagnosed with breast cancer between 1992 and 2009.

The team, led by Richard J. Bleicher, MD, found a 9% increased risk of death from all causes for each 30-day delay in the time from diagnosis to surgery.

The link between time to surgery and risk of death from all causes was only statistically significant for patients with earlier stages of cancer, the researchers noted. In the study, delays seemed to affect prognosis for patients with stage 1 and stage 2 cancers, but not for those with stage 3 cancers.

The findings were similar when Dr. Bleicher's team conducted a second analysis of data involving more than 115,700 American women ages 18 and older, who were diagnosed with breast cancer between 2003 and 2005.

Even after adjusting for a number of other factors, a longer time to surgery was still associated with increased risk of death, the researchers found.

This is "the most comprehensive study of the subject ever performed, and includes two extraordinarily large groups from two of the largest cancer databases in the United States," said Dr. Bleicher, associate professor of surgical oncology. "The findings from the analysis answer a question that nearly every patient asks: 'Will my prognosis be affected by the time it takes me to get to surgery?'"

Long delays were rare: Only 1.2% of patients in the first analysis and 1.5% of those in the second analysis had surgery more than 90 days after their breast cancer diagnosis, the researchers noted.

Study #2

In a second study, researchers at the University of Texas MD Anderson Cancer Center in Houston tracked outcomes for nearly 25,000 patients in California who were diagnosed with invasive breast cancer (stages 1 to 3).

The researchers wanted to see if survival was affected by the time elapsed between breast cancer surgery and the initiation of follow-up chemotherapy.

The women averaged 53 years of age and the median time to chemotherapy after their breast cancer surgery was 43 days, reported a team led by Mariana Chavez MacGregor, MD, assistant professor of breast medical oncology at the University of Texas MD Anderson Cancer Center.

The researchers found no differences in outcomes for patients whose chemotherapy began anywhere between 31 days and 90 days after their surgery.

However, women whose post-op chemo started 91 days or longer after their surgery did fare worse. Those women had a 34% higher risk for death from any cause, and a 27% higher risk for death linked to breast cancer, compared to women whose chemo started sooner, the researchers said.

"Given the results of our analysis, we would suggest that all breast cancer patients that are candidates for adjuvant chemotherapy should receive this treatment within 91 days of surgery or 120 days from diagnosis," said Dr. Chavez MacGregor and colleagues.

"Administration of chemotherapy within this frame is feasible in clinical practice under most clinical scenarios, and as medical oncologists, we should make every effort not to delay the initiation of adjuvant chemotherapy," they added.

Both studies were published in *JAMA Oncology*.

Expert Reaction

Experts in breast cancer care agreed that timing is important to patient outcomes.

"Though these two studies are retrospective, and not the highest level of evidence, they nonetheless support the notion that delays of beyond 30 days in both time to surgery and time to adjuvant chemotherapy after breast surgery should be kept to a minimum as much as possible," said Charles L. Shapiro, MD, director of Translational Breast Cancer Research at Mount Sinai Health System in New York City.

Another expert said that a patient's medical team must work together to ensure that treatments occur in a timely manner.

"The best way to treat breast cancer is with a team approach," said Frank Monteleone, MD, chief of breast services and director of the Breast Health Center at Winthrop-University Hospital in Mineola, New York.

"Radiologists, breast surgeons, radiation oncologists and medical oncologists need to work together to ensure that the time between diagnosis, surgery and oncology treatment is done in the quickest time possible," he said. "Also important is a supportive staff, including nurse navigators and social workers, to identify and reduce or eliminate barriers that will delay patients from receiving the care they need."

Lauren Cassell, MD, chief of breast surgery at New York City's Lenox Hill Hospital, agreed. "There's nothing wrong with a little helping hand in navigating the process, particularly for a patient who may be overwhelmed by her diagnosis," she said.

For more information on breast cancer surgery, visit Breastcancer.org at *breastcancer.org/treatment/surgery*.

The New Test That May Save You from Chemo

Laura van 't Veer, PhD, leader, Breast Oncology Program, University of California, San Francisco Helen Diller Family Comprehensive Cancer Center.

Jose Baselga, MD, PhD, physician-in-chief and chief medical officer, Memorial Hospital at Memorial Sloan-Kettering Cancer Center, New York City.

Stephanie Bernik, MD, chief, surgical oncology, Lenox Hill Hospital, New York City.

Victor Vogel, MD, MHS, director, Breast Medical Oncology/Research for Geisinger Health System, Danville, Pennsylvania.

Presentation, American Association for Cancer Research meeting, New Orleans.

Many breast cancer patients receive chemotherapy they don't need, according to the results of a long-awaited clinical trial.

A genetic test called MammaPrint determined that nearly half the women slated for chemotherapy based on standard clinical assessments didn't really need to undergo the challenging treatment.

After surgery to remove their tumors, breast cancer patients with a MammaPrint score recommending against chemotherapy had a 95% survival rate, said co-researcher Laura van 't Veer, PhD, the test's inventor.

"That's very high, and we showed that it doesn't differ between those who are treated and those who are not treated by chemotherapy," said Dr. van 't Veer, leader of the breast oncology program at the University of California, San Francisco Diller Family Cancer Center.

The clinical trial involved nearly 6,700 women at 111 medical centers in nine countries. It "represents what we in medicine call the highest level of evidence," AACR President Jose Baselga, MD, PhD, said.

"This study is telling us in a very clear way we can spare many women chemotherapy," said Dr. Baselga, chief medical officer of Memorial Hospital at Memorial Sloan Kettering Cancer Center, in New York City.

Previously, doctors guessed whether a woman needed chemo by measuring the tumor, examining its cells under a microscope, and using genetic testing to determine whether the tumor would respond to hormone therapy, Dr. Baselga said.

The MammaPrint test looks at a panel of 70 genes within the tumor itself to assess its aggressiveness and the odds it will come back without chemotherapy, Dr. van 't Veer said.

"Our test looks under the hood, at the engine of the tumor," she said. "The biology tells more about the tumor than simply examining its size, because you're really looking into the tumor."

MammaPrint has been on the US market since FDA approval in 2007. But many cancer doctors have waited for the results of this clinical trial to see how well it works, Dr. Baselga said.

Although the results should be considered preliminary until published in a peer-reviewed medical journal, Dr. Baselga said, "This is the result we were hoping for."

In the clinical trial, researchers sorted breast cancer patients into four groups, based on whether MammaPrint testing or traditional clinical assessment recommended chemotherapy.

MammaPrint reduced chemotherapy prescriptions by 46% among the more than 3,300 patients in the trial categorized as having a high risk of breast cancer recurrence based on common clinical and pathological criteria, the researchers said.

Further, just over 2,700 patients who had a low MammaPrint risk score but a high clinical risk score wound up with a 94.7% five-year survival rate, whether they got chemo or not, the researchers said.

Stephanie Bernik, MD, chief of surgical oncology at Lenox Hill Hospital in New York City, said the results of this study were eagerly anticipated.

"If we can select those patients that don't need chemotherapy, unneeded treatment can be avoided and we will be one step closer to making sure treatment for breast cancer is tailored to the individual," she said.

MammaPrint testing will be particularly valuable for young women with breast cancer, said Victor Vogel, MD, director of Breast Medical Oncology/Research for the Geisinger Health System in Pennsylvania.

Young women have been more likely to receive chemotherapy in standard breast cancer care, even though it can destroy their fertility and leave them open to long-term health problems, Dr. Vogel said.

"In my training, if you had a young woman with breast cancer, she got chemotherapy," Dr. Vogel said. "But now we can be selective, and we know there's a very large number of young women with small hormone-responsive tumors who do not need chemotherapy."

Dr. Vogel said he frequently uses the MammaPrint test in his practice, and found that it helps all patients regardless of how they fare on it.

"It works both ways," he said. "It reassures the people who don't need chemotherapy, and when you get a big score that says there would be benefit, it encourages the patient they're doing the right thing by taking chemotherapy."

MammaPrint is covered by Medicare and is reimbursed by most large health insurers in the United States, Dr. van 't Veer said.

The test is expected to save health care dollars, Dr. Baselga said.

"You are saving all the money for chemotherapy that would be used for no reason, and you are protecting women from chemotherapy that is toxic and they don't need," he said.

For more on breast cancer treatments, visit the American Cancer Society at Cancer.org.

1 in 4 Breast Cancer Lumpectomies Requires Follow-Up Surgery

Art Sedrakyan, MD, PhD, professor, health care policy and research, Weill Cornell Medicine, New York City.

Anthony Echo, MD, assistant professor, plastic surgery, Houston Methodist Hospital.

JAMA Surgery, online.

Women with early-stage breast cancer who opt for a breast-conserving surgery known as a lumpectomy have a one in four chance they will need a second operation within 90 days, researchers report.

"The chance of getting a second surgery has gone down a little, but it is still high and it is substantial," said study author Art Sedrakyan, MD, PhD. He is a professor of health care policy and research at Weill Cornell Medicine in New York City.

About Lumpectomy

In a lumpectomy, the tumor tissue, along with a margin of surrounding tumor-free tissue, is removed. However, if the tissue in the margin is not completely free of tumor cells, a second operation is needed.

The Study

The researchers evaluated data on nearly 90,000 women who had lumpectomies in hospitals and ambulatory surgery centers in New York. The rates of re-operation were highest among those aged 20 to 49 and lowest in those aged 65 and older.

During the study period, which ran from 2003 through 2013, the overall rate of re-operation within 90 days was almost 31%, Dr. Sedrakyan said. It declined from nearly

Chemo Dangers

Fish Oil Chemo Warning

Fish oil could cause chemo resistance, according to recent research. In animal models, fatty acids in fish oil and fatty fish, such as herring or mackerel, were found to interfere with the metabolism of certain chemotherapy drugs. These resistance-inducing fatty acids are also found in human blood after consumption of fish oil and fatty fish. If you're on chemotherapy: Ask your doctor if it's safe for you to take a fish oil supplement or eat fatty fish.

Emile Voest, MD, PhD, professor of medical oncology, Netherlands Cancer Institute, Amsterdam.

Chemo Might Harm More Than Help

Chemotherapy might hurt more than help end-stage cancer patients. Doctors often prescribe chemo to patients expected to live six months or less to shrink tumors and make them feel better—but side effects such as nausea and vomiting can make them feel worse. And if cancer has progressed despite two or more courses of chemotherapy, the chance that another regimen will work is very small. Self-defense: Question your doctor on the pros and cons.

Holly G. Prigerson, PhD, is director of the Center for Research on End-of-Life Care, Weill Cornell Medical College, New York City.

40% in 2003 through 2004, to 23% from 2011 through 2013, the study found.

"Having a second surgery after you think you've solved all your problems is stressful," Dr. Sedrakyan said.

"Patients operated on by higher-volume doctors had a lower chance of getting this re-operation," Dr. Sedrakyan said. High-volume surgeons were defined as those who had 34 or more cases a year, on average, while low-volume surgeons had 13 or fewer cases. The lowered risk with high-volume doctors was about 33%, the study findings showed.

The study appeared in the journal *JAMA Surgery*.

Implications

The question of how often women need a repeat surgery is critical for a number of reasons, Dr. Sedrakyan explained. These reasons include letting women know the risk of re-operation if they choose breast-conservation surgery. Doctors also need to know the risk so they can come up with guidance to help reduce that risk, he said. He believes the data, while gathered only from one state, New York, would be applicable to other regions of the United States.

Possible Explanation

Anthony Echo, MD, an assistant professor of plastic surgery at Houston Methodist Hospital in Texas, agreed.

The decline found in re-operation rates in the study is probably due to a number of factors, Dr. Echo said. They include better training of breast surgeons and the team approach now used at many hospitals.

"There is much more knowledge," Dr. Echo said. And some radiologists and pathologists now dedicate their practices to breast cancer, he added.

The team approach may indeed help explain the decline, along with better techniques, Dr. Sedrakyan said. In addition, new guidelines from the Society of Surgical Oncology and the American Society for Radiation Oncology specifying when re-operation is needed may further reduce the second surgery rates, the study authors suggested.

The Link Between Thyroid and Breast Cancer

Raymon Grogan, MD, assistant professor, surgery, and director, endocrine surgery research program, University of Chicago Medicine.
Carol DeSantis, MPH, director, breast and gynecological cancer surveillance, American Cancer Society.
Cancer Epidemiology, Biomarkers and Prevention.

Women who survive either breast or thyroid cancer may be at increased risk for the other tumor type, according to a new analysis.

About Thyroid Cancer

Thyroid cancer cases have nearly tripled in the United States over the past 30 years, and breast cancer is the most common cancer among women, according to background notes with the study. Thanks to medical advances, more women are surviving each cancer, said study lead author Raymon Grogan, MD, director of the University of Chicago's endocrine surgery research program.

The Study

University of Chicago researchers reviewed 37 published studies. Nineteen of the studies analyzed breast cancer patients and their risk of thyroid cancer. Another 18 looked at thyroid cancer cases and their incidence of breast cancer.

The researchers then combined these data and calculated the odds of a woman having thyroid cancer after breast cancer and vice versa.

They found that breast cancer survivors were 1.55 times more likely to develop thyroid cancer than women who hadn't had breast cancer. And, female thyroid cancer survivors were 1.18 times more likely to get breast cancer than women who hadn't had thyroid cancer, researchers said.

"This is a real risk," said Dr. Grogan. "People who have had one of these cancers need to be aware that they are at higher risk for developing the other cancer," he said.

The report was published in the journal *Cancer Epidemiology, Biomarkers and Prevention*.

Possible Explanations

In addition, the researchers combed through the studies to find reasons why these cancers seemed related. One explanation was that women who survive either cancer were more likely to be screened and examined so that other cancers were found early.

Another possible connection was that breast and thyroid cancers share hormonal risk factors. There is some evidence that exposure to estrogens and to thyroid-stimulating hormones may contribute to both cancers, Dr. Grogan said.

A third theory points to radiation therapy, which has been shown to increase the risk for lung, esophageal and blood cancers, and sarcomas. Also, earlier research found that radioactive iodine, used to treat thyroid cancer, may play a small role in the development of other cancers, including breast cancer, but that is not clear, Dr. Grogan said.

Finally, it is possible that a genetic mutation might be responsible for the connection, Dr. Grogan said.

Expert Commentary

Carol DeSantis, MPH, director of breast and gynecological cancer surveillance at the American Cancer Society, said the connection between thyroid and breast cancer is known.

She said her concern with this new report is that by lumping together so many studies that differ in their methods and findings, it's impossible to come up with a single number that accurately reflects the risk of having one cancer after having had the other.

"The review of different studies is helpful to see that there is that link, but combining them all together, I am not sure who that would be applicable to," DeSantis said.

Dr. Grogan said the research team tried to control for those differences as best they could.

Advice

DeSantis said that cancer survivors should be aware of the increased risk of developing other cancers.

"Generally, cancer survivors are at risk for developing a second cancer," she said. "Breast cancer survivors are at risk for blood cancers, uterine cancer, ovarian cancer and other cancers. Likewise, thyroid cancer survivors are at risk for a number of other cancers, including breast cancer."

Doctors need to be more aware of the link between the two cancers, Dr. Grogan said.

"It should just become one of the common discussions between a patient and her doctor," he said. "It doesn't change the recommendations for screening, but people need to be aware and be screened at the appropriate time."

You, HRT and Ovarian Cancer

Hormone replacement therapy (HRT) is linked to ovarian cancer risk. In a recent analysis of more than 21,000 postmenopausal women, those who used either oral or patch HRT to ease menopause symptoms, even for the commonly recommended limit of less than five years, were 20% more likely to develop ovarian cancer than those who never used HRT.

If you are considering HRT: Talk to your doctor about your cancer risk.

Valerie Beral, DBE, MD, director, Cancer Epidemiology Unit, University of Oxford, UK.

Regular Screening Can Help Catch Ovarian Cancer Before It's Too Late

Currently, most cases are detected only at an advanced stage.

But: A recent study found a 20% reduction in ovarian cancer deaths when postmenopausal women with no known malignancies or family history of ovarian cancer were screened annually for seven or more years. The screening—an ultrasound and the CA-125 (Cancer Antigen-125) blood test—already is used in high-risk women with certain gene mutations or an extensive family history of ovarian or breast cancer.

Anil Sood, MD, director of the Blanton-Davis Ovarian Cancer Research Program, University of Texas MD Anderson Cancer Center, Houston.

Lifesaving Ovarian Cancer Treatment

Maurie Markman, MD, an oncologist and president of Medicine and Science at Cancer Treatment Centers of America, which has hospitals in Atlanta, Chicago, Philadelphia, Phoenix and Tulsa. CancerCenter.com

Three major US studies have concluded that a treatment known as intraperitoneal (IP) therapy often extends the lives of women diagnosed with ovarian cancer. One study found that IP therapy reduces the risk for death within the 10 years following treatment by 23%.

Yet according to some estimates, fewer than half of ovarian cancer patients receive IP therapy, which involves pumping chemotherapy drugs directly into the abdominal cavity. Many patients are not even told about it.

Why is IP therapy not more widely used? *Several reasons…*

•**Pharmaceutical companies are not pushing it.** IP therapy uses generic drugs,

Low-Dose Aspirin Protects Against Ovarian Cancer

Low-dose aspirin reduces risk for ovarian cancer. Women who took low-dose aspirin (less than 100 milligrams) daily to protect against cardiovascular disease were 34% less likely to develop ovarian cancer. This may be especially important to women with BRCA genetic mutations, which raise the risk for both breast and ovarian cancers.

Caution: Aspirin has potential side effects—discuss the risks and benefits with your doctor.

Analysis of 12 studies of aspirin use by researchers at the National Cancer Institute, Bethesda, Maryland, published in *Journal of the National Cancer Institute.*

so there's no big company promoting it to doctors.

•**The procedure is time-consuming, unprofitable and unfamiliar to many doctors.** Some oncologists do not provide IP therapy simply because they have no experience with it. They have little economic incentive to learn—pumping chemotherapy drugs into the abdomen takes significantly more time and effort than simply setting up a traditional IV. (IP therapy is used in conjunction with intravenous delivery of chemotherapy drugs, not instead of it.)

•**There are side effects.** IP therapy can cause increased discomfort for patients, including painful abdominal bloating during treatment. The process also is more invasive than traditional IV delivery—typically a catheter is inserted into the abdomen, which occasionally leads to infection. But any side effects are temporary, and any infection is likely to be treatable.

If you are diagnosed with ovarian cancer: Ask your oncologist if IP therapy is an option. If your oncologist doesn't seem to be well-informed about IP therapy or simply says he/she doesn't do it, ask for a referral to an oncologist who does use the therapy. If your oncologist cannot provide such a referral, contact the American Cancer Society

(*Cancer.org*) and/or the American Society of Clinical Oncology (*ASCO.org*) and ask for a referral to a gynecological oncologist in your area who has experience with IP therapy.

Two Heart Medications That Might Help Treat Ovarian Cancer

A popular heart medication may help ovarian cancer patients. In a recent retrospective study, researchers found that ovarian cancer patients who took "nonselective" beta-blockers, such as *carvedilol* (Coreg) and *propranolol* (Inderal), while undergoing treatment for ovarian cancer lived more than twice as long as patients who did not use the drugs.

Possible reason: The medications inhibit mechanisms that are involved in the growth and spreading of tumors.

Anil Sood, MD, director of Blanton-Davis Ovarian Cancer Research Program, University of Texas MD Anderson Cancer Center, Houston, and senior author of a study published in *Cancer*.

Itching After a Shower and Other Surprising Cancer Symptoms

Eugene Ahn, MD, hematologist and oncologist at Cancer Treatment Centers of America (CTCA) and medical director for clinical research in integrative oncology at CTCA at Midwestern Regional Medical Center in Zion, Illinois. CancerCenter.com

Certain cancer symptoms almost always prompt a visit to the doctor. A breast lump. A mole that changes in size, shape or color. Blood in the stool.

But there are other symptoms that most people ignore.

Startling new finding: In a study published in *British Journal of General Practice,* nearly half of people with a warning sign of cancer decided not to see a doctor about it, often because they thought the symptom was insignificant.

For the following symptoms, your first step is to visit your primary care physician who can perform the appropriate tests and/or refer you to a specialist.

If you have any one of these symptoms in isolation, the likelihood of you having cancer is less than 1%. That doesn't mean you should dismiss the symptom. But it does mean that you shouldn't panic if it shows up.

• **Heartburn.**

Most likely cause: Gastroesophageal reflux disease (GERD).

But it could be a sign of: Esophagus or stomach cancer. Symptoms of heartburn can include burning pain or discomfort in the stomach, upper abdomen, chest and/or throat…and/or excessive burping, bloating or nausea after eating. If those symptoms are chronic, it's time to see a doctor for a work-up. You might have Barrett's esophagus, a precancerous condition that is triggered by chronic inflammation and increases the risk for esophageal cancer. Or you might have H. pylori, a bacterial infection of the stomach that increases your risk for stomach cancer (and ulcers)—but is easily treatable with a two-week treatment that includes antibiotics and possibly a proton-pump inhibitor.

What to do: Ask your doctor if you need an esophagogastroduodenoscopy (EGD), in which an endoscope is used to explore your esophagus, stomach and duodenum (the first section of the small intestine). A biopsy can be taken during the procedure if there is suspicious-looking tissue.

• **Itching after a hot shower.**

Most likely cause: Dry skin or a contact allergy to a cleansing product.

But it could be a sign of: Polycythemia vera, a common myeloproliferative disorder, a type of blood cancer. In the early stages of this cancer, histamine-containing mast cells (cells behind allergic reactions) become hypersensitive, causing the skin to react to hot water.

49

What to do: If you're over age 40 (when this cancer most commonly occurs), ask your doctor for a complete blood count (CBC), which will detect an elevation of red blood cells, a feature of polycythemia vera.

• **Eating ice.**

Likely cause: Iron deficiency.

But it could be a sign of: Gastrointestinal cancers, bladder cancer or any cancer that leads to blood loss. Called pica, this phenomenon—a compulsion to eat ice, sand, soil, clay, paper or chalk or to chew on something metallic—usually occurs during pregnancy and can be a sign of iron deficiency. But iron deficiency also can signal chronic internal blood loss, sometimes from cancer.

What to do: Ask your doctor about a blood test for iron deficiency. If you have an iron deficiency, work with your doctor to determine the cause.

• **Unbearable pain in a bone when touched.**

Most likely causes: Trauma, rheumatological disease or infection.

But it could be a sign of: Bone metastases (the spread of an original, primary tumor into the bone). This symptom is a hallmark of bone cancer.

What to do: If you have unexplained pain that tends to increase over a month—particularly if it's sensitive to the touch—talk to your doctor about imaging studies, such as a CT scan, a bone scan, an X-ray or an MRI.

• **Diarrhea plus facial flushing.**

Likely cause: Irritable bowel syndrome (IBS).

But it could be a sign of: Neuro-endocrine tumor, metastasized to the liver. Diarrhea alone rarely leads to a diagnosis of cancer, but diarrhea and flushing of the face are a unique pair of symptoms that could indicate a neuroendocrine tumor—a type of cancer arising from the hormone-producing cells in the body.

What to do: Talk to your doctor about possible imaging (CT, PET or MRI) to potentially detect liver metastases and primary tumor.

• **Reddened skin on the breast.**

Likely cause: Skin infection.

But it could be a sign of: Breast cancer. A lump is not the only warning sign of breast cancer. Redness of the breast—particularly if the skin also is thickened, with the texture of an orange peel—is a sign of inflammatory breast cancer, a rare and aggressive form of the disease that can be missed by a mammogram, an ultrasound or an MRI.

What to do: Ask your doctor about a breast biopsy, the best way to detect this type of cancer.

Important: If the doctor diagnoses the redness as an infection and treats it with antibiotics, and the redness doesn't resolve or worsens, return quickly for a follow-up examination.

• **Blood clot.**

Likely causes: Leg or arm injury, such as a sprained ankle…recent hospitalization or surgery…a long period of inactivity, such as a plane ride.

But it could be a sign of: Breast, pancreatic, ovarian and many other cancers. A blood clot (a symptom of deep vein thrombosis, or DVT) is a common problem, affecting 900,000 Americans yearly. But DVT is not commonly understood as a potential early warning sign of cancer and so is often overlooked as a cancer symptom, even though as many as one in 10 patients with an unexplained blood clot may have some type of cancer.

What to do: If you have a blood clot (typically signaled by a sudden, painful swelling of an arm or a leg) without any of the common triggers (see common causes above), talk to your doctor about a workup for cancer. This is an early warning sign that often is missed.

• **Bloating.**

Likely cause: Eating too much or too fast.

But it could be a sign of: Ovarian cancer. Bloating is a common symptom that is rarely a sign of cancer. But persistent bloating can be a sign of cancer in the peritoneal cavity, a common feature of advanced ovarian cancer, particularly if accompanied by a persistent, dull ache in the abdomen and unexplained weight loss (a symptom of advanced cancer).

What to do: Your doctor may recommend a CT scan or a transvaginal ultrasound. If the results are negative, ask about getting a laparoscopy, in which a thin, lighted tube is put through an incision in the belly to look at the abdominal and reproductive organs. A CT scan or a transvaginal ultrasound can easily miss ovarian cancer.

•**Quitting smoking easily.**

Likely cause: You decided to quit, and you succeeded.

But it could be a sign of: Lung cancer. A chronic smoker who suddenly finds it unusually easy to quit may be experiencing a strange physiological symptom of lung cancer—inexplicably losing the desire to smoke. Usually, non-small-cell lung cancer is diagnosed three to four years after a chronic smoker easily quits, and small-cell lung cancer (a more aggressive type) is diagnosed about six months after quitting.

What to do: If you have been a lifelong smoker who suddenly finds it easy to quit, talk to your doctor about having a chest CT scan for lung cancer. You also would benefit from routine annual surveillance even if the scan is negative.

Lung Cancer Is On the Rise Among Nonsmokers

Timothy Burns, MD, PhD, assistant professor of medicine in the department of medicine, division of hematology/oncology, at the University of Pittsburgh Cancer Institute, where his laboratory focuses on discovering targeted therapies for lung cancer.

People who have never smoked often assume that they'll never get lung cancer. But they can—and the prevalence of these cases is increasing at a troubling rate.

Update: Two important recent studies show that rates of lung cancer among so-called "never-smokers" (less than 100 ciga-

rettes smoked in a lifetime) are mysteriously skyrocketing—in one study, from 9% to 20% of all such malignancies.

But it's not all bad news.

The recent discovery of genetic mutations called "oncogenes" that drive lung cancer in never-smokers has fueled the development of powerful medications that are often more effective and have fewer side effects than conventional chemotherapy.

Bonus: These new drugs are taken orally rather than intravenously, as is more common with conventional chemotherapy.

Testing for Mutations

If you're one of the roughly 24,000 never-smokers diagnosed with lung cancer each year in the US, it's crucial for you (as well as current and former smokers) to be tested for a genetic mutation that might be driving your disease.

Shockingly, many of these patients are not tested despite the recommendations of national cancer organizations. This is due, in part, to the lack of awareness of many community oncologists in the US.

The most accurate test uses a tissue biopsy to screen for a handful of critical mutations that predict a more than 70% chance of responding to FDA-approved drugs. If the size and location of the tumor make a biopsy impossible, the oncologist should order a blood or urine test to check for mutations.

Important: If possible, get your genetic testing at one of the 45 medical institutions designated by the National Cancer Institute (NCI) as a "Comprehensive Cancer Center" (check *Cancer.gov/research/nci-role/cancer-centers/find*). You will get the most accurate testing at one of these centers and the most reliably up-to-date information on the latest cutting-edge medicine and clinical trials. A medical oncologist near you can administer the treatment. If you're not able to travel to an NCI-designated center, a tissue sample from a biopsy performed at your local medical facility can be sent to certain institutions (such as the Mayo Clinic and Johns Hopkins) that offer molecular testing.

Key Genetic Mutations

If you have a genetic mutation, a targeted medication can be used to treat the lung cancer. (Patients who do not test positive for a mutation receive standard cancer care, including conventional chemotherapy and/or radiation.)

Genetic mutations may include...

•**Epidermal growth factor receptor (EGFR).** This is the most common mutation in never-smokers with lung cancer, occurring in about 40% of these patients. Several FDA-approved drugs called EGFR-inhibitors can counter this mutation, including *gefitinib* (Iressa)...*erlotinib* (Tarceva)...and *afatinib* (Gilotrif). Additionally, *icotinib* (Conmana) is in clinical trials.

•**Anaplastic lymphoma kinase (ALK).** About 5% to 8% of lung cancer patients (most of these never-smokers) have this genetic mutation. The FDA-approved drug is *crizotinib* (Xalkori) for ALK-positive patients who have never received lung cancer treatment.

Time for a Different Drug

Even when a genetic mutation is identified, eventually a new mutation is generated and the tumor starts growing again—a phenomenon called acquired resistance. This typically occurs after about a year of treatment. Therefore, patients on these therapies undergo regular CT scans at two- to three-month intervals to make sure their disease is not growing.

Best approach: When your tumor develops acquired resistance, it's important to have another biopsy so that your doctor can determine which drug is right for you. Two months after starting a second-line drug, the patient will undergo a new CT scan to make sure it is shrinking the tumor.

Important: The patient should alert the physician if he/she is taking any over-the-counter supplements—some can have life-threatening interactions with the targeted therapies.

Early Detection

The cause of lung cancer in never-smokers is unknown, but it is believed that up to 50% of cases are due to exposure to radon, a naturally occurring radioactive gas, and/or secondhand smoke. A distant third is indoor air pollution, such as particles from wood-burning stoves and cooking fumes from stir-, deep- or pan-frying. *Main risks...*

•**Radon.** Get your home tested. If levels are high (4 pCi/L or above), hire a state-licensed "radon mitigation contractor" to reduce levels to 2 pCi/L or below by installing a pipe that vents the gas outdoors.

•**Secondhand smoke.** Avoid it whenever possible.

•**Indoor air pollution.** If you have a wood stove, get a high-efficiency particle arresting (HEPA) air filter...if you fry food, vent the fumes—they may contain harmful carcinogens.

Important: If you are a never-smoker who has one or more of the symptoms of lung cancer—a persistent cough, chest pain, shortness of breath and/or sudden weight loss...or if you've had pneumonia that's persisted for months in spite of several rounds of antibiotics—ask your doctor to test for lung cancer.

Unfortunately, never-smoker lung cancer often has no (or only vague) symptoms that doctors may not immediately suspect as a malignancy. For this reason, it is usually diagnosed when the cancer has spread to the bone, brain, liver and/or other organs. At that point, the most that can be done is to control the disease, giving the patient as much as three to five or more extra years of life if the disease is treated. As new therapies continue to emerge, the goal is to make never-smoker lung cancer a chronic disease and to someday provide a cure.

Surgery Helps Lung Cancer Patients

Surgery helps some advanced-lung-cancer patients. Some patients with Stage 3b non-small-cell lung cancer lived an average of almost 10 months longer if, in addition to chemotherapy and radiation, they had surgery to remove diseased lung tissue. Surgery recipients lived 26 more months, on average, compared with 16 months for those who had only chemotherapy and radiation.

Study of more than 9,000 patients by researchers at Washington University School of Medicine, St. Louis, published in *The Annals of Thoracic Surgery*.

When a CT Scan Could Save Your Life

A CT scan follow-up program after surgery for lung cancer significantly increases survival rates.

Details: About 400 patients who received CT scans of the thorax (chest) and upper abdomen every three months for two years and then every six months for three more years had a survival rate during the study of 67.8% versus a survival rate of 55.7% for those who did not receive CT scans.

If you have had surgery for lung cancer: Ask your doctor about getting regular CT scans.

Niels-Chr. G. Hansen, MD, pulmonologist, Odense University Hospital, Denmark.

5 Widespread Myths About Sunscreen

Barney Kenet, MD, a board-certified dermatologist and dermatologic surgeon at New York-Presbyterian/ Weill Cornell Medical Center and in private practice, both in New York City. He is author of *Saving Your Skin* and *How to Wash Your Face*.

It used to be that summer didn't officially begin until that first sunburn.

What's changed: Even though dermatologists have cautioned for years that burned—or even suntanned—skin can lead to skin cancer, far too many people are failing to heed that warning. In fact, only about 20% of men and 43% of women use sunscreen

regularly, according to a new survey by the Centers for Disease Control and Prevention.

Why do so few of us take advantage of this basic form of skin protection? Part of the problem is that there are so many misconceptions about sunscreens and skin cancer.

Among the most common myths…

MYTH #1: If you wear sunscreen, you'll develop vitamin D deficiency.

Truth: Our skin needs to be exposed to sunlight in order for our bodies to manufacture vitamin D. Deficiencies of this crucial vitamin are now being linked to everything from bone loss and multiple sclerosis to heart disease and dementia.

It's true that if you were perfectly covered in sunscreen every minute of every day, then you could, theoretically, develop a vitamin D deficiency. This, however, isn't a reality for most people.

Dr. Kenet's take: To produce sufficient vitamin D, you need only about 10 to 15 minutes of sun exposure three times a week on your arms or face (without sunscreen). If you are worried because you live in an area where you get limited sun exposure, ask your doctor for a blood test to measure your vitamin D level. If your level is low, you may need to take a vitamin D supplement.

MYTH #2: Only fair-skinned people develop skin cancer.

Truth: While it is true that fair-skinned people are at highest risk for melanoma, the deadliest form of skin cancer, olive-skinned and dark-skinned people are also at risk. Among African-Americans, for example, melanomas mainly occur on parts of the body that are not pigmented, such as the palms of the hands, the soles of the feet and the skin beneath the nails.

Dr. Kenet's take: No matter what your skin tone, use sunscreen to help protect against skin cancer. Be sure to cover areas that frequently get overlooked—the back, behind the ears and the backs of the legs.

If you have dark skin, you might not need to wear sunscreen on a daily basis, but I advise using it when you are spending time outdoors in intense sunlight.

MYTH #3: Sunscreen is all you need to avoid skin cancer.

Truth: Sunscreen is just one tool in skin cancer prevention.

Dr. Kenet's take: When it comes to skin protection, think "belt and suspenders"—that is, no single approach will guarantee safe skin, so do as much as possible.

Reduce your exposure to ultraviolet (UV) radiation by avoiding outdoor activities during the peak UV-risk hours of 10 am to 4 pm.

Hide your skin from the sun by seeking shady areas...using a wide-brimmed hat that shades your face and ears...and wearing a tight-weave, long-sleeved shirt. Also, consider wearing clothing made with UV-protective fabric. Check *Coolibar.com*...and *SunPre cautions.com.*

Important: Don't forget sunglasses—ocular melanoma is a real risk, especially for people with light (blue or green) eyes. One in four Americans rarely or never wears sunglasses, according to a new survey. Be sure your sunglasses block out 99% to 100% of both UVA and UVB rays.

Important: Skin cancer can develop on the lips, too, so use a lip balm that includes sun protection factor (SPF). It doesn't have to be anything fancy—ChapStick Ultra Lip Balm with SPF 30 works great.

MYTH #4: When it comes to SPF, the higher the better.

Truth: Sunscreens with SPF 15 filter out 93% of UVB rays (the primary cause of sunburn)...SPF 30 filters 97%...and SPF 50 filters 98%. There is very little difference between the protection offered by SPF 30 and SPF 50+.

People often mistakenly assume that a high-SPF product that blocks sunburn is adequate, not realizing that it may not protect them from the effects of UVA exposure, which is more closely associated with skin cancer. "Broad-spectrum" products provide protection against both UVB and UVA exposure.

Dr. Kenet's take: For maximum sun protection, purchase a broad-spectrum sunscreen with at least SPF 15, then be sure to reapply it every two hours (use a golf ball–size dollop—roughly one ounce). And yes, that means you'll go through a bottle of sunscreen very quickly!

Note: People who have lupus or a family history of skin cancer should use an SPF of at least 30.

It is a good idea to wear sunscreen year-round. Apply it before you get dressed (this helps reduce the chance that you'll miss a spot).

MYTH #5: It's fine to choose any form of sunscreen, as long as it's broad-spectrum and has an SPF of at least 15.

Truth: That's true in theory, but the form of the sunscreen can make a big difference in whether you actually use it.

Dr. Kenet's take: Spray-on sunscreens can be practical for people playing golf or tennis, for example, who need to reapply quickly and often. Because concerns have been raised about potential dangers due to inhaling spray-on sunscreens, these products shouldn't be sprayed on the face. Instead, spray the sunscreen on your hands and then apply it to your face.

Gel sunscreens are water-based and easy on the skin for people who are prone to acne. However, gel sunscreens are not good if you plan to spend a lot of time in the water or tend to get very sweaty. For these people, sunscreens containing titanium dioxide and/or zinc oxide work well (they do leave a white coating on the skin).

Secrets to Getting the Best Colonoscopy

Douglas K. Rex, MD, a Distinguished Professor of Medicine at Indiana University School of Medicine and director of endoscopy at Indiana University Hospital, both in Indianapolis. DouglasKRex.com

It's estimated that if every person age 50 and older had a colonoscopy, 64% of people with colorectal cancer would have never developed the disease.

But since you are going to the trouble to get this test (and we all know the bowel-cleansing prep is no picnic), then it also makes sense to make sure you're getting the best possible screening. *How to ensure that you get the maximum cancer protection from your colonoscopy...*

How Good Is Your Doctor?

One of the most important aspects of a colonoscopy is the doctor's ability to detect a type of polyp called an adenoma—the doctor's so-called "adenoma detection rate" (ADR). This varies widely depending on the doctor's skill.

If your doctor has a low ADR, you're more likely to get colon cancer before your next colonoscopy. Gastroenterologists are more likely to have good ADRs than primary care physicians and general surgeons who might perform colonoscopies, but there's a wide range of performance within each group.

Precisely defined, a doctor's ADR is the percentage of screening colonoscopies in patients age 50 or older during which he/she detects one or more adenomas.

My advice: Look for a doctor with an ADR of 20% or higher in women and 30% or higher in men (who have more adenomas)...or a "mixed-gender" rate of 25% or higher—in other words, the doctor detects at least one adenoma in 25% of the screening colonoscopies he conducts.

Startling recent finding: A 10-year study published in *The New England Journal of Medicine* evaluated more than 300,000 colonoscopies conducted by 136 gastroenterologists—and found that for every 1% increase in ADR, there was a 3% reduction in the risk of developing colorectal cancer before the next colonoscopy. This means that having your colonoscopy performed by a doctor with a high ADR (as described earlier) is a must for optimal screening. But how does a patient ask about his doctor's ADR without seeming to question the physician's competence?

My advice: Ask about your doctor's ADR on the phone, during the colonoscopy scheduling process, when you are talking to an administrator or a nurse. If that person doesn't know, request that someone get back to you with the number. That will make your query less confrontational.

However: Even your doctor may not know his own ADR. Monitoring of ADRs is endorsed by several professional medical societies, such as the American Society for Gastrointestinal Endoscopy and the American College of Gastroenterology, but there is no law mandating that doctors must track it. Or your doctor may refuse to disclose his ADR—a response you should find concerning. If you don't get the information you need from your doctor, it's probably a good idea to find a new one.

Also important: Make sure your colonoscopy is being performed with a high-definition colonoscope, the current state-of-the-art in colonoscopy. Inquire about this when you ask about a doctor's ADR.

A Better Bowel Prep

Another key to a truly preventive colonoscopy is the preparation. Before the procedure, a patient drinks a defecation-inducing liquid (prep) that cleanses the rectum and colon of stool so that the doctor can clearly see the lining. In some patients, a four-liter prep (about one gallon), or even more, is best for optimal cleansing. If you don't have a condition associated with slow bowel motility, such as chronic constipation, or use constipating medications such as opioids, you may be eligible for one of the regimens that requires only two or three liters of fluid. (A pill preparation is also available, but it is seldom used because it can cause kidney damage.) Ask your doctor what regimen will give you the best combination of excellent cleansing and tolerability.

A common mistake: Many people think that they can drink the prep one to two days before the procedure and then drink nothing but clear fluids (such as Gatorade, apple juice or water) until the day of the colonoscopy.

But even during the prep, the small intestine (the section of bowel after the stomach and before the colon) continues to produce chyme, a thick, mucousy secretion that sticks to the walls of the ascending colon—so that seven to eight hours after drinking the prep the colon is no longer completely clean.

Best: A split prep, with half the prep ingested the day before the procedure and half ingested four to five hours before (the middle of the night when the colonoscopy is scheduled for the morning…or the morning when the colonoscopy is scheduled for the afternoon).

Scientific evidence: Split preparation improves ADR by 26%, according to a study in *Gastrointestinal Endoscopy*.

Also helpful: Drinking the prep can be difficult, even nauseating. How to make it more palatable…

Chill the liquid thoroughly, and drink it with a straw. Follow each swallow with ginger ale or another good-tasting clear liquid. Suck on a clear menthol lozenge after you drink the prep. And if you throw up the prep, wait 30 minutes (until you feel less nauseated) and then continue drinking the prep as instructed—it can still work.

Several recent studies have found that eating a fiber-free diet all or part of the day prior to colonoscopy allows for better cleansing of the colon. Some doctors advise avoiding high-fiber foods such as corn, seeds and nuts for about a week before a colonoscopy. Ask your doctor what he advises for you.

Pancreatic Cancer? Only 1 in 5 Patients Gets This Critical Test

Mayo Clinic research to be presented at the annual meeting of the Western Surgical Association in Napa, California.

Pancreatic cancer is deadly—only 7% of patients survive five years after diagnosis. But giving just-diagnosed patients an inexpensive blood test can help doctors choose the treatment that is most likely to improve their chances.

The test measures CA 19-9—a tumor "biomarker" found in the blood of 90% of the population. When researchers at the Mayo Clinic analyzed data on 97,000 pancreatic cancer patients in the National Cancer Data Base, they found that having elevated levels of CA 19-9 predicted a worse outcome from therapy.

The good news: Having chemotherapy before surgery instead of the usual practice of having it afterward eliminated the elevated biomarker's negative effect. That is, these patients did as well as patients without the elevated risk. The test is widely available and costs less than $200.

Esophageal Cancer Is Rising Fast

Michael S. Smith, MD, medical director of the Esophageal Program and an associate professor of medicine in the Section of Gastroenterology at Temple University School of Medicine in Philadelphia.

With the incidence of some cancers (such as lung cancer) now declining, you might assume—or at least hope—that this promising trend applies to all malignancies. But this isn't the case for a certain type of esophageal cancer. The rate of this malignancy has increased by nearly six-fold in recent decades, making it one of the fastest-growing cancers in the US.

The New Risks

A generation ago, most US patients with esophageal cancer had a type of malignancy known as squamous cell carcinoma. Largely due to smoking and drinking, it mainly affects the upper two-thirds of the esophagus and remains the predominant type worldwide. Now, as the incidence of esophageal squamous cell carcinoma has declined in the US, another form, known as adenocarcinoma, affecting primarily the lower third of the esophagus, has dramatically increased. Interestingly, there's also a different set of risk factors for this cancer.

How anatomy plays a role: We all know that what we eat and drink passes through the esophagus, the tube that connects the throat to the stomach. What goes down, however, is less of a problem than what comes up. *What to watch for…*

• **Heartburn.** The upsurge of acid and other digestive juices into the esophagus from the stomach can cause tissue damage that can lead to cancer.

One in five American adults suffers from frequent heartburn and/or damage to the esophagus due to chronic reflux, also known as GERD (gastroesophageal reflux disease). The classic symptoms include heartburn and reflux (the sensation of food or fluid rising from the stomach into the chest). But the true number may be higher because many people have atypical GERD, where they have other symptoms—such as hoarseness, an unexplained cough or the feeling of a lump in the throat—but not the characteristic burn. Others have an even more dangerous form, silent GERD, which has no symptoms at all.

Even though GERD is a cancer risk factor, don't worry too much if you have heartburn only once or twice a month (but be sure to mention it at your annual physical). Do consult a doctor if you have heartburn once or more a week…or if you have any of the other atypical symptoms mentioned above. You may be advised to have an endoscopy, in which a long flexible tube with a camera and light at one end is inserted through the mouth into the esophagus, stomach and upper part of the small intestine to look for signs of damage from GERD, such as scar tissue formation, or Barrett's esophagus (next column), a precancerous condition.

What you can do: The foods that can trigger heartburn vary from person to person, so try to identify and avoid your food triggers. And don't eat within two hours of lying down. For occasional relief, you can try an antacid such as Tums or Maalox or an acid-suppressing drug such as *ranitidine* (Zantac) or *famotidine* (Pepcid). But using these drugs more than once every few weeks is a sign that you need to see your doctor soon—before you do more damage to your esophagus.

• **Barrett's esophagus.** If you have frequent or severe episodes of GERD, you could be at risk of developing Barrett's esophagus. This precancerous condition, in which the chronic onslaught of digestive fluids causes tissue-damaging cell changes, increases risk for esophageal adenocarcinoma by 40 times. Barrett's esophagus should be monitored closely by a physician.

What you can do: Even with the dietary advice above, you will likely need a strong acid-reducing drug called a proton-pump inhibitor (PPI). PPIs include *omeprazole* (Prilosec) and *lansoprazole* (Prevacid). Endoscopic ablation or even surgery may be required in advanced cases.

• **Weight gain.** This could be the main reason for the increase in esophageal cancer. Being overweight or obese adds intra-abdominal pressure, which increases the chance that stomach contents will be pushed up into the esophagus.

What you can do: Eat healthier foods. Also, you may have heard it before, but it really is helpful to eat smaller, more frequent meals—the less you put in the stomach at a time, the harder it is for the contents to back up into the esophagus and do damage. And try exercising regularly—even walking after dinner will help empty the stomach.

• **Alcohol.** You may assume that the "burn" of alcohol going down damages the esophagus. But small amounts of alcohol do not cause cell damage. The real problem is alcohol's role in triggering GERD.

What happens: Alcohol relaxes the lower esophageal sphincter (LES), the ringlike muscle at the junction of the stomach and esophagus. This muscle keeps the bottom end of the esophagus closed, which helps prevent reflux. The more you drink, the more the LES relaxes—and the more likely you are to have an upsurge of stomach contents.

What you can do: If you're prone to heartburn, limit your alcohol consumption. Women should have no more than one drink a day, and men should have no more than two. And don't drink any alcohol within two hours of lying down.

• **Coffee.** Years ago, researchers noticed a high incidence of esophageal cancer in parts of the world where hot beverages are frequently consumed and speculated that this practice may be behind the high cancer rate. Subsequent research did not support this hypothesis—with a caveat. Coffee is usually served hot, and it can play a role in GERD... but heat isn't the issue. Rather, the caffeine in coffee, like alcohol, relaxes the LES and makes reflux more likely.

What you can do: Limit coffee to two or three cups a day—or even less if you keep having reflux. Have it early in the day, and not before bedtime. You might want to switch to decaf, although it too contains some caffeine and may affect those who are sensitive. Any caffeinated beverage can trigger reflux—and so can chocolate and peppermints!

4 Secret Cancer Fighters

The late Mitchell Gaynor, MD, founder and president of Gaynor Integrative Oncology in New York City. He was a board-certified oncologist, internist and hematologist and a clinical assistant professor of medicine at Weill Cornell Medical College. He wrote *The Gene Therapy Plan: Taking Control of Your Genetic Destiny with Diet and Lifestyle.* GaynorWellness.com

The new science of epigenetics shows that it is possible to "upregulate" (trigger) the "expression" (activity) of powerful anticancer genes using a whole-foods diet, regular exercise, restful sleep, stress reduction—and concentrated nutritional and herbal compounds.

These natural compounds can activate genes that tell the body to turbocharge the immune system so that it can locate can-

cer cells...kill those cells...douse chronic, low-grade inflammation, which generates "growth factors" that fuel cancer...decrease the liver's production of insulin-like growth factor one (IGF), the most deadly "tumor promoter"...reduce a tumor's cancer-spreading blood supply...and even improve the effectiveness of chemotherapy.

In addition to taking vitamin D daily, I recommend these four powerful anticancer supplements for preventing or controlling cancer or stopping its recurrence. Take one, two or all four. At the dosages recommended, they are very safe. Of course, always check with your doctor before taking any new supplement.

Magnolia Extract

This herbal supplement from the bark of a magnolia tree contains *honokiol*, which has anticancer functions—it is anti-inflammatory and anti-angiogenic (limiting blood supply to tumors), and it targets many biochemical compounds that "signal" cancer to start and to grow, such as nuclear factor-kappaB and epidermal growth factor receptor.

Scientific research: More than 200 studies show that honokiol (and *magnolol*, another compound in magnolia bark) can fight cancer. In a recent cellular study, published in *International Journal of Oncology,* honokiol activated a gene that "suppressed" the spread of kidney cancer and deactivated two genes that allow kidney cancer cells to invade and colonize the surrounding tissue (metastasize).

Typical dosage: 200 mg, daily.

Suggested product: Magnolia Extract from NutriCology.

Artichoke Extract

This extract from artichoke leaves contains rutin, quercetin, gallic acid and chlorogenic acid—all of which have been shown in laboratory studies to kill a variety of cancer cells, including colon, breast and liver cancers, and leukemia. Artichoke extract also contains cynarin, which decreases inflammation. Plus, the extract has been shown in people to improve insulin sensitivity, the body's ability to utilize the glucose-regulating hormone insulin. When insulin is used efficiently, the body makes less insulin—and less cancer-sparking IGF.

Recent study: A cellular study published in *Asian Pacific Journal of Cancer Prevention* showed that artichoke extract triggered tumor suppressor genes.

Typical dosage: 320 milligrams (mg), once daily.

Suggested product: Artichoke Extract from Enzymatic Therapy.

Black Cumin Seed Oil

Many years ago, a patient of mine with prostate cancer started taking black cumin seed oil (Nigella sativa) with honey, three times a day, on the recommendation of a naturopathic physician. His Gleason score (a measure of the severity of prostate cancer) went from nine on a scale of one to 10 (an aggressive, invasive cancer with poor prognosis) to six—essentially, a precancerous lesion. Amazed, I started investigating this compound, which has been used in Turkish cooking for millennia—and started taking it myself, adding the seed to blended shakes and the oil to foods as seasoning. I recommend that patients use the oil—rich in *thymoquinone,* which is found in few other foods—either in their diets or as a supplement.

Compelling research: Researchers at Barbara Ann Karmanos Cancer Institute at Wayne State University School of Medicine in Detroit reviewed hundreds of cellular and animal studies on thymoquinone and cancer and concluded that the compound is anti-inflammatory...stops cancer cells from dividing and spreading by triggering their death...limits the formation of blood vessels that nourish the tumor (angiogenesis)...and "sensitizes" cells to chemotherapy.

Example: In a recent animal study, published in *Archives of Medical Science,* researchers found that thymoquinone "decreased the expression" of both BRCA1 and BRCA2 genes—genes that increase the risk for breast cancer three- to five-fold and the risk for ovarian cancer as much as 30-fold.

Typical dosage: 500 mg, twice daily.

Suggested product: Black Seed Cumin Seed Oil from Amazing Herbs.

Bee Propolis, Bee Pollen and Royal Jelly

Bee propolis (a waxlike material used by bees to repair holes in hives) is rich in caffeic acid phenethyl ester (CAPE), chrysin and cinnamic acid, compounds that affect cancer genes. Studies show they are immune-strengthening, anti-inflammatory and anti-angiogenic and can reduce the growth of many cancers, including colon, prostate and kidney. Bee propolis also has been used clinically to reduce mouth sores caused by chemotherapy and radiation.

Recent study: In a cellular study on prostate cancer from the University of Texas Medical Branch, researchers found that CAPE boosted the cancer-killing power of chemotherapeutic drugs.

Another cellular study shows that bee pollen can inhibit vascular endothelial growth factor (VEGF), which helps create blood supply to tumors.

Royal jelly (a milky secretion produced by worker bees) contains several epigenetic factors. It has been shown to suppress the blood supply to tumors.

Typical dosage: 500 mg, once daily.

Suggested product: Triple Bee Complex from Y.S. Organic Bee Farms, which contains bee propolis, bee pollen and royal jelly.

Caution: People who are allergic to bee stings should not take bee products.

Antioxidants Linked to Cancer

Sean Morrison, PhD, director of the Children's Medical Center Research Institute at UT Southwestern in Dallas. He led the team of scientists who conducted a recent study investigating the effect of antioxidants on melanoma cells.

Several studies have strongly suggested that antioxidants might significantly accelerate the spread of cancer among people who have the disease and increase the odds of getting cancer among people in high-risk groups. This might come as a shock to anyone used to reading about the health benefits of antioxidants such as vitamins C and E and beta-carotene. Research has suggested that antioxidants might protect our cells from certain types of damage, slowing the aging process and providing some defense against serious health problems, including heart disease.

Why would antioxidants also promote cancer? The most likely explanation is that they provide the same protection to cancer cells that they do to normal, healthy cells. In fact, cancer cells appear to benefit even more than normal cells. One study of more than 35,000 men over age 50 found that taking large doses of vitamin E increased their risk for prostate cancer by 17%...another study of more than 18,000 former smokers and workers exposed to asbestos found that taking large doses of beta-carotene and retinol (a form of vitamin A) increased their risk for lung cancer by 28%.

Bottom line: I would not take antioxidant supplements if I had been diagnosed with cancer...or was at high risk for cancer, perhaps because of family history or a long-term smoking habit. There is not enough evidence to state whether people who currently are healthy and not in a high-risk group are better or worse off if they take antioxidant supplements regularly. But everyone should continue to consume foods that contain antioxidants, such as berries, nuts and leafy green vegetables.

Getting the Most Out of Integrative Cancer Care

Dwight McKee, MD, a medical oncologist based in Aptos, California, who is also board-certified in nutrition and integrative and holistic medicine. He is coauthor of the soon-to-be-released book *After Cancer Care: The Definitive Self-Care Guide to Getting and Staying Well for Patients After Cancer*.

Cancer is a complex disease—elusive and difficult to control, let alone cure. To get the best possible outcome, you want to have all hands on deck.

More than the conventional approach: While modern oncology has given us powerful weapons to fight cancer—drugs, surgery and radiation that attack tumors head on—the most effective integrative cancer therapies focus on the cancer patient, bolstering his/her natural defenses to help suppress tumor growth. Combining these approaches not only fills in gaps but also creates a powerful synergy.

Build Your Defenses

While there are a multitude of integrative approaches now available for cancer patients, ranging from acupuncture and massage to aromatherapy and music therapy, it's crucial to fortify your body's defenses to fight the inflammation associated with cancer. *Here's how...*

●**Diet.** Strive for a plant-based diet (especially cruciferous vegetables and berries—both are extremely rich in cancer-fighting nutrients) with plenty of whole grains, nuts and omega-3–rich fatty fish (omega-3s have been linked to reduced cancer risk). Cut back on animal proteins and sugar—these foods are associated with cancer-promoting inflammation.

●**Exercise.** Try to get 150 minutes weekly of moderately vigorous exercise (such as brisk walking) to help optimize your body's own cancer-fighting abilities. An ideal regimen could include some aerobic activity (such as cycling)...some stretching (such as yoga or tai chi)...and some strength training (with hand weights or resistance bands).

●**Stress reduction.** The first weeks after diagnosis are likely to be the most stressful of your life.

There are myriad ways to control stress, including meditation, hypnosis, yoga and tai chi, but one method that seems particularly effective is progressive muscle relaxation, which involves systematically relaxing all the muscle groups in the body, one after another. Twenty minutes daily has been shown to provide major benefits to people with cancer.

For a free video demonstrating progressive muscle relaxation, go to: CMHC. utexas.edu/stressrecess/Level_Two/progressive.html.

●**Herbs and supplements.** While adopting the inflammation-fighting lifestyle practices described earlier, anti-inflammatory herbs, such as curcumin and boswellia, can be powerful aids.

In addition, a typical herb-and-supplement regimen for a colon cancer patient, for example, may include some combination of the following: Vitamin D, green tea extract, resveratrol, grape seed extract, probiotics and omega-3 fatty acids.

Important: For specific advice on herbs and supplements, work with a skilled, experienced complementary/alternative doctor or herbalist (see the box below).

Getting Rid of the Tumor

While conventional methods, such as surgery, radiation and chemotherapy, can be quite effective, they have important downsides, too. For example, chemotherapy and radiation not only have harsh side effects, including nausea and hair loss, but they also suppress the immune system at a time when it should be working overtime to fight the cancer.

Newer alternatives: The immune-suppressing effects of chemo and radiation can be avoided with thermal ablation. With this approach, doctors insert a needle into the tumor, often guided by computed tomography (CT) imaging, to kill the cancer cells with heat (radiofrequency or microwave ablation) or freezing (cryoablation). Irreversible electroporation (the NanoKnife) uses electrical pulses to kill cancer cells by disrupting their cell membranes. These methods are also much less invasive and traumatic than surgery.

Right now, ablation is mainly used for tumors that can't be treated with conventional

---

Getting the Help You Need

It's risky for cancer patients to try to treat themselves with integrative approaches. Some therapies, including certain herbs, such as St. John's wort, may even interfere with conventional treatment. But finding oncologists, herbalists and other health-care professionals who are knowledgeable about the latest approaches in integrative cancer care is also challenging.

To find a health-care professional who specializes in integrative oncology: Ask your doctor for a referral or consult the Society for Integrative Oncology, *IntegrativeOnc. org.* When you find an experienced integrative professional, ask him/her to work with your primary oncologist in coordinating your care.

surgery, due to their location or number, and for isolated metastases in the lung and liver. But ablation and electroporation have the potential to replace a considerable amount of surgery.

Immunotherapy

Scientists are actively developing new medications that help undo the tumor's ability to produce chemicals that inactivate the body's cancer-fighting immune cells.

Examples: Ipilimumab (Yervoy) and *pembrolizumab* (Keytruda) have been approved for the treatment of melanoma. Clinical trials to investigate their use against a wider range of malignancies, including certain kinds of lung cancer, and bladder, colon and metastatic prostate cancer, are also under way. For details on clinical trials using these drugs, check ClinicalTrials.gov.

Because these drugs target molecular mechanisms driving cancer, they are far less toxic than conventional chemotherapy. The drugs are, however, extremely expensive (costing up to $150,000 a year). If insurance won't cover the drug and a clinical trial is not available, sometimes the pharmaceutical manufacturer will donate it to a patient without the financial resources to purchase it so that it can be administered by his/her oncologist.

The Radical New Cancer Treatment That Could Save Your Life

Louis Weiner, MD, director, Lombardi Comprehensive Cancer Center, Georgetown University, Washington, DC.

James P. Allison, PhD, department of immunology and immunotherapy platform, The University of Texas MD Anderson Cancer Center, Houston.

Too often we read about a new theoretical approach to cancer treatment that saves lives in one or two studies...only to wait and wait for it to materialize in the practice of cancer medicine. This time is different.

"No chemotherapy drug works so well on so many patients," says Louis Weiner, MD, director of the Lombardi Comprehensive Cancer Center at Georgetown University. "This is not theoretical or another case of over-hyping, overpromising and underdelivering. These drugs are working."

Dr. Weiner is talking about a new way to fight cancer by using the body's own immune system to wage war on cancer cells. Many leading cancer experts believe this new approach, cancer immunotherapy, could revolutionize how we treat many forms of cancer. When it comes to certain cancers, the revolution has already begun. In fact, former President Jimmy Carter, currently in his early nineties, claims to be cancer-free while using one of these drugs.

6 Things You Need to Know About the New Cancer Immunotherapy

Here are the details on this latest form of cancer immunotherapy...

1. It treats the body's immune system so the immune system can fight the cancer. T cells are the immune system's main line of defense, but they're not always effective against cancer cells. In the 1990s, cancer researchers identified a class of molecules in the body that are known as immune checkpoints. These molecules keep T cells from attacking normal cells, but cancer cells can hijack them for their own purposes. "Cancer cells employ immune checkpoints to turn off killer T cells that would otherwise recognize and destroy a cancer that was growing in somebody's body," Dr. Weiner says. Drugs that block these checkpoints so T cells can do their job are called immune checkpoint inhibitors, he explains. "They're the game changers."

2. It still has side effects, but early results suggest a less toxic experience. "All of us would love to see a day when very toxic chemotherapy agents that cause hair loss, low blood counts, fatigue, etc., are no longer the backbone of therapy for cancer," Dr. Weiner says. "With checkpoint inhibitors, there will potentially be fewer side effects and certainly different ones." So far, the most common side effects caused by checkpoint inhibitors already in use include fatigue, cough, nausea, skin rash and itching. But more serious side effects including severe diarrhea, colitis and intestinal inflammation (even perforation) have also been reported.

3. It can be very effective and long-lasting. Consider the effects of checkpoint inhibitors against end-stage Hodgkin's disease, where patients have already received every imaginable therapy and were running out of hope. "More than 90% of these patients went into complete remission, and these remissions were durable," Dr. Weiner says. When checkpoint inhibitors are combined against metastatic melanoma—the most deadly form of skin cancer—as many as half of those cancers are completely eliminated, with benefits that have lasted 10 years so far. He adds, "You've taken a disease that was destined to end somebody's life very quickly, and you've completely changed it."

4. It works against many forms of cancer. In a viewpoint recently published in *JAMA*, James Allison, PhD, who pioneered the use of immune checkpoint inhibitors against cancer, wrote: "The therapy does not target the tumor cell but rather engages a target on the patient's immune system. Thus, there is no inherent reason that it would not be successful against a wide variety of tumors." At this time, checkpoint inhibitors are FDA-approved only for treating certain types of melanoma and lung cancer. But studies show they also work against no fewer than 20 different cancers including certain forms of kidney cancer, triple negative breast cancer, stomach cancer, Hodgkin's disease, bladder cancer and head and neck cancer.

5. It is very expensive. "It can cost tens of thousands of dollars or more to have a course of therapy with these drugs, especially if you start combining them with other expensive cancer therapies," Dr. Weiner says.

6. It is still evolving. One promising innovation in cancer immunotherapy that's currently being researched is chimeric antigen receptor (CAR) T-cell therapy. Here, a patient's T cells are genetically engineered to produce antibodies against a specific type of cancer. When these T cells proliferate, they pass their cancer-killing modifications along. So far, says Dr. Weiner, this experimental treatment has had "stunning results" against a hard-to-treat and deadly form of leukemia called acute lymphocytic leukemia.

What to Do Now

While many checkpoint inhibitors are in development, currently only three have been approved by the FDA…

•**Opdivo** (*nivolumab*) and **Keytruda** (*pembrolizumab*) are approved for advanced-stage non-small cell lung cancer that has spread and that is not responding to conventional platinum-based chemotherapy, and for advanced melanoma.

•**Yervoy** (*ipilimumab*) is approved for melanoma that has spread within the body (metastatized) or that cannot be removed by surgery.

Until new drugs for different cancers make it through the FDA approval process—or the existing approved ones get future approvals for different cancers—these are the only three of this type of cancer treatment that insurance companies or Medicare are likely to pay for. If you have the financial wherewithal, you may be able to have your doctor prescribe the approved drugs off-label and pay for them yourself.

For everyone else, however, there is another potential option. If there is an immunotherapy cancer drug in development for a cancer that you are being treated for, ask your oncologist whether there is a clinical trial that you can get into.

How to Get into a Cancer Clinical Trial...

Toni Kay Mangskau, a social worker and clinical trials referral coordinator at the Mayo Clinic Cancer Center in Rochester, Minnesota.

About 20% of newly diagnosed adult cancer patients in the US are eligible for clinical trials, studies for which people volunteer to test new drugs or other treatments. Yet only about 3% to 5% actually participate.

Why? Most people assume that clinical studies are an option for only the sickest patients for whom there are no effective treatments. Not true! The only requirement for many studies is having a specific type of cancer or being in a certain age group or other demographic category. Also, many people assume that one group in a study receives a placebo. The fact is that a placebo is not used in the vast majority of studies. In treatment studies, some patients are given the drug/procedure under investigation...others are given the best available standard treatment.

Here's what else you need to know about clinical trials...

What's Available?

At any given time, thousands of clinical trials are under way. The National Cancer Institute website alone lists more than 12,000 trials that are looking for participants. The studies that get the most attention are those that look at breakthrough cancer treatments, but that's just the tip of the iceberg. Other trials compare single drugs with combination treatments...find new uses for old drugs...study new surgical techniques or radiation treatments, etc.

For some studies, all you have to do is give researchers permission to review your medical records.

Example: Researchers at the Mayo Clinic Cancer Center learned from chart review studies that patients with chronic lymphocytic leukemia responded better to treatments when they had normal blood levels of vitamin D.

Random Selection

Typically, a computer will assign a participant to a group in a clinical trial. One group will be given the new drug/treatment. The control group will be given a standard treatment.

If you're randomly assigned to the control group, you'll still get the same treatment that you likely would have gotten if you hadn't joined the study. Those in the "active" group will get something that's expected to be at least as good—and possibly better.

The Risks

New drugs/procedures can have side effects or other complications that the researchers didn't anticipate. Should you take the risk?

It's a valid concern, particularly if it's an early-phase study, with a lot of unknowns. But most treatment studies already have a long history. Cancer drugs typically have been studied for at least six years in the laboratory before they make it to clinical trials with humans. It may take another eight years before drugs are approved—or not—by the FDA.

Researchers may not know everything about the drug/treatment, but they know a lot by the time these studies begin. It's always possible that the therapy being researched in the clinical trial is going to be less effective than the standard treatment. But typically study data is reviewed while the study is under way—and a study could be stopped because of side effects or because a treatment is not showing effectiveness.

My advice: If you are considering joining a particular study, ask the researchers how familiar they are with the treatment being researched. Some treatments have been used for other purposes for decades—they're unlikely to bring too many surprises. The diabetes drug *metformin*, for example, now is being studied as a treatment for breast and ovarian cancers. Doctors are knowledgeable about the drug and the probable side effects.

Moderate Exercise Can Boost Cancer Treatment

Regular activities that use 30% to 60% of a patient's aerobic capacity—not less and not more—can make radiation treatment for cancer more effective by enhancing oxygen delivery and blood flow to the tumors. Examples of this type of exercise are a brisk walk or a slow jog. Too much exercise may have a negative impact by shutting down blood flow to the tumor region or harming the immune system. Each patient should talk to his/her doctor for specific recommendations.

Study led by researchers at Kansas State University, Manhattan, published in *Journal of the National Cancer Institute*.

How to Participate

•**Talk to your oncologist.** In one poll, patients reported that 70% of their doctors never mentioned a clinical trial as an option. So ask. Even if your doctor isn't personally involved in a clinical trial, he/she can talk you through the issues—the pros and cons of participating...where to look for studies that involve your type of cancer...and what the studies are likely to involve.

Helpful: For a list of cancer clinical trials, go to *Cancer.gov/clinicaltrials.*

•**Make the decision early.** One of the first things you should ask your oncologist is how quickly you must make a decision about treatment options. Some studies accept only patients who haven't started other treatments.

Important: If you decide to participate in a study, you can change your mind later. Patients can quit a study at any time.

•**Is it practical?** Even if you would like to participate, you may find that it's not a good fit.

Example: A study might require weekly tests at a medical center hundreds of miles away. That's not practical for most people. But other studies may involve monthly vis-its at a site closer to home. Or there may be times when routine blood work or imaging may be done at your local doctor's office and results sent to the study team.

Study participants typically get more face time with doctors—along with additional checkups, tests, etc.—than patients who don't participate in studies. One study found that 95% of those who participated in one clinical study said that they would consider doing so again.

•**Check the costs.** Many tests and treatments will be paid for by the study sponsor—but that doesn't mean all of your care is free. In most cases, you (or your insurer) still will be responsible for "routine" care costs—for example, routine blood work or scans. Travel expenses are rarely covered.

Under the Affordable Care Act, some health plans are required to cover the routine costs of study participants. Check with your insurance company, or contact your state's Health Insurance Commission.

The 4 Phases of a Study

Before joining a clinical trial, ask about the study phase. This will give you some idea of how much is known about the treatment.

•**Phase 0 is the earliest stage.** Small doses of a drug are tested in just a few people to find out if it reaches the tumor, how it's metabolized, etc. A participant won't benefit from a phase 0 study, but future patients might.

•**Phase 1 studies are used to determine the highest drug dose that can be given safely and identify possible side effects.** Sometimes, these are referred to as "dosing" studies. Researchers also may make sure that the treatment has some benefit, such as slowing tumor growth.

•**Phase 2 trials involve slightly larger numbers of patients.** The goal is to see if the treatment actually works—for example, if it causes a tumor to shrink. If enough patients benefit and side effects aren't too much of a problem, the drug then may go on to the final stage.

• **Phase 3 studies look at anywhere from hundreds to thousands of patients.** These are the treatment studies that most cancer patients join. If the drug is clearly effective, an application for approval is submitted to the FDA.

Cervical Cancer Can Be Prevented

Shyam Kalavar, MPH, cytologist, Food and Drug Administration, Silver Spring, MD.

Marion Gruber, PhD, director, Office of Vaccines Research and Review, Food and Drug Administration, Silver Spring, MD.

U.S. Food and Drug Administration, news release.

Although cervical cancer claims the lives of an estimated 4,000 American women every year, the disease is largely preventable, according to the U.S. Food and Drug Administration (FDA).

What's more, if the disease is diagnosed early, cervical cancer is often curable, the agency said.

"It's important to understand, however, that cervical cancer is also preventable. There are three FDA-approved vaccines that protect against the disease," said Shyam Kalavar, an expert in the microscopic examination of cells for the FDA.

About Cervical Cancer

Cervical cancer forms in the cervix, or the lower part of the uterus that connects to the vagina. Human papillomavirus (HPV) causes cervical cancer, the FDA said, but not everyone who has HPV develops cervical cancer.

PAP Test

Cervical cancer often doesn't cause symptoms, but can be detected during routine Pap tests, also called a Pap smear. The Pap test involves cells taken from the cervix. These cells are examined in a lab for signs of abnormalities that could lead to cancer, Kalavar said.

Pap smears are not 100% accurate and a small number of cancers may be overlooked in any one test, but it takes several years for cervical cancer to develop from abnormal cells. The FDA pointed out that by having routine Pap smears, changes in cervical cells can be detected early enough for women to receive the treatment they need.

HPV Test

Women with an abnormal Pap smear must undergo more testing for cervical cancer, which may include an HPV test. Having both tests reduces the likelihood that abnormal cells are missed, the agency said.

There are more than 100 different types of HPV, the FDA said. Some of these viruses aren't harmful. The HPV test checks for the presence of the types of HPV most likely to cause cancer. Some women may also need to have a biopsy of their cervix, the FDA noted.

HPV Vaccine

The HPV vaccines don't help treat cervical cancer, but they are all effective in protecting against the two types of HPV that cause about 70% of cervical cancers, according to the FDA. One vaccine—Gardasil 9—also offers protection against five additional HPV types that cause about 20% of cervical cancers. People must be vaccinated before being infected with HPV to be fully protected, the FDA said.

"These vaccines are preventative and work like other vaccines that prevent diseases caused by viruses and bacteria: they prompt the body to produce antibodies to protect against infection," said Marion Gruber, MD, director of the FDA's Office of Vaccines Research and Review.

"Women, including those who have been vaccinated, should continue to get Pap tests because they are essential to detect cervical cancer and precancerous changes," Dr. Gruber said.

Chapter 3

STROKE: RISKS, SYMPTOMS, AND SECRETS TO RECOVERY

Is It a Migraine, Low Blood Sugar, a Seizure...or a Stroke?

They're called stroke mimics. The symptoms are similar to a stroke—slurred speech, a weakness on one side of your body and confusion—but what you're experiencing is actually low blood sugar, a migraine or another condition. If you know you have diabetes, suffer from migraines, have a seizure disorder or other conditions, you may be tempted to ignore possible stroke symptoms.

That's a big mistake.

Reason: When you're having a stroke, minutes—even seconds—count. Getting emergency treatment with blood clot–dissolving medications—typically tissue plasminogen activator (tPA)—or other therapies can mean the difference between life and death and can dramatically affect recovery. To learn more about stroke mimics, we spoke with Edward Jauch, MD, director of the division of emergency medicine at the Medical University of South Carolina.

MIMIC #1: **Low Blood Sugar (Hypoglycemia)**

When blood sugar dips too low, a common problem for people who take medication for diabetes, the symptoms mimic a stroke—confusion, feeling dizzy or light-headed, slurred speech and/or muscle weakness.

Clues that it may be hypoglycemia, not stroke...

Symptoms may build up slowly, rather than occur suddenly, as they do with a stroke. If you do a finger prick and discover your blood sugar is low, and if symptoms resolve after eating a glucose tablet or drinking a half cup of fruit juice, it's likely not a stroke.

But if you have any doubts, call 911. Be sure to tell the EMS professionals that the patient is a diabetic so they can rule out hypoglycemia with a finger-prick test—and maybe save a trip to the ER. It's actually standard practice to test everyone's glucose right away, whether or not they have diabetes, but it's not always followed, says Dr. Jauch.

MIMIC #2: **Hemiplegic Migraine**
You may remember when the newscaster Serene Branson frighteningly lost her speech during a live broadcast, and everyone

Edward Jauch, MD, professor and director, division of emergency medicine; professor, department of neurosciences, comprehensive stroke program; and director, acute stroke trials, Medical University of South Carolina, Charleston.

thought she had had a stroke. Well, it turned out to be a hemiplegic migraine. This type of migraine can cause loss of speech, weakness and other strokelike symptoms.

Clues that it may be a migraine, not a stroke…

• **You know you get migraines,** the pain is familiar, and an aura precedes the symptoms.

• **The headache comes on gradually,** over several minutes or longer, intensifies to a peak and tends to be throbbing or a dull ache.

• **You have known triggers** such as stress, caffeine, foods, weather changes, etc.

• **You have visual disturbances such as seeing flashing lights or wavy lines.**

Signs that it may be a stroke, not a migraine…

• **You're older than 50, and you've never had a migraine.** Migraines don't tend to develop after age 50.

• **The headache comes on suddenly and is the worst headache of your life.**

• **You have visual disturbances that involve loss of part of your visual field**—you may bump into things because you don't see them, for example.

As always, when in doubt, call 911. It's particularly important for people who get migraines frequently to pay attention to possible stroke symptoms. "There's a small increased risk for stroke in people who have migraines, but we are still researching if treatment of a migraine reduces stroke risk," says Dr. Jauch.

MIMIC #3: A Seizure

Some seizures leave people with neurological symptoms such as difficulty speaking or a weakness in one or more limbs often on one side of the body, known as Todd's paralysis. "When you have a seizure, your brain turns off, just like when you shut down a computer," Dr. Jauch explains. "When you turn the computer back on, it takes a while to boot up. Your brain, too, may take some time to get back to normal."

Clues that it may be a seizure…

• **The patient has a history of seizures, a bite mark on the side of the tongue**—or confusion that gradually improves.

• **Typically symptoms subside with time…from a few minutes to a few hours.**

Clues that it may be a stroke: If there is confusion, it is persistent and doesn't improve.

If you're concerned that it's a stroke, time isn't on your side. EMS guidelines state that the ER team should consider stroke if someone has a seizure and has symptoms of neurological deficits, such as weakness, numbness or language issues, particularly if the patient doesn't have a history of seizures. Sometimes, seizures are symptoms of a stroke.

MIMIC #4: Bell's Palsy

Bell's palsy causes facial drooping, but it's not because of a stroke. It's typically caused by a viral infection such as shingles or the flu or Lyme disease that leads to an inflammation or infection in the facial nerve (called the seventh cranial nerve). It can also cause your eyelid to droop, drooling, dryness of the eye or mouth or excessive tearing in one eye. Though this is easy for the pros to diagnose, patients often confuse it with a stroke.

Clues that it may be Bell's palsy…

• **It typically causes significant facial distortion including the forehead.** Facial symptoms are your only symptoms.

Clues that it may be a stroke…

• **You're older than 60, when Bell's palsy becomes less common.**

• **You have other stroke symptoms, not just facial droop.**

Not sure? You know what to do—call 911.

MIMIC #5: A Brain Tumor

Brain tumors can also cause symptoms that mimic stroke, such as headache, confusion, nausea, weakness and disturbance in the way you walk.

Clues that it's a brain tumor rather than a stroke…

Symptoms are headaches that are worse in the morning, when coughing, exercising or changing position.

Both are serious ailments, of course, so these symptoms, whatever the cause, require immediate attention. For any of these unexplained symptoms, you would likely be given a CT scan, which would pick up the tumor versus signs of a stroke.

What Happens If I Think It's a Stroke and It's Not?

Stroke mimics confuse even health-care professionals. In one study, about 20% of the time when neurologists thought patients were having a stroke, the cause was a different condition. The result can be getting a CT scan and treatment when it's not needed, with all the anxiety that entails. But the risk for harm is much lower than having a stroke and not getting it promptly treated.

Here's what you can do: Help health-care professionals by giving them the right information. Let them know if the symptoms came on suddenly (common in strokes) or more gradually (uncommon), and let them know when the symptoms began or when the person was last known to be normal. If the patient has diabetes or is subject to frequent migraines or has a seizure disorder, tell the EMS professionals right away. Also let them know if the person takes any form of regular medications. It'll help them sort things out quicker.

How to Speed Up Stroke Treatment

Everyone should know the classic signs of a stroke, made easy to remember with the acronym, FAST...

Face drooping. One side of the face may droop or become numb. Ask the person to smile, and check to see if the smile is uneven.

Arm weakness. One arm only may be weak or numb. Ask the person to raise both arms, and check to see if one arm drifts downward.

Speech problems. Speech may be slurred, or the person may have trouble speaking or being understood. Ask the person to re-peat a simple sentence, such as "The sun is shining."

Time, as in, act quickly! If you think you or someone you're with is having a stroke, call 911 immediately. "We know that if you use the ambulance, you will get to the hospital faster, you see a doctor faster, you get a CT scan faster, you're more likely to get tPA, and you're more likely to get it faster." After calling 911, check the time so that the first responders know when symptoms started. When the ambulance arrives—and again when you get to the ER—say the word stroke if you think that's what you or the patient is having. Don't just say, "my arm is numb" or "I'm dizzy." Says Dr. Jauch, "The sooner someone says, 'I think I'm having a stroke,' the sooner health-care providers can start the proven system called the "Stroke Chain of Survival.""

Stroke Alert for Migraine Sufferers

Elizabeth Loder, MD, MPH, chief, Division of Headache and Pain, Brigham and Women's Hospital, Boston.

Souvik Sen, MD, MPH, neurologist, University of South Carolina School of Medicine.

Haseeb Rahman, MD, neurology resident, Houston Methodist Hospital, Texas.

American Stroke Association annual meeting, Los Angeles.

Migraine sufferers may face an increased risk of stroke if they suffer from visual symptoms called auras or if they take the female hormone estrogen, a pair of recent studies suggests.

About the Studies

People who have migraine headaches with auras may be 2.4 times more likely to have a stroke caused by a blood clot, compared to migraine patients who don't see auras, says one study presented at the American Stroke Association's annual meeting, in Los Angeles.

And, women with more severe migraines who take hormone-replacement therapy may be 30% more likely to suffer a clot-based stroke than women not taking medication containing estrogen, according to a second paper presented at the meeting.

The two risk factors could combine to pose a dangerous mix for some women, said Elizabeth Loder, MD, MPH, chief of the headache and pain division at Brigham and Women's Hospital in Boston.

Estrogen, a female hormone, is contained in birth control pills and hormone-replacement therapy.

It's important to note, however, that the recent research only found associations between migraines with aura, estrogen therapy and stroke risk. It did not prove cause-and-effect.

The two studies focused on strokes caused by blood clots, which account for about 87% of all strokes in the United States, according to the American Stroke Association.

Study #1

One study took a closer look at migraines with aura, which have been established by earlier research as a risk factor for stroke, according to the researchers.

About one in five migraine sufferers experiences visual symptoms before and during a headache, said study author Souvik Sen, MD, MPH, a neurologist at the University of South Carolina School of Medicine. These symptoms can include flashes of light, blind spots, or seeing zigzag or squiggly lines.

In a 25-year ongoing study of nearly 13,000 adults in four US communities, researchers identified 817 participants who had suffered a blood-clot stroke.

They found that migraine patients who experience aura symptoms seem more likely to suffer a blood-clot stroke than typical migraine sufferers. Specifically, people who have migraine with aura appear to be three times more likely to have a stroke caused by a clot that forms in the heart, dislodges and travels to the brain, the study authors said.

They also seem twice as likely to have a stroke caused by a clot that develops in a clogged part of the blood vessel supplying blood to the brain.

Future research needs to look into blood flow patterns in the brains of migraine-with-aura patients, Dr. Sen said.

"When they have the vision symptoms, it could be an effect of the migraine on the blood vessels of the brain," Dr. Sen said.

Study #2

The other study focused on another known risk factor for stroke—medications containing estrogen.

"Estrogen, which is contained in hormone-replacement therapy and in certain kinds of combination birth control pills, increases the likelihood of blood clots," and thus increases stroke risk, Dr. Loder said.

Researchers analyzed data for more than 82,000 women 50 to 79 years old from the Women's Health Initiative, a study begun by the US National Institutes of Health in the early 1990s. All reported having some degree of migraines, and about 45% were using hormone replacement.

At a follow-up visit three years later, women completed a questionnaire to determine if their migraines had gotten better or worse.

Women who experienced worsening migraines while taking hormone-replacement therapy appeared to be 30% more likely to have a clot-based stroke than migraine sufferers who either stopped taking or never took hormone-replacement therapy, researchers concluded.

Advice

Study lead author Haseeb Rahman, MD, a neurology resident at Houston Methodist Hospital in Texas, said the findings suggest women on hormone-replacement therapy should notify their doctor of any migraine symptoms.

"You should not simply ignore an increasingly bad migraine," said Dr. Rahman, who worked on the study with a research team from the Zeenat Qureshi Stroke Institute in Minneapolis. "You should also tell your doc-

Strokes Affecting More Pregnant Women

The rate of stroke is falling among Americans ages 65 and older, but it increased by 47% in women during pregnancy or after childbirth from the mid-1990s to 2010–2011 (latest data available).

Possible reasons: Increasing obesity among women of childbearing age...inactivity of people in their 20s, 30s and 40s...and older maternal age.

Analysis of data from nearly 82 million hospitalizations of pregnant women by researchers at Massachusetts General Hospital, Boston, published in *Obstetrics & Gynecology*.

---

tor if you're getting migraines for the first time while on hormone-replacement therapy."

"Women who have migraine with aura probably want to think more carefully about the potential risk of stroke associated with using estrogen," Dr. Loder said. "I would not go so far as to say they should never use it, but they should think more carefully about it."

However, Dr. Loder noted that the increased risk is "certainly higher than we would like it to be, but it's not terribly high," given that just 2,063 women experienced clot-based strokes out of more than 82,000 female migraine sufferers.

"Other risk factors like smoking and high blood pressure are much more important," Dr. Loder said. "It's important to put the risk into context."

Migraine sufferers or women taking estrogen should address more important risk factors, Dr. Loder said, by quitting smoking, controlling their blood pressure, treating their diabetes or lowering their cholesterol.

For more information about stroke prevention, visit the website of the American Stroke Association, *strokeassociation.org*, and search "prevent stroke."

Pregnancy After 40 May Boost Risk of Stroke

Adnan Qureshi, MD, director, Zeenat Qureshi Stroke Institute, St. Cloud, Minnesota.

David Liebeskind, MD, professor, neurology, and director, Neurovascular Imaging Research Core, Ronald Reagan UCLA Medical Center, Los Angeles.

Presentation, American Stroke Association's annual meeting, Los Angeles.

Women who become pregnant at age 40 or older may face a greater risk of a "bleeding" stroke later in life, new research suggests.

"Women who have a pregnancy after the age of 40 appear to have a higher chance, 15 or 20 years down the line, of having a stroke, particularly the hemorrhagic type of stroke, which is bleeding in the brain," said lead researcher Adnan Qureshi, MD. He is director of the Zeenat Qureshi Stroke Institute, in St. Cloud, Minnesota.

However, the study only uncovered an association between later pregnancies and potential stroke risk. It did not prove cause-and-effect.

Study Details

Dr. Qureshi and colleagues reviewed data from more than 72,000 women, aged 50 to 79, enrolled in the Women's Health Initiative, a large-scale study launched to look at ways to prevent health problems in women.

The researchers zeroed in on more than 3,300 women who had a pregnancy after the age of 40. The investigators looked at their rates of stroke, heart attack and death from cardiovascular disease over the next 12 years, and then compared them with women who had a pregnancy at a younger age.

Hemorrhagic stroke was 60% more likely to occur in women who had a pregnancy after age 40, the study authors reported. The findings held even after taking into account age, race, the presence of congestive heart failure, high blood pressure and other factors that might boost stroke risk.

The risk of a stroke caused by a clot ("ischemic stroke"), a heart attack and death from cardiovascular disease also rose in those who were pregnant after age 40. However, after taking other factors into account, the increased risks for those events were no longer statistically significant, Dr. Qureshi added.

For all but the hemorrhagic strokes, risk factors such as high blood pressure explained the increased risk, Dr. Qureshi said. But pregnancy later in life seems to be a risk factor for hemorrhagic stroke by itself, he said.

Dr. Qureshi said he can't explain the possible link with certainty. It's known that women who become pregnant later in life have a higher risk of developing high blood pressure and diabetes during pregnancy. So, perhaps women who get pregnant later are predisposed to these problems, he suggested.

Or, "the pregnancy itself in later life may cause stress on the cardiovascular system," Dr. Qureshi added.

Expert Comment

The link between later pregnancies and stroke risk is a new topic in the medical community, said David Liebeskind, MD. He is director of the Neurovascular Imaging Research Core at the Ronald Reagan UCLA Medical Center in Los Angeles. However, "you would want to see confirmatory evidence" from additional studies, he said.

Dr. Liebeskind also reiterated that the researchers behind the new studies did not prove a cause-and-effect relationship between later pregnancies and stroke risk. "It doesn't mean that if you become pregnant above a certain age, you are going to have a hemorrhagic stroke," he said. "This is simply an association that has been found."

In future studies, researchers must "provide a rational basis for the underlying biology," Dr. Liebeskind said. "If it reaches that stage, perhaps there are underlying things that could be managed," he suggested. Or, ongoing research may identify a specific group of women who are vulnerable to stroke if they become pregnant after age 40.

Dr. Qureshi said that the finding suggests that women, when planning later-life pregnancies, should be aware of these risks. Once pregnant, they should be carefully monitored, as guidelines already recommend, he added.

"What the study suggests is, perhaps that rigorous monitoring should continue for years afterwards," Dr. Qureshi said.

The study findings were presented at the American Stroke Association's annual meeting, in Los Angeles.

See page 77, "How to Survive the Worst Type of Stroke," for more information on hemorrhagic strokes.

More Evidence Smog May Raise Stroke Risk

Longjian Liu, MD, PhD, associate professor, epidemiology and biostatistics, Drexel University, Philadelphia.

Presentation, American Stroke Association, International Stroke Conference, Los Angeles.

As levels of air pollution rise, so too does the risk for stroke, a new study suggests.

Researchers used data from the United States and China. These two countries are the biggest producers of greenhouse gases in the world, and are responsible for one-third of global warming, according to study lead author Longjian Liu, MD, PhD.

"Cities with poorer air quality have significantly higher prevalence of stroke, compared with cities that have a better air quality," said Dr. Liu, an associate professor of epidemiology and biostatistics at Drexel University in Philadelphia.

The differences are particularly striking in winter and summer, Dr. Lui added. "Winter and summer have higher concentrations of air pollution than spring and fall, and death from strokes is significantly higher in winter," he said.

It's important to note, however, that this study was only designed to look for an association between air pollution and stroke. It did not prove a cause-and-effect relationship.

The results of the study were presented at the annual meeting of the American Stroke Association (ASA), in Los Angeles.

Stroke is the fifth-leading cause of death in the United States, killing nearly 129,000 Americans each year, and is a leading cause of disability, according to the ASA. In addition, stroke is the second-leading cause of death worldwide, after heart disease.

Study Details

For the study, Dr. Liu's team collected data on air quality between 2010 and 2013. The data came from more than 1,000 counties in 49 US states and from 120 cities in 32 provinces in China, the study authors said.

The researchers looked at a type of pollution known as particulate matter. These tiny bits of air pollution come from cars, power plants, forest fires and other sources, according to the U.S. Environmental Protection Agency (EPA). Such particles that are less than 2.5 micrometers in diameter (PM2.5) pose the greatest health risks because they are so small—⅓₀th diameter of a human hair—and can easily lodge in the lungs.

The investigators found that across the United States and China, the total number of stroke cases rose 1.19% for each 10 micrograms per cubic meter increase in PM2.5.

In addition, the researchers found regional differences in PM2.5 levels linked to the number of strokes.

High Risk Regions

The American South had the highest average annual PM2.5 levels, while the West had the lowest, according to Dr. Liu. The South, known as the "stroke belt," had the highest prevalence of stroke at 4.2%, compared with the West, which had the lowest at 3%, Dr. Liu said.

Temperature also seemed to have an effect on air quality and the risk of stroke, he said. Seasonal variations in air quality can be partly attributable to climate changes, he explained.

"In the summer, there are lots of rainy and windy days, which can help disperse air pollution. High temperatures create a critical thermal stress that may lead to an increased risk for stroke and other heat- and air quality-related illnesses and deaths," Dr. Liu said.

Although patients can't control air quality, these study findings provide evidence for policy makers and public health officials to develop better models for monitoring and predicting climate changes so patients can better protect themselves, Dr. Liu suggested.

"Air pollution, extreme cold in winter or extreme heat in summer are risk factors for stroke," he said. "Patients, specifically older adults, who live in areas with poor air quality should pay specific attention to the risk of stroke that may be caused by both air pollution and extreme cold or heat," Dr. Liu said.

The Vitamin That Cuts Stroke Risk More Than 20%

According to a large study, supplements of the B vitamin decrease incidence of a first stroke in people with high blood pressure by 21%. People with normal blood pressure are likely to benefit, too. A standard daily multivitamin should provide adequate folic acid.

Better: Getting the vitamin from food, especially broccoli, beans (cooked from dried) and dark, leafy greens.

Also: Enriched grain products.

Meir Stampfer, MD, DrPH, professor of medicine at Harvard Medical School, Boston, and coauthor of an editorial published in *JAMA*.

3 Foods That Help Prevent Stroke

According to recent research, people who had a stroke were more likely to have low blood levels of vitamin C than people who had not had a stroke. A deficiency of vitamin C may raise blood pressure, a risk factor for stroke. Also, vitamin C helps your body build collagen, which is important for blood vessel health.

Best: Get at least 75 milligrams (mg) of vitamin C a day.

Best sources of vitamin C: Red peppers (118 mg per cup)…broccoli (78 mg per cup)…oranges (63 mg per fruit).

Study of 65 people by researchers at Pont-chaillou University Hospital and University of Rennes, France, presented at the American Academy of Neurology's 66th annual meeting in Philadelphia.

Avoid a Stroke by Avoiding Shingles

Maria A. Nagel, MD, department of neurology, University of Colorado School of Medicine, Aurora. Her expert commentary and the study on shingles and stroke appeared in *Current Neurology and Neuroscience Reports*. The study, titled "Risk of Stroke Following Herpes Zoster: A Self-Controlled Case-Series Study," by researchers on the faculty of epidemiology and population health at the London School of Hygiene and Tropical Medicine, United Kingdom, was published in *Clinical Infectious Diseases*.

The chronic pain and unsightly rash of shingles is bad enough, but now there's increasing evidence that you're at much higher risk for stroke in the first few weeks following the onset of a shingles attack. Protect yourself by knowing which shingles symptom is most associated with stroke and how you can lower your risk for shingles and shingles-related stroke.

The Ghost of a Childhood Scourge

Shingles, also known as herpes zoster, is caused by varicella zoster virus (VZV)—the same virus that causes chicken pox. Decades after infection, when a person's immune system is weakened by age, disease or medications, the virus can reactivate. Shingles'

main symptoms are shooting pain, burning, numbness, itchiness and a rash and blisters on one side of the body, which usually last about two weeks but can become chronic.

Shingles usually affects the skin, but the virus can also affect blood vessels, the brain, eyes and spinal cord, leading to inflammation of the brain (encephalitis), inflammation of the membranes around the spinal cord and brain (meningitis), blindness or stroke. The new study examined more than 6,500 patients and showed that the risk for stroke increased by 63% during the first month following the first symptoms of shingles. The increased risk gradually lessened—to 42% during the second and third months and to 23% during months four through six.

One specific form of shingles greatly increased stroke risk. Herpes zoster ophthalmicus (HZO)—where the shingles rash occurs around one or both eyes—turned out to be a telltale risk factor for stroke in the study. Patients with HZO had a greater than three-fold increased risk for stroke. That's because HZO is a sign that the herpes virus has reactivated from a cluster of neurons in the head called the trigeminal ganglia. When the virus reactivates here, it not only travels along nerve fibers that go straight to the area around the eye, but also has potential to travel along nerve fibers directly to blood vessels in the brain.

Best Defense Against Shingles

Getting the shingles vaccine (Zostavax) is no guarantee that you won't get shingles, but it does cut your risk in half. The U.S. Centers for Disease Control and Prevention recommends the vaccine for adults 60 years of age and older, but it is FDA-approved for anyone over 50.

The vaccine is not recommended for every older adult. *Avoid it if you…*

• **Are allergic to gelatin,** the antibiotic *neomycin* or any other component of the vaccine.

• **Have a weakened immune system,** either due to a medical condition such as diabetes, kidney failure, sickle-cell anemia, cirrhosis or HIV infection…because you are receiving treatments that modify or suppress your immune system such as chemotherapy or radiation or are on immunosuppressive therapies for an autoimmune disease such as rheumatoid arthritis, multiple sclerosis and Crohn's disease…or take certain medications including corticosteroids, *infliximab* (Remicade), *adalimumab* (Humira) and *etanercept* (Enbrel).

Best Defense If You Get Shingles

If you do get shingles, even after vaccination, take action. Antiviral therapy such as *acyclovir* (Zovirax), *valacyclovir* (Valtrex) or *famciclovir* (Famvir) not only relieves symptoms, but can lower your risk for stroke. In the study on stroke and shingles, patients who were treated with antiviral therapy for shingles were still at increased stroke risk but at a much lower rate—28%—than patients who did not receive antiviral therapy.

Shingles patients should be treated with a full two-week course of antiviral therapy, taking into consideration their kidney function and any medical conditions that need to be monitored while on antiviral therapy. The rash usually resolves within two weeks or less if antivirals are used, but pain can persist for up to three months.

If you haven't already been vaccinated for shingles, this study is a good reason to stop procrastinating. If shingles does happen to erupt, discuss antiviral therapy with your doctor instead of just toughing it out—especially if you develop a rash around your eyes. Also, be on the lookout for strokelike symptoms, such as drooping or numbness on one side of the face, weakness or numbness in an arm or leg, slurred speech or sudden loss or dimness of vision, in the first few months after a shingles outbreak. If these occur, seek urgent medical care and be sure to let your doctor know about your recent history of shingles.

Hiccups Can Be More Than Just Annoying

Anil Minocha, MD, professor of medicine and chief of gastroenterology, Overton Brooks VA Medical Center, Shreveport, Louisiana, and the author of *Dr. M's Seven-X Plan for Digestive Health.*

"I'm a 56-year-old woman who has recently been getting hiccups more frequently—sometimes for 15 minutes or so. Should I worry?"

Hiccups, those annoying chest spasms, are usually caused by gulping air…drinking carbonated or alcoholic beverages…or stress.

What happens: The diaphragm muscle that separates the chest from the abdomen involuntarily contracts, which causes the vocal cords to close suddenly, triggering the "hic" sound. Most episodes of hiccups are brief and don't require medical follow-up.

Folk wisdom abounds, but certain remedies do cure hiccups.

Examples: Close your ears with your fingers while drinking water through a straw. Biting on a lemon also works!

But if your hiccups are persistent and painful, you need to see your doctor. Hiccups can be a sign of many conditions, including gastroesophageal reflux disease (GERD), kidney disease or a brain or esophageal tumor.

Hiccups, accompanied by chest pain, can also be a little-known early symptom of stroke in women. Other symptoms of stroke that are unique to women may include shortness of

The Dangers of Sleeping Too Much

Sleeping more than eight hours a night is linked to stroke. It is unclear if oversleeping causes cardiovascular concerns that can lead to stroke or if it is an indicator of other health issues. Oversleeping has also been linked to diabetes, obesity and other health problems.

Study of nearly 10,000 people, ages 42 to 81, over 10 years by researchers at Cambridge Institute of Public Health, University of Cambridge, UK, published in *Neurology.*

breath and whole-body numbness. If your hiccups are painful and unrelenting and you are also experiencing traditional stroke symptoms—such as blurred vision, severe headache, arm weakness, facial drooping, confusion and/or speech difficulty—call 911.

An Irregular Heartbeat Can Cause a Stroke

Hugh Calkins, MD, a professor of medicine and the Nicholas J. Fortuin MD Professor of Cardiology at The Johns Hopkins University School of Medicine, and director of Cardiac Arrhythmia Services and Electrophysiology Laboratory at The Johns Hopkins Hospital, both in Baltimore.

If you have a type of irregular heartbeat known as atrial fibrillation (or "A-fib"), your increased risk for stroke and other serious conditions can be a frightening prospect to live with.

Good news: New guidelines to improve treatment for people with A-fib—the first such recommendations in nearly 10 years—have recently been released by the American College of Cardiology, the American Heart Association and the Heart Rhythm Society. The guidelines are important because they help ensure that A-fib patients are receiving the highest standards of care.

What Goes Wrong

A-fib is a rapid and irregular heartbeat triggered when the upper chambers of the heart (atria) quiver erratically, sometimes faster than 300 times per minute.

Symptoms may include the sensation of a pounding or fluttering heart, chest pain, intense fatigue, shortness of breath for no apparent reason and/or sudden dizziness. However, in some cases, A-fib can be "silent"—with no symptoms at all.

A-fib is usually suspected based on a person's symptoms and a physical exam. It is also sometimes discovered when a person undergoes routine heart tests, such as an electrocardiogram (ECG or EKG)…a stress test…or an echocardiogram. A definitive diagnosis of A-fib requires some type of ECG monitoring, which shows A-fib.

New treatment approaches…

Is Medication Right for You?

Stroke is the number-one problem caused by A-fib—but prescribing a blood-thinning medication (anticoagulant) to prevent stroke isn't always straightforward—each drug has possible side effects that must be balanced against its benefits.

Fortunately, decision-making about drugs for A-fib just got a lot easier for doctors. Guidelines now endorse the use of a new medical calculator—the exact name is "CHA2DS2-VASc Score for Atrial Fibrillation Stroke Risk"—that includes several specific stroke risk factors, such as vascular disease and female gender, to more accurately predict who is likely to suffer a stroke and whether treatment with a blood thinner is right for the patient. Older risk calculators did not include these specific risk factors.

What to do: If you have been diagnosed with A-fib, tell your doctor that you want to check your stroke risk with the CHA2DS2-VASc Score to determine whether or not you should be on a blood-thinning medication to prevent a stroke. The calculator and instructions on how to use it are available online at many websites, including *ClinCalc.com/cardiology/stroke/CHADSVASC.aspx*.

The Blood Thinner Question

The new guidelines also recommend for the first time that doctors treating patients with A-fib consider prescribing one of three blood-thinning drugs that have entered the marketplace in the last five years—*dabigatran* (Pradaxa), *rivaroxaban* (Xarelto) and *apixaban* (Eliquis). A fourth new blood thinner called *edoxaban* (Savaysa) has been released since these guidelines were published and will be included in the next update. Although more expensive than *warfarin* (Coumadin), the standard blood thinner, these drugs may offer some advantages over it.

See appendix page 315 "The Truth About Blood Thinners" for more information.

Beyond Stroke Prevention

The frequency of A-fib symptoms can be eliminated or reduced with antiarrhythmic medication, such as *flecainide* (Tambocor) or *propranolol* (Inderal), or catheter ablation. With this procedure, a catheter (thin, flexible tube) is inserted through a vein in the groin and snaked into the heart. Radiofrequency energy is used to destroy "aberrant pacemaker" cells that send out irregular impulses that trigger A-fib.

For best results: The most successful outcomes occur in medical centers where the procedure is performed regularly. Guidelines also recommend that an electrophysiologist (a cardiologist who specializes in treating electrical problems of the heart) perform a minimum of two A-fib ablation procedures each month to maintain competency. There is no substitute for experience, for both the physician and ablation center, when it comes to complex cardiac procedures.

Help for A-Fib Patients at Risk for Stroke

Atrial fibrillation patients at the highest risk for stroke can be identified with a cardiac MRI, says Hiroshi Ashikaga, MD, PhD. People suffering from the common heart-rhythm disorder atrial fibrillation (A-fib) already have five times higher risk for stroke.

Recent finding: A-fib patients with a specific alteration in the function of the heart's left atrium have slower blood flow and are at even higher risk for blood clots and future stroke.

Hiroshi Ashikaga, MD, PhD, assistant professor of medicine and biomedical engineering at Johns Hopkins University School of Medicine, Baltimore.

How to Survive the Worst Type of Stroke

Edward C. Jauch, MD, director of the division of emergency medicine at the Medical University of South Carolina in Charleston, where he is also a professor in the department of neurosciences, the associate vice-chair for research in the department of medicine and director of Acute Stroke Trials, ongoing clinical research into the optimal treatment approaches for stroke.

If someone asked you for a quick definition of a stroke, you would probably say that it is caused by a blood clot...and requires quick treatment with a clot-dissolving drug. These points are true for the most common strokes, called ischemic strokes, but there's another type of stroke that doesn't get nearly as much attention.

The "other" stroke: A hemorrhagic, or bleeding, stroke is entirely different from an ischemic stroke—and usually more devastating. Fortunately, new research has uncovered potentially lifesaving advice for people who suffer this type of stroke. *The facts you (and your loved ones) need...*

The Grim Statistics

Up to 20% of the nearly 800,000 new or recurrent strokes that occur each year in the US are hemorrhagic strokes, but they account for 40% of stroke deaths.

What makes these strokes so dangerous? Hemorrhagic strokes result from bleeding into or around the brain, a catastrophic event that damages brain tissue. In addition, as the pooled blood degrades, it releases iron from red blood cells. Iron is toxic for brain tissue.

Worst Headache of Your Life

While most people can identify the main symptoms of an ischemic stroke (for example, facial drooping...numbness or weakness on one side of the body...and/or trouble speaking), the red flags for hemorrhagic stroke are not as well known.

77

With hemorrhagic strokes, a sudden, intense headache is usually the main symptom. Sometimes mild headaches can be a warning sign a few days or weeks before this type of stroke.

Important: Headache sometimes occurs with an ischemic stroke, but it's usually accompanied by other symptoms, such as those described above. With a hemorrhagic stroke, additional symptoms may include nausea, vomiting and/or loss of consciousness. Symptoms can overlap, however, with both types of stroke, and only an imaging test can tell the difference.

If you have a severe headache that's unusual for you: Call 911. This is particularly true if you have stroke risk factors such as smoking, high blood pressure or diabetes.

A lifesaving new finding: For people suffering a subarachnoid hemorrhage (a type of hemorrhagic stroke described below), treatment at a comprehensive stroke center was associated with a 27% reduced risk for death, compared with care at a hospital that did not provide specialized stroke care. Comprehensive stroke centers have specialists who are trained to deal with these strokes and 24-hour access to a neurosurgeon (if needed).

For the nearest comprehensive stroke center: Go to the National Stroke Association website, *stroke.org/emergency-stroke-center-locations.* A family member can ask the ambulance driver to take you there.

How Bleeding Strokes Occur

There are two main types of hemorrhagic stroke...

• **Subarachnoid hemorrhage.** About half of hemorrhagic strokes occur in the subarachnoid space, between the inner and middle layers of tissue that cover the brain.

What happens: Most subarachnoid hemorrhages are caused by a ruptured aneurysm, a bulge in an artery wall that tends to develop after age 40, due to years of high blood pressure. It can also be congenital (present at birth). An aneurysm that doesn't bleed isn't necessarily a problem—you can have one for decades and not know it unless it shows up during an imaging test for some other condition.

But once an aneurysm "bursts" and bleeds, you will likely have a "thunderclap" headache that gets progressively worse—and may be followed by a brief loss of consciousness. You may also have blurred vision or loss of vision and/or pain behind and above one eye. Permanent brain damage or death can occur within hours or even minutes. Get to an ER.

Next steps: This type of stroke can be quickly identified with a CT scan or an MRI, and with magnetic resonance angiography (MRA) and/or cerebral angiography (a catheter is used to inject a dye, which illuminates blood vessels in the brain). *Once the damaged artery is identified, there are two main choices...*

• Clipping, the traditional approach, is done under general anesthesia. A surgeon creates an opening in the skull (craniotomy), locates the aneurysm and seals it off with a titanium clip that remains on the artery permanently.

• Endovascular coiling is a newer approach. With this minimally invasive technique, there is no incision in the skull. A tiny catheter is inserted into an artery in the groin, then threaded through the vascular system (with the aid of a special type of X-ray) until it's inside the aneurysm. Then, a flexible platinum coil is placed within the aneurysm to stop the bleeding.

Which technique is better? It depends on the location and size of the aneurysm, as well as the overall health of the patient. One large study found that the risk for disability or death in patients who were treated with coils was almost 27% lower than in those who were clipped. However, the study found a greater risk for the brain to bleed again with coils versus clipping.

• **Intracerebral hemorrhage.** Intracerebral hemorrhages cause bleeding within the brain. They're often caused by decades of high blood pressure, which can damage small blood vessels. They can also be caused by excessive doses of blood thinners taken for cardiovascular disease…or bleeding disorders (such as hemophilia).

Along with a severe headache, symptoms might include weakness, paralysis, a loss of speech or vision and sometimes mental confusion. Headache and high blood pressure are more common with this type of stroke than with ischemic stroke, but only a CT scan or MRI can provide an accurate diagnosis.

In some cases, surgery or endoscopic drainage may be helpful to remove blood that's causing excess pressure. *Next steps…*

•Lower systolic (top number) blood pressure to below 140. This will reduce brain bleeding.

•Reverse the medication's effects in patients with strokes that are caused by blood thinners. This can be done, for example, by giving an intravenous solution that contains clotting factors, platelets or other products that help blood clot.

Survivors of hemorrhagic stroke should receive rehabilitation care to aid their recovery.

Effective New Poststroke Treatment for Women

Promising new treatment cuts poststroke disability in women.

Preliminary study: 42% of female patients who received IV uric acid in addition to the usual treatment, the clot-busting drug tPA, were relatively free of disability three months after a stroke compared with 29% of women given tPa and no uric acid. Little difference was found among men.

Theory: Men tend to have higher blood levels of uric acid.

Ángel Chamorro, MD, PhD, director of the Comprehensive Stroke Center, Hospital Clinic, University of Barcelona, Spain, and senior author of a study of 411 patients, published in *Stroke.*

Moving More Means Better Stroke Recovery

Julie Bernhardt, PhD, head, stroke division, Florey Institute of Neuroscience and Mental Health, Victoria, Australia.
American Stroke Association, news release.

It may be good for hospitalized stroke patients to be taken out of bed for frequent but short periods of movement, researchers report.

The Study

The study authors from Australia looked at more than 2,100 patients in a hospital stroke unit and found that getting them out of bed and moving around soon after their stroke benefited them.

The more often this was done, the better their physical recovery and their chances of regaining their independence three months after their stroke, according to the study.

But researchers found the sessions were only effective when kept short. Increasing the length of each session reduced the likelihood that patients would be independent within a few months.

Some experts have raised concerns about the safety of getting patients out of bed soon after a stroke, but the researchers found no evidence that doing so increased the risk of serious problems.

Conclusion

Early and frequent out-of-bed movement helped reduce the risk of serious complications in patients between the ages of 65 and 80, according to lead author Julie Bernhardt, head of the stroke division at the Florey Institute of Neuroscience and Mental Health in Victoria, and colleagues.

The study was presented at the American Stroke Association's annual meeting, in Los Angeles.

For more information about recovering from a stroke, visit the US National Institute of Neurological Disorders and Stroke website, *ninds.nih.gov*, and search "stroke rehabilitation."

Physical Therapy: A Path to Stroke Recovery

Even a year after surviving a severe stroke, intense physical therapy helps patients recover a surprising amount of arm function.

Recent study: 39 patients (a year or more poststroke) who did physical therapy involving exercises, electrical stimulation and/or a robotic device five hours a day, five days a week for 12 weeks doubled or nearly doubled their ability to do everyday activities, such as placing the affected arm into a sweater sleeve.

Janis Daly, PhD, professor of neurology, University of Florida College of Medicine, Gainesville.

Stroke's Aftermath Often Worse for Women and Minorities

Richard Libman, MD, vice chairman, neurology, Long Island Jewish Medical Center, New Hyde Park, New York.
American Stroke Association, news release.

Anyone can be laid low by stroke, but a recent study finds that the road back to health may be tougher for female and minority patients.

Research led by Dr. Cheryl Bushnell, professor of neurology at Wake Forest School of Medicine in Winston-Salem, North Carolina, found that male and white stroke survivors tended to fare best in terms of their physical function a few months after their stroke.

The study involved 129 patients who were asked about their mobility, arm strength and ability to do daily tasks three months after a

Stroke–Cancer Link

Stroke survivors may have higher risk for cancer. Among 3,247 ischemic stroke survivors who started out cancer-free, 2% were diagnosed with cancer within two years—a 40% higher rate than the norm for older US adults.

Possible reasons: The same risk factors that lead to stroke may also make cancer more likely—for example, smoking or unhealthful eating habits. Or an underlying condition such as chronic low-grade inflammation may make both stroke and cancer more likely.

Study of 3,247 ischemic stroke survivors by researchers at Zeenat Qureshi Stroke Institute, St. Cloud, Minnesota, presented at a meeting of the American Stroke Association's International Stroke Conference 2015.

stroke or mini-stroke—also known as a transient ischemic attack, or TIA.

The patients received scores ranging from zero (worst) to 100 (best).

The overall average score was just over 81. However, men had an average score of 85.7 while women had an average of 75.8—an indication that men did better in regaining physical function.

When it came to race, white patients had an average score of 85.4, while nonwhite patients had an average of 69.4, Dr. Bushnell's team found.

Patients who had suffered a prior stroke or mini-stroke tended to have had lower scores than those who had suffered a first stroke or mini-stroke, the researchers noted.

According to the researchers, the findings highlight the need to improve physical rehabilitation among stroke survivors who are women or members of racial minorities.

The findings didn't surprise one expert in stroke care.

"It is incumbent upon all of us involved in stroke research and treatment to clarify the reasons for worse outcome," Richard Libman, MD, vice chair of neurology at Long Island Jewish Medical Center in New Hyde Park, New York said.

Women Smokers at Higher Risk for Brain Bleed

Joni Lindbohm, MD, physician, neurosurgery and public health, University of Helsinki, Finland.

Ralph Sacco, MD, chairman, neurology, University of Miami Miller School of Medicine.

Stroke, online.

S trokes characterized by bleeding inside the lining of the brain are more common among smokers, especially women, researchers report.

These serious strokes—called *subarachnoid* hemorrhages—are eight times more common among women who smoke more than a pack a day compared to nonsmokers, Finnish researchers found.

Even light smoking tripled a woman's risk for this type of stroke, the study found.

"There is no safe level of smoking, and naturally, the best option is never to start," said lead researcher Joni Lindbohm, MD, of the University of Helsinki.

Subarachnoid hemorrhages often affect younger people and "can be quite devastating in terms of disability and death, with fatality rates around one in five," said Ralph Sacco, MD, chairman of neurology at the University of Miami Miller School of Medicine, who wasn't involved in the study.

This type of stroke usually results from a bleeding aneurysm in the brain. An aneurysm is a small weak spot in a blood vessel that can burst at any time.

Study Details

For the study, Dr. Lindbohm and colleagues collected data on nearly 66,000 adults listed in Finnish national surveys since 1972. Participants were followed for an average of 21 years, until they had a first stroke, died, or until the end of 2011.

The researchers found that among light smokers—one to 10 cigarettes a day—women were three times more likely to have subarachnoid hemorrhage, and men were twice as likely to have one compared to nonsmokers.

Among those who smoked 11 to 20 cigarettes a day, women were four times more likely and men two times more likely to suffer this type of stroke.

But those who quit smoking significantly reduced their odds of having a subarachnoid hemorrhage. After six months without smoking, their risk fell to the level of nonsmokers, the researchers reported.

These Strokes More Common in Women

Subarachnoid hemorrhage is more common among women than men. The reasons why are unclear, Drs. Lindbohm and Sacco said. "Cigarette smoking and high blood pressure are two important modifiable risk factors for subarachnoid hemorrhage," Dr. Sacco said.

Dr. Lindbohm said that heavy-smoking females with unruptured aneurysms in their brain are a high-risk population, and their aneurysms should be treated.

For more on subarachnoid hemorrhage, visit the Brain Aneurysm Foundation at *BA found.org*.

The Simple Treatment That Improves Stroke Recovery

R esearch on stent retrievers was halted early because patients showed such significant benefit—including a 70% increase in functional independence 90 days after a stroke.

How the retrievers are used: The stent is inserted into an artery in the groin and guided to the brain clot. The stent grabs the clot and is pulled out. Side effects may include bleeding in the brain—but the benefits outweigh the risks.

Igor Rybinnik, MD, medical director of the Comprehensive Stroke Center at Robert Wood Johnson University Hospital, Rahway, New Jersey.

Chapter 4

LUNG HEALTH AND ALLERGIES

Secondhand Smoke Tied to Infertility and Early Menopause

Smoking and being exposed to secondhand smoke may trigger early menopause and infertility in women, a recent study suggests.

Other research has linked smoking with higher rates of infertility and perhaps earlier menopause. However, "secondhand smoke is less researched," especially among never-smoking women, said study author Andrew Hyland, PhD, chair of health behavior at Roswell Park Cancer Institute, in Buffalo, New York.

About the Study

In the study, Dr. Hyland and his colleagues evaluated women enrolled in the Women's Health Initiative, a large study launched in 1991 to look at a variety of health issues in more than 160,000 generally healthy, postmenopausal women.

Dr. Hyland's team looked at information about age of menopause and fertility, along with tobacco exposure, among some of the women enrolled in the study. The investigators evaluated information available on about 88,000 women to look at the fertility effects. They also looked at information on about 80,000 to examine onset of natural, or non-surgical, menopause.

Both smoking and exposure to secondhand smoke were linked to fertility issues and early menopause (before the typical age of 50), the researchers found.

Study Findings

Compared with never smokers, current or former smokers were 14% more likely to be infertile and 26% more likely to have early menopause. Early menopause has been linked with a higher risk of death from all causes, Dr. Hyland pointed out.

Among never smokers, those exposed to the highest level of secondhand smoke (such as living with a smoker for 10 years or more) were 18% more likely to have fertility problems and early menopause, the study found.

Female smokers reached menopause about 22 months before those who never smoked or never were exposed to smoke. Those ex-

Andrew Hyland, PhD, chair, department of health behavior, Roswell Park Cancer Institute, Buffalo, New York.

Patricia Folan, director, Center for Tobacco Control, North Shore-LIJ Health System, Great Neck, New York.

Tobacco Control, online.

posed to the highest level of passive smoke reached menopause 13 months earlier than those not exposed, the findings showed.

The study was published in the journal *Tobacco Control*.

Implications

But the study cannot prove cause and effect, Dr. Hyland added. "This is an observational study looking at data already collected," he said. "It [the link] could be something associated with early development and exposure as a young child."

Smoke interacts with hormones and can have adverse effects as well, he added.

Expert Commentary

The findings are a valuable reminder to avoid all smoke, said Patricia Folan, director of the Center for Tobacco Control at North Shore-LIJ Health System in Great Neck, New York.

"This study provides additional motivation and incentive for women of all ages to avoid smoking and exposure to secondhand smoke, as well as to quit smoking," she said. Both are associated with premature birth, low birth weight, infant death and certain birth defects, she added.

"This evidence, in addition to the data from the current study, offers health care providers, particularly ob-gyn practitioners, the information needed to counsel women about the hazards of smoking and secondhand smoke, and to encourage cessation," Folan said.

To learn more about the risk of secondhand smoke, visit the website of the American Cancer Society, *cancer.org*. Search "secondhand smoke."

Air Pollution Harms Unborn Children

Prenatal exposure to air pollution is tied to changes in the structure of an unborn child's brain and intellectual deficits and behavior problems later in childhood. The higher the mother's exposure to polycyclic aromatic hydrocarbons (PAHs)—pollution caused by burning gasoline, diesel fuel, home-heating oil and coal—the greater the damage to the unborn child.

Study of 40 pregnant women in their third trimester by researchers at Institute for the Developing Mind at The Saban Research Institute of Children's Hospital Los Angeles, published in *JAMA Psychiatry*.

Study Shows the Best Way to Quit Smoking

Nicola Lindson-Hawley, PhD, post-doctoral researcher, Nuffield Department of Primary Care Health Sciences, University of Oxford, UK.

Michael Fiore, MD, MPH, MBA, professor, University of Wisconsin, Madison.

Annals of Internal Medicine, online.

What's the best way to kick a smoking habit? New research suggests quitting all at once beats a more gradual approach.

Smoking Is a Serious Risk to Women

According to the American Lung Association, smoking and tobacco use pose a serious risk of death and disease for women. Annually, cigarette smoking kills an estimated 201,770 women in the US. And although more men smoke than women, women share a larger burden of smoking-related diseases.

Female smokers are nearly 22 times more likely to die from chronic obstructive pulmonary disease (COPD), which includes emphysema and chronic bronchitis, compared to women who never have smoked.

Aside from lung cancer, women who smoke also have an increased risk for developing cancers of the oral cavity, pharynx, larynx (voice box), esophagus, pancreas, kidney, bladder and uterine cervix. They also double their risk for developing coronary heart disease, according to the U.S. Department of Health and Human Services.

Smoking is still the leading preventable cause of death for both male and female Americans. And for every person who dies due to smoking, another 30 people are living with smoking-related illness, the government agency reports.

The good news is that stopping smoking greatly reduces the risk of smoking-related diseases, the CDC notes.

Study Details

The study found that after four weeks, nearly half of those who quit "cold turkey" were still not smoking. But, among people who quit gradually over two weeks, only 39% were smoke-free at four weeks, researchers said.

The latest research included just under 700 adult smokers from England. The study participants smoked an average of 20 cigarettes a day. More than nine in 10 of the participants were white. The average age of the smokers was 49, and half were women.

The study volunteers were randomly assigned to quit smoking abruptly or to cut down gradually by 75% over two weeks.

Before the day they quit, the gradual quitters used nicotine patches plus short-term products such as gum and lozenges; the abrupt quitters used only nicotine replacement patches. All of the participants received counseling assistance from nurses and short-term nicotine replacement medications after the quit day.

The researchers followed up at four weeks and six months after the experiment started. Blood testing was used to confirm whether smokers had actually quit.

At four weeks, 39% of those who'd gradually quit had stopped smoking compared to 49% of those who stopped abruptly. At six months, 16% of the gradual quitters and 22% of the abrupt quitters were still non-smokers, the study found.

"Most people thought cutting down would suit them better," said study lead author Nicola Lindson-Hawley, PhD, post-doctoral researcher with the University of Oxford in the United Kingdom. "But whatever they thought, it turned out they were better to try to quit abruptly."

The percentages of smokers who successfully quit may seem quite low, but Dr. Lindson-Hawley said those percentages are normal.

Findings from the study were published online in the *Annals of Internal Medicine*.

Even With Therapy Aids, Quitting Remains Difficult

Unfortunately, quitting smoking for good is no easy task. And no wonder...Research has suggested that nicotine is as addicting as drugs such as heroin and cocaine, the CDC says.

Smokers who try to quit often suffer from stress, hunger and weight gain, according to the CDC. These all contribute to low quit rates. Strategies such as using nicotine replacement therapy and getting counseling can help, however. And many people do succeed in quitting, even if it takes several attempts.

Experts on Quitting Weigh In

Michael Fiore, MD, a professor at the University of Wisconsin-Madison who's helped develop federal guidelines about quitting smoking, pointed out that the percentages from the study are still higher than quitting without support from counseling or medication.

Why might quitting abruptly be better? Those who try to quit gradually, Dr. Fiore said, often succumb to "the challenges of life even when they have very good intentions and a lot of structure."

This Is How to Quit

What should smokers take from the study results? They should try quitting abruptly first, Dr. Lindson-Hawley said. However, "many people feel that they cannot quit smoking all at once. If the decision is between cutting down or not trying to quit at all, then quitting gradually is still a viable approach."

Dr. Fiore said physicians should let patients try to quit gradually if they prefer that approach. "If I see them two months later and they crashed and burned, now I say, 'You've learned from that, let's try this quick-cessation thing.'"

For more about smoking cessation, visit the US Centers for Disease Control and Prevention at *CDC.gov*.

Air Pollution: The Invisible Killer

Study titled "Ambient Particulate Matter Air Pollution Exposure and Mortality in the NIH-AARP Diet and Health Cohort" by researchers at New York University School of Medicine, University of California, Berkeley, Washington University School of Medicine, St. Louis, and National Cancer Institute, Bethesda, Maryland, published in *Environmental Health Perspectives*.

Fine particulates kill. They're so tiny—less than 2.5 micrograms (about 1/10,000th of an inch). Because they're too small to be coughed out of your lungs like other irritants, these deadly particles, which often contain toxic compounds such as mercury and arsenic, slip deep into the tissues of the lungs…and eventually into the bloodstream.

Environmental researchers have been concerned about them for years. But now a large new study of more than 500,000 Americans reveals just how nasty they are. People who live in areas with the highest levels were 3% more likely to die from any cause, 10% more likely to get heart disease and, among non-smokers, 27% more likely to get respiratory diseases, compared with people who live in the cleanest areas.

Want to know where your part of the country stands? There's a NASA map for that. Visit *www.nasa.gov* and search "health sapping pollution"…click on the bottom-right-column map of the US.

What E-Cigarettes Really Do to Your Lungs

Study titled "Endothelial Disruptive Proinflammatory Effects of Nicotine and E-cigarette Vapor Exposures" by researchers at Indiana University School of Medicine, Indiana University-Purdue University and Richard L. Roudebush Veterans Affairs Medical Center, all in Indianapolis, and The Johns Hopkins University, Baltimore, and City University of New York, published in *American Journal of Physiology—Lung Cellular and Molecular Physiology*.

Let's face it—debates over e-cigarettes won't be over anytime soon. Users (and, of course, manufacturers) say that they are safer than "real" cigarettes and they help people quit smoking. And unlike the treasure trove of damning health evidence about "real" cigarettes—the latest even adds schizophrenia to the list—research about the health effects of electronic cigarettes is truly in its infancy.

But don't let that fool you, because one thing is becoming clear—inhaling nicotine…along with the other compounds in e-cigarettes such as formaldehyde…is far from harmless for your lungs. You should be aware that vaping (inhaling the vapor) causes temporary constriction in the lungs and that the vapor contains carcinogenic nitrosamines, which newer research has confirmed.

The latest news: Researchers have shown that vaping may damage the cell barrier that protects the lining of the lungs, called the endothelium. In the study, the researchers exposed human and mouse cells and live mice to an e-cigarette solution that either contained nicotine or was nicotine-free. The result with either solution was not only loss of the endothelial cell barrier, but also lung inflammation and an impairment of cell growth, a sign of cell stress. It's just a short-term lab study, to be sure, but if sustained, that kind of damage is associated with risk for lung diseases such as asthma and chronic obstructive pulmonary disease (COPD).

Note that it wasn't just the nicotine that caused harm in the study, either. Even the

E-Cigarette Vapor Dangerous for Children

E-cigarette vapor may cause respiratory infections in children. The vapor may trigger a strong immune response in epithelial cells that line and protect the inside of the lung. Once exposed to the vapor, these cells become more susceptible to infection.

Study by researchers in the department of medicine, National Jewish Health, Denver, published in *PLOS ONE.*

nicotine-free e-cigarette solutions were found to include lung-harming substances, such as the compound *acrolein*. This substance, which is present in e-cig vapor, damages the endothelial cells in the lungs.

Should You Ever Use E-Cigarettes?

Such short-term lung damage might be acceptable if we knew that e-cigs help people quit smoking. Some studies have found that they do...others have found they are no help at all.

To be fair, there's no question that vaping is less harmful than inhaling cigarette smoke, which is one of the most toxic substances that humans have ever come to use regularly. Even the biggest opponents of e-cigarettes acknowledge that. So if you switch from smoking cigarettes to vaping e-cigarettes, you're likely doing less harm to your lungs. If doing so helps you quit entirely, that's a win-win.

But don't fool yourself into thinking that vaping is a safe alternative to tobacco. It harms you. And if your children or grandchildren who don't smoke cigarettes think that vaping is a cool and safe habit to pick up, let them know that they're playing with addictive electronic fire.

Asthma and Motherhood: What You Need to Know

European Respiratory Journal, news release.

Women with asthma may take longer to get pregnant and have a lower pregnancy rate than those without the lung disease, new research suggests.

The study included 245 women, aged 23 to 45, who had unexplained fertility problems and were undergoing fertility treatment. Ninety-six of the women had been diagnosed with asthma.

The women were followed until they had a successful pregnancy, stopped treatment or the study ended. The median time for women without asthma to get pregnant was about 32 months compared to more than 55 months for those with asthma. Median means half took more time to conceive; half, less.

About 60% of women without asthma got pregnant, compared with just under 40% of those with asthma, the findings showed. The gap between the two groups increased with age, according to the study published in the *European Respiratory Journal.*

The trial finding adds new weight to evidence suggesting a link between asthma and fertility, lead author Dr. Elisabeth Juul Gade said in a journal news release. Dr. Gade is with the department of respiratory medicine at Bispebjerg University Hospital in Copenhagen, Denmark.

"We have seen here that asthma seems to have a negative influence on fertility as it increases time to pregnancy and even more so with age," she said. "We do not yet know the causal relationship; it may be complex with different types of asthma, psychological well-being, asthma medication and hormones all playing a role."

Dr. Gade said doctors should encourage women with asthma to become pregnant at an earlier age and step up their asthma treatment before conceiving.

"Patient education is also of paramount importance as adherence to treatment may be enhanced if patients are informed of this link," Dr. Gade said in the news release.

While the study found an association between asthma and difficulty conceiving, it did not prove cause-and-effect.

Natural Remedies for Asthma Relief

Jamison Starbuck, ND, a naturopathic physician in family practice and a guest lecturer at the University of Montana, both in Missoula. She is also a past president of the American Association of Naturopathic Physicians and a contributing editor to *The Alternative Advisor: The Complete Guide to Natural Therapies and Alternative Treatments.* DrJamisonStarbuck.com.

Asthma is a disease that begins in childhood, right? Well, not always. Though many adult asthma sufferers have struggled with the condition since childhood, research shows that up to 40% of new asthma patients are over age 40 when they have their first asthma attack. Some of my patients are surprised when I explain to them the role that a naturopathic physician can play in helping them prevent and control mild-to-moderate asthma. While patients with severe or unresponsive moderate asthma need conventional medical attention, natural medicine has a lot to offer.

First, it's important to recognize which adults are at increased risk of developing asthma. This includes people who suffer from frequent and recurrent upper respiratory infections, such as colds, sinusitis and the flu. When these illnesses occur too frequently (once a month or more often), inflammation can damage the respiratory tract—a perfect setup for asthma. Asthma is also closely linked to allergies (due, for example, to certain food preservatives, such as sodium bisulfate, and inhaled irritants, such as pollen and mold) as well as exposure to pollutants and toxins, including cigarette smoke. Re-

search now shows that severe stress can also trigger an asthma attack.

There's no one-size-fits-all approach to treating asthma. In general, I recommend approaches for my patients that will reduce inflammation and enhance their lung and immune health. Asthma-fighting supplements that I recommend (all can be used with asthma medication, if needed)...*

• **Fish oil.** Research has found that these oils reduce bronchial inflammation that often accompanies asthma.

Typical dose: 2,000 mg daily.

• **Antioxidants.** Vitamin C—2,000 mg per day—and vitamin E—400 international units (IU) daily. Both improve immune health and reduce the allergic response that so often triggers an asthma attack.

• **Magnesium.** Use of this mineral (300 mg to 500 mg daily) can reduce bronchospasm (a tightening of the airways that makes breathing more difficult).

• **Botanicals.** One of my favorites is astragalus. It supports both lung and immune health.

Typical dose: Use one-quarter teaspoon of tincture in two ounces of water, daily until asthma symptoms improve. Repeat when needed.

Also helpful: Deep-breathing exercises and/or yoga help prevent asthma attacks by calming the nervous system and increasing lung capacity.

Because all asthma patients have different needs, I recommend seeing a naturopathic doctor (ND) to help create a personalized natural regimen. To find an ND near you, consult The American Association of Naturopathic Physicians, *naturopathic.org.* But remember, not all asthma can be well controlled with natural medicine. If you have more than mild-to-moderate asthma, you should also be under the care of an allergist or pulmonologist and not shirk any prescription drugs, such as inhalers, that he/she has prescribed for you.

*Consult your doctor to find out if this asthma-fighting protocol is right for you.

Combining natural medicine with prescription medication (when needed) gives you the best chance of keeping your asthma well controlled!

Can Salt Rooms Really Help Asthma?

Leonard Bielory, MD, chair of the American College of Allergy, Asthma & Immunology (ACAAI) Integrative Medicine Committee, professor and director, STARx Allergy & Asthma Center, Springfield, New Jersey, research associate, Rutgers University, Center of Environmental Prediction, New Brunswick, New Jersey.

At the very same time that we're being inundated with advice on restricting salt intake, we're also hearing about a new type of therapy based on the claim that spending time in a salt room, breathing in moist, salty air, can help ease chronic respiratory problems such as asthma while also clearing up skin issues such as acne or psoriasis. Based on a centuries-old Eastern European curative therapy, spalike salt rooms are beginning to appear around the country. Are the benefits for real?

The Salt Room Experience

The quasi-medical term for this treatment is "halotherapy." It involves sitting in a smallish room lined with blocks of salt mined from ancient salt caves. A generator (like a steam vaporizer) emits vapor containing about one-half cup of salt during a 45-minute session. People remain clothed for the treatment but often bring a clothing change for afterward since the salt tends to leave a residue.

It sounds like "a day at the beach"—but does halotherapy help your health in any meaningful way? To find out, we spoke with asthma and allergy specialist Leonard Bielory, MD, chair of the American College of Allergy, Asthma & Immunology (ACAAI) Integrative Medicine Committee and director, STARx Allergy and Asthma Center in Springfield, New Jersey.

Nice But...

Dr. Bielory calls salt rooms a "nice concept"—but voices some concerns. He agrees that the salt particles may help skin conditions such as acne or eczema but he worries that salt therapy may prove detrimental to some people with asthma. He pointed out that asthma is the result of constriction in the respiratory tract, which can be caused by excess mucus or by spasms. Breathing salt-infused air might help break up mucus and therefore help some folks to breathe better, but others may find that the salt is an irritant that triggers spasms.

Dr. Bielory's objections don't stop there. There's no way to guarantee the purity of the air in the rooms, he said—pointing out that, theoretically at least, salt attracts certain bacteria and that each person coming for treatment brings a fresh supply of additional bacteria that might evolve in the environment. Other worries relate to the length of time and at what temperature it is safe to stay in the rooms, and whether salt rooms may be dangerous for people with other health conditions, such as cardiac problems.

Offering a different perspective, *Health Insider* contributing medical editor Andrew L. Rubman, ND, was less dismissive. While agreeing with some of Dr. Bielory's concerns, he pointed out that this therapy has hundreds of years of successful use in Europe behind it, and he knows naturopathic physicians who treat patients with inhaled salt therapy for such things as chronic bronchitis, asthma and chronic fatigue syndrome. "There is potential benefit for some patients under the supervision of a skilled doctor with experience," he said. Dr. Rubman agrees with Dr. Bielory that medical oversight is imperative because there is potential for harm.

Is it worth a try? Maybe, but don't be casual about it. If you are interested in exploring the use of halotherapy for a particular medical concern, make sure you find a doctor "worth his salt":...in other words, one who knows the way around this particular block.

Play Your Way to Stronger Lungs

Missy Von Luehrte, RN, a pulmonary rehabilitation nurse, El Camino Hospital, Mountain View, California. John Schamen, MD, Ontario Aerobics Center, Canada. Vivian Low, MPH, RN-BC, clinical manager of the pulmonary-rehabilitation program at El Camino Hospital.

Blowing the blues is good for your lungs. So is just about anything else you play on a harmonica. Whether your tastes run to "Love Me Do," "Sweet Home Chicago" or that 19th-century nonsense ditty "Oh! Susanna," as little as 10 minutes a day playing a harmonica may give you better breathing. In fact, what they're calling "harmonica therapy" is gaining steam in pulmonary-rehabilitation programs across the country for people with asthma, COPD and even lung transplants. But don't let the word "therapy" put you off. Playing the harmonica is a ton of fun, and it's good exercise for healthy lungs, too.

Whether your lungs are compromised or in good shape, you should try it—here's why.

Toe-Tapping Music-Making Clinical Therapy

How does harmonica playing strengthen the lungs? Experts say that it mimics the inspiratory (inhaling) and expiratory (exhaling) breathing exercises taught by pulmonary rehabilitation staff.

When you play a harmonica, you create sounds by the resistance of your breath against the instrument's reeds. Unlike, say, the clarinet, you're working against that reed resistance when you're exhaling and when you're inhaling. That strengthens the diaphragm (the largest muscle of the respiratory system), encourages deep breathing, and may help clear mucus from the lungs. While scientific studies haven't specifically validated therapeutic harmonica playing, it mimics...and encourages...the breathing exercises that have been shown to improve lung function.

Lung specialists around the country believe in it. "We use harmonicas for all patients with pulmonary disease," says Missy Von Luehrte, RN, pulmonary rehabilitation nurse at El Camino Hospital in Mountain View, California. It's not only effective but fun and relaxing, easy to learn and an inexpensive, easy-to-carry instrument, she says. Patients like it, too. Says Vivian Low, MPH, RN-BC, clinical manager of the pulmonary-rehabilitation program at El Camino Hospital, "Anecdotally, in all the programs across the United States that have used harmonica with lung patients, the patients feel that they are strengthening their breathing."

For People with Healthy Lungs, Too, It's Internal Power Lifting

Some experts believe that playing a wind instrument such as the harmonica can benefit everyone, especially as we age. After about the age of 30, most people begin to lose lung function. By age 50, even people with healthy lungs may lose 50% of their younger capacity, says John Schaman, MD, Ontario Aerobics Center, a cardiac rehabilitation center in Ontario, Canada. "There is considerable anecdotal evidence that those who use their lungs in more extraordinary ways have less decline," he says.

Sure, you can get deep breathing in other ways, such as meditation practice and yoga, and that's great. What harmonica adds is resistance, says Von Luehrte. "It's like lifting weights for your lungs."

Do You Need a Special Type of Harmonica?

Some experts recommend harmonicas specifically developed for lung therapy. The Pulmonica (*pulmonica.com*) for example, is designed to create more resistance than a standard harmonica, promoting the clearance of secretions. It makes a pleasant sound, but you can't as easily use it to play songs. The Seydel Medical Harmonica *harmonicaMD. com*, which Dr. Schaman helped develop, uses chords rather than single notes, so it may be easier for some people to learn than a standard harmonica.

Others prefer everyday harmonicas. Pulmonary nurse Von Luehrte thinks devices such as the Pulmonica and the Seydel can take the fun out of a simple, joyful musical experience, making harmonica play more like other physical therapy exercises and less of a relaxing, social activity. And while playing chords may be easier and create more resistance, it hasn't been shown that one way of playing is better, healthwise, than another.

So go play...a minimum of 10 minutes a day—more is better. Many pulmonary centers across the country have harmonica therapy groups, which can make it a more social—and musical—experience. Plus the instructors can teach patients the basics of proper breathing and playing. Some senior centers are getting into the act, too. The most important skill to learn is to breathe with your diaphragm to help your lungs expand, according to nurse Low. If you want to explore a musical approach, check out the book and CD *Harmonica for Fun and Health* to get you started. Or you can Google "harmonica therapy" or "learn to play harmonica" to find a number of instructional sites.

Next topic for research inspired by a Steven Foster song: Is there therapeutic value to playing a banjo—on your knee?

Foods for Better Breathing

A diet high in fiber—especially from fruits and vegetables—can protect against such lung conditions as chronic obstructive pulmonary disease (COPD) and asthma.

New study: Spirometry tests found that among more than 1,900 adults, those who ate the most fiber every day had the best lung function.

Possible reason: Inflammation underlies many lung diseases, and fiber has anti-inflam-

matory properties. Fiber also changes the composition of the gut microbiome, which may release lung-protective compounds.

Corinne Hanson, PhD, RD, associate professor of medical nutrition, University of Nebraska Medical Center, Omaha.

Exercise Can Extend Lives of People with COPD

Marilyn Moy, MD, assistant professor, Harvard Medical School, Boston.
Alan Mensch, MD, chief, pulmonary medicine, Northwell Health's Plainview Hospital, Plainview, New York.
Len Horovitz, MD, pulmonary specialist, Lenox Hill Hospital, New York City.
ERJ Open Research, news release.

Regular exercise could help boost the survival of people who've left the hospital after battling chronic obstructive pulmonary disease (COPD), a recent study finds.

"We know that physical activity can have a positive benefit for people with COPD and these findings confirm that it may reduce the risk of dying following hospitalization," study lead author Marilyn Moy, MD, assistant professor of medicine at Harvard Medical School, said in a news release from *ERJ Open Research*.

Background on COPD

COPD includes emphysema, chronic bronchitis or a combination of the two, and is often related to smoking. Common symptoms include difficulty breathing, chronic cough, wheezing and phlegm production. Over time, the condition can prove fatal.

One expert, Alan Mensch, MD, noted, "COPD is estimated to affect up to 7% of adults and is a leading cause of death worldwide."

He explained that "difficulty breathing often leads to a sedentary lifestyle in COPD patients, resulting in deconditioning of multiple organ systems, including the heart and muscles.

"Improving muscle function with exercise has been demonstrated to decrease the use of health services in patients with COPD," said Dr. Mensch, who is chief of pulmonary medicine at Northwell Health's Plainview Hospital in Plainview, New York.

Study Details

The study's authors said that the risk of hospital readmission and death is especially high after a person has been hospitalized for COPD.

Could exercise help lower that risk? To find out, Dr. Moy's team looked at the medical records of almost 2,400 people in California who were hospitalized for COPD.

The researchers found that those who did any amount of moderate to vigorous physical activity were 47% less likely to die in the 12 months after hospitalization than inactive patients.

In fact, even low levels of physical activity reduced the risk of death by 28%, the researchers reported.

Dr. Moy's team published their findings in the journal *ERJ Open Research*.

Because of the observational nature of the study, the findings can't prove cause and effect. However, the researchers believe that tracking physical activity levels might be a good way for doctors to pinpoint those COPD patients at high risk for death after hospitalization.

Respiratory Diseases Linked to Cancer

Common respiratory diseases are linked to lung cancer. People who have chronic bronchitis or emphysema were 30% to 50% more likely to have lung cancer than people without the disease. Co-occurring bronchitis, emphysema and pneumonia were associated with twice the lung cancer risk. This in-

creased cancer risk may be related to chronic inflammation.

Ann Olsson, PhD, MPH, epidemiologist, International Agency for Research on Cancer, Lyon, France, and coauthor of an analysis of seven studies, published in *American Journal of Respiratory and Critical Care Medicine*.

What Really Works to Clear Your Sinuses

Study titled "Medical Therapies for Adult Chronic Sinusitis: A Systematic Review" by Luke Rudmik, MD, MSc, director of the Endoscopic Sinus and Skull Base program, and colleagues, University of Calgary, Canada, published in *The Journal of the American Medical Association*.

If you're one of the millions of Americans who suffer from chronic sinusitis, with that nasal discharge, painful pressure and congestion that builds up in your head and just won't go away, you may have tried just about anything to get relief—antibiotics, decongestants, pain relievers, saline sprays, steroid sprays, steroid pills…you name it. You may have even considered surgery.

You can stop now. We know what really works.

A Misunderstood Condition

Sinus passages are small, hollow air-filled spaces in your face that drain into your nose. After a cold, you might feel nasal congestion for a few days or a week, and then it goes away. But for some people the condition turns into a constant stuffy nose, pain and pressure in the face, postnasal drip, and a reduced sense of smell. You have trouble sleeping, which makes you tired during the day. You're just miserable. When this lasts three months or more, it's chronic sinusitis. It affects 3% to 7% of the population.

When you just can't take it anymore, you might run to your doctor for an antibiotic. It's a common treatment that many doctors still rely on. But most of the time, antibiotics just don't work.

Here's why: While chronic sinusitis was until recently believed to be basically an infection, it's now recognized as primarily an inflammatory disease...similar to asthma.

To find out what works best, researchers at University of Calgary in Canada and the Medical University of South Carolina performed a systematic review of more than 40 clinical studies. They found out that antihistamines, antibiotics and other common treatments didn't work very well.

Here's what probably will: A combination of saline nasal irrigation and prescription corticosteroid sprays.

A Great Combination

Saline irrigation doesn't mean those low-volume saline nasal sprays or mists you can buy in the pharmacy—which only help a little—but a product such as a neti pot. These vessels look like tiny tea pots or squeeze bottles, and they make it easy to pour salt water into one side of your nose and let it drain out the other side. They've been used for centuries but have only recently become a part of mainstream Western medicine. Saline irrigation helps clean the sinuses by removing mucus and irritants that contribute to inflammation. According to the new analysis, saline irrigation improves sinusitis symptoms—and quality of life.

Cortocosteroid nasal sprays are prescription-only topical medicines that reduce inflammation and reduce symptoms such as nasal congestion and nasal discharge. Steroid sprays by themselves have been shown to be more effective than nasal irrigation by itself.

While there haven't been studies of the two approaches together, these were the only two treatments that scored the highest rating (A-1) based on the American Heart Association Grade of Evidence and Recommendation Grading Scale. They also work in a true complementary fashion—nasal irrigation clears out the sinus passages while corticosteroids fight the inflammatory process.

Based on the strength of the evidence, the researchers recommend a combination of the two treatments as the best first therapy for most people with chronic sinusitis.

Finding Out What Works for You

If you're concerned about using a steroid medication, it's important to realize that a topical spray is much safer than a steroid pill. Corticosteroid sprays are considered safe for all adults, although pregnant women should discuss this treatment option with their physicians before using it. It typically takes two to three weeks before symptoms start to improve, and that depends on how severe your sinusitis is. Some patients use the sprays for a few months during seasons when their symptoms are the worst, while others need to be on them indefinitely.

As for using a neti pot, you can do that once or twice a day. However, some research has found that using a neti pot every day can lead to more infections—after all, there's a reason your body produces mucus, which has antimicrobial properties. So removing your mucus all the time isn't ideal. "It comes down to balancing the benefit with potential risks," says Luke Rudmik, MD, clinical associate professor at University of Calgary in Canada and the lead author of the study. "If you don't have symptoms, you may not want to use a neti pot preventively. You can use it when you do get symptoms, such as when you have a cold. But if you have daily symptoms of chronic sinusitis, then the benefit of using daily saline irrigations often outweighs the small risks."

Since several other conditions can mimic sinusitis, including sinus migraines, if your symptoms don't improve after about two to three months, check back in with your doctor to rule out other conditions. If you're seeing your primary care doctor, he or she may send you for a CT scan of your sinuses or to an otolaryngologist for more detailed evaluation.

Finally, no one study can replace individualized medical care. For example, many people with chronic sinusitis have nasal polyps—noncancerous, teardrop-shaped growths that form in the nose or sinuses. For them, according to Dr. Rudmik, the best treatment is often to take an oral corticosteroid pill (such as prednisone) for one to three weeks, to take a course of the antibiotic doxycycline for three weeks or to use a leukotriene receptor antagonist (such as montelukast/Singulair), a drug that blocks inflammation.

If you don't want to use any medications at all, there's no harm in trying a neti pot for a few weeks and seeing if that works for you. Make it part of your preventive strategy. Since sinus infections typically follow a cold or other upper respiratory infection, use your neti pot at the first sign of an infection coming on. Avoid cigarette smoke, which can irritate nasal membranes, and consider getting a humidifier at home to increase the moisture in the air.

But if preventing colds plus saline irrigation isn't enough help for a chronic sinus condition, talk to your doctor about adding a corticosteroid spray to the mix.

Surgery Not Always Best for Chronic Sinusitis

Surgery may not be the best treatment for chronic sinusitis. Some patients do well with an ongoing course of treatments involving nasal sprays, antibiotics and antihistamines. Patients with chronic sinus infections who continued medical treatment for 13 months instead of opting for surgery had an annual cost of lost productivity that fell to $2,700 from $3,400, on average…their absenteeism from work fell from five days to two…and they went to work sick an average of 15 days rather than 17. For patients with more severe chronic sinusitis, surgery remains a better option. Ask your doctor for details.

Luke Rudmik, MD, clinical associate professor of endoscopic sinus and skull base surgery, University of Calgary, Alberta, Canada, and leader of a study published in *JAMA Otolaryngology-Head & Neck Surgery.*

The Embarrassing Sleep Apnea Symptom No Woman Should Ignore

Study titled "Association of Obstructive Sleep Apnea Risk Factors with Nocturnal Enuresis in Postmenopausal Women," by Patrick Koo, MD, assistant professor of medicine, Alpert Medical School of Brown University, Pawtucket, Rhode Island, and colleagues published in *Menopause.*

Chances are, you already know the symptoms of obstructive sleep apnea (OSA), which apply to both women and men—snoring, snorting, choking, gasping for air and going to the bathroom several times a night.

But if you're a postmenopausal women, there's a new symptom to watch out for.

It's something that you may never have experienced before menopause, or if you did, it happened when you were a kid—nocturnal enuresis (bed-wetting).

A New Symptom

Patrick Koo, MD, assistant professor of medicine at Alpert Medical School of Brown University, and his colleagues analyzed data from 161,808 postmenopausal women who were part of the Women's Health Initiative study. They found that the more traditional risk factors a woman had for OSA, the more likely she was to also urinate during her sleep.

In fact, women who had all six OSA risk factors included in the study—obesity, frequent snoring, restless sleep quality, sleep fragmentation, daytime sleepiness and high blood pressure—were seven times more likely to also wet the bed than women who had no risk factors.

Here's a likely explanation of how it happens. With OSA, the soft tissue around your airway closes up when you relax during sleep, so you are gasping for air. "This 'sucking' motion causes the heart to stretch and release a protein that increases urine production," explains Dr. Koo. Combine that with changes in the urinary tract in postmenopausal women, which make it easier to leak urine when the bladder is full, and the result can be bed-wetting during sleep.

A Dangerous Condition That's Often Undiagnosed

Bed-wetting is embarrassing, of course, but it could be a positive thing if it helps more women discover that they have OSA, which robs the body of oxygen during sleep, contributing to high blood pressure, heart attack, stroke and early death.

Here's why: Studies show that women tend to underreport common symptoms to their doctors, such as snoring, fatigue or frequent awakenings to urinate. "Either they're embarrassed to tell others that they snore or wake up multiple times a night to urinate, or they're not aware that these are symptoms of OSA," says Dr. Koo. Worse yet, the OSA symptoms women may bring up to their doc, such as sleeping problems or low energy during the day, are often misdiagnosed. Doctors tend to assume they're signs of depression or insomnia, which are more common in women than in men.

For these reasons, too many women aren't getting the treatment they need for a dangerous health condition—especially after menopause, when the incidence of sleep apnea jumps in women. OSA affects 18 million Americans. It's estimated that 2% of women have the condition, but in reality, the incidence is very likely higher, especially after menopause.

Getting Help

If you find yourself wetting your bed—even if you're not sure if you snore—ask your doctor to evaluate you for obstructive sleep apnea.

If you are diagnosed with OSA, your doctor may prescribe a continuous positive airway pressure (CPAP) machine—a mask you wear when you go to bed that's attached to a machine that ensures that you get the right amount of oxygen. There are other solutions as well, including an easier-to-use mandibular

Sleep Apnea May Worsen Depression

Nearly 300 depressed women and men with sleep apnea who successfully received continuous positive airway pressure (CPAP) treatment for their sleep disorder reported that they no longer had feelings of depression after three months.

Why: Disrupted sleep cycles can worsen depression.

If you have symptoms of depression and snore or have disturbed sleep: Ask your doctor to evaluate you for sleep apnea.

David Hillman, MD, clinical professor, The University of Western Australia, Perth.

advancement device (MAD), which fits in the mouth like an orthodontic dental retainer.

Discovering that you have sleep apnea—and getting the right treatment for it—can bring a host of benefits. You'll reduce your risk for high blood pressure, heart disease and stroke. You'll breathe better, sleep more soundly and have more energy during the day. For many women, it may also mean keeping the sheets dry.

Papain: The Dark (and Allergenic) Side of a Skin-Care Ingredient

Study titled "Papain Degrades Tight Junction Proteins of Human Keratinocytes In-Vitro..." by researchers at the Medical University of Vienna, Austria, published in *Journal of Investigative Dermatology*.

What's sweet to your gastrointestinal tract may not be so kind to your skin. Papain, an enzyme derived from the papaya fruit, has long been relied upon, in supplement form, to aid the digestive process, especially the breakdown and absorption of proteins. It's generally considered to be a safe digestive aid, although there can be some allergic reactions, especially in people allergic to mangoes or kiwis. If most people can put the stuff inside their bodies, you might figure there should be no problem putting it on skin, right? Well, think again!

Removing Dead Skin...and Causing Allergies

The cosmetic industry uses papain in many different skin-care products, shampoos and conditioners and even in enzymatic contact lens cleaners to remove protein deposits. When it's applied to the skin, it helps remove dead cells from the surface, revealing fresh, healthy cells that lie beneath and improving skin texture and appearance. It may also open clogged pores. No wonder it's used in exfoliating products such as facial scrubs, body cleansers, facial masks and peels. In hair-care products, papain conditions and softens dry or damaged hair, but there's a dark side.

In a recent study, researchers in Vienna, Austria, put papain directly on the skin of mice as well as on human skin cells in the petri dish. *Within a short time (30 to 120 minutes), the papain*…

•**Compromised the integrity of the skin barrier** by degrading the "tight junctions" that join skin cells together. That makes it easier for other compounds…including nasty ones…to penetrate your skin's natural protective barrier.

•**Increased water loss,** contributing to drier skin.

•**Induced vasodilation**—a widening of blood vessels—which can cause skin to become warm, red and itchy.

•**Stimulated the release of inflammatory cells in the skin** (which can lead to irritation)…including mast cells, which release histamine as part of allergic reactions.

After repeated exposure, the mice developed antibodies to papain—a sure sign of an allergic response. (Papain, it turns out, is structurally very similar to a very common dust mite allergen.) All of these effects are problematic on their own but, adding insult to injury, compromising the skin barrier function could allow other chemicals to penetrate the skin more deeply, setting the stage for further irritation or allergic responses. This is a particular concern for people who have eczema, whose skin is already susceptible to bacteria, fungi and viruses.

The researchers' conclusion: Papain has all the characteristics of a strong allergen.

The FDA, it turns out, already strongly warned manufacturers against selling unapproved ointments that contain papain as a treatment for serious skin conditions such as diabetic ulcers and traumatic wounds, based on allergic reactions. That was back in 2008. The new research makes us wonder if its place in everyday cosmetics should be revisited, too.

Take-home message: If you have sensitive skin or you're prone to skin redness or irritation, especially after using new products, read product ingredient lists and steer clear of skin- and hair-care products that contain papain. The allergy is related to latex allergies, the researchers find, so that if you're allergic to latex, you should avoid papain-containing products as well. (Look for other names as well—papainase, papaine, summertrin, tromasin, vegetable pepsin, velardon.)

If your skin is at all sensitive, you are prone to allergic skin reactions or you have a skin condition such as eczema, there's no need to take a chance on papain.

What It Really Means If You're Allergic to Mango

"I got a terrible allergic rash when I ate an unpeeled mango. A friend told me this might mean I have other allergies, too. Is this true?"

Yes. It sounds like you are allergic to mango tree sap, which is on the skin of the fruit. The sap contains an oil called urushiol (also in poison ivy and poison oak). Urushiol can cause mild to severe skin reactions, including hives, blistering and/or itching.

In some instances, it is the fruit of the mango that triggers a reaction, which can range from mild to extremely severe, causing gastrointestinal discomfort, itching in the mouth, swelling, hives and, in rare instances, throat swelling. People with this allergy may also react to cashews and pistachios, and similar fruits, such as papaya.

Mango sensitivity has also been linked to latex allergies, so your health-care providers should be advised to use nonlatex gloves.

An allergist can determine if you are allergic to the mango peel or fruit as well as check for other food sensitivities with skin or blood tests.

Michael Lewin, MD, an allergist in New York City and Wilton, Connecticut. He is a leading expert in sublingual immunotherapy.

High Price of Manicures

The late Mitchell Gaynor, MD, founder and president of Gaynor Integrative Oncology in New York City. He wrote and lectured extensively on environmental pollution and human illness.

There has been a lot of media coverage about toxins in nail salons and the effect that these chemicals can have on the people working at the salons.

But weekly salon goers also should take precautions to reduce exposure to the toxic trio—toluene, formaldehyde and dibutyl phthalate—often found in typical nail products used at salons. These toxins have been linked to serious health conditions including kidney problems, asthma-like attacks, breast and prostate cancers, and abnormal fetal development. The thing to remember is that when it comes to toxins, it's not just about what you inhale but also about what touches your skin.

When you get that weekly mani/pedi, your skin—an absorbent surface—comes into contact with these chemicals. And while no one has studied toxin levels in people who frequent salons, the levels could be high.

But there are ways to protect yourself. Choose a salon with a good exhaust system to reduce the amount of toxins you inhale during your visit. Read the labels of the products that the salon uses, and if toxin-free versions of polishes, hardeners and removers are not available, consider bringing your own. This helps you and your manicurist.

Finally, consider skipping the salon and polishing your nails at home with toxin-free products, such as those from Scotch Naturals, Zoya and Acquarella.

The Allergy-Fighting Diet

Leo Galland, MD, director of the Foundation for Integrated Medicine in New York City. He is coauthor of *The Allergy Solution: Unlock the Surprising, Hidden Truth About Why You Are Sick and How to Get Well.* DrGalland.com

The right diet can help relieve your allergies whether you're allergic to pollen, dust, mold, certain foods or other allergens. And it can relieve symptoms that you might not even know come from allergies—including fatigue, weight gain and depression. The key is to use foods to improve your immune response. *Here's how…*

Boost Your T-regs

Immune cells known as regulatory T-cells, or T-regs, limit inflammation and dampen the allergic response. The cells don't function properly in people with allergies, which can lead to a host of allergic symptoms.

If you know you're allergic to something, avoidance is an obvious solution. But many people don't know what they're allergic to—or even if they are allergic. You can use dietary changes to increase T-regs and dampen any allergic response.

***STEP 1*: Three-Day Power Wash**
I advise patients to completely give up the foods that commonly aggravate allergies. These include dairy (including yogurt), wheat, seafood, eggs, soy, nuts, peanuts, yeast (found

in bread, alcohol, vinegar, commercial fruit juice and commercial soups and sauces) and nightshade vegetables (such as tomatoes, bell peppers, potatoes and eggplant).

This is not meant to be a permanent diet. You have to give up these foods for three days (unless you discover that you're allergic to a particular food, in which case you'll give it up altogether). Taking a break from likely offenders resets the immune system—it clears your body of potential allergens and lets you start with a clean slate.

For three days, you'll consume only the soup and the smoothie (see below) that I developed for blunting the immune response (you'll also drink oolong tea). Have the smoothie for breakfast and a midafternoon snack. The soup is lunch and dinner. Eat until you are satisfied but not too full. Have your doctor look at the recipes to make sure that they are appropriate for you.

• **Immune Balance Smoothie.** In a blender, combine one cup of strawberries, one medium avocado, one cup of chopped arugula, one-half head of chopped romaine lettuce, two tablespoons of ground chia seeds and one cup of brewed green tea. If desired, add one medium banana.

Blend until smooth. The smoothie will become thicker and creamier if you refrigerate it after blending.

If you happen to be allergic to any of the ingredients, just leave it out.

• **Immune Balance Soup.** This is one of the Galland family's favorite recipes.

Sauté three cups of sliced carrots in three tablespoons of extra-virgin olive oil for 10 minutes. Add one cup of chopped parsley, two cups of chopped scallions (green parts only), 12 ounces of chopped broccoli, three ounces of chopped baby kale, one teaspoon of turmeric powder and one-quarter teaspoon of ground black pepper. Add salt to taste. Cook and stir for one minute. Add 12 cups of water, and bring to a boil. Cover and simmer for 20 minutes.

Add one tablespoon of shredded daikon radish just before serving.

• **Organic oolong tea.** I emphasize this tea for a specific reason. It's very high in catechins, which are flavonoids that inhibit allergic reactions—they're even stronger than the compounds in green tea. One study found that a majority of patients with allergic eczema who didn't respond to medications had significant improvements after drinking oolong tea for one to two weeks. Drink four cups daily (no more) during the Power Wash and a cup or two daily after that.

STEP 2: Reintroduction

After three days, continue to enjoy the homemade smoothie and soup and organic oolong tea as you gradually reintroduce foods from your regular diet—a new food or food group each day. Start with foods that are less likely to provoke allergic reactions such as rice or free-range poultry, and gradually move toward the more allergenic foods such as nuts, seafood, eggs and dairy products, one group at a time. Keep notes about what you're eating and symptoms (if any) that you experience—including symptoms you don't typically associate with allergies (see list on page 98). This will help you determine whether particular foods—or ingredients in packaged foods—are triggering symptoms.

I've found that patients who give up problem foods for at least six months can sometimes eat them again, in small amounts, without having symptoms return. This doesn't apply to things such as sodas, candies or other junk foods, including commercially prepared pastries. These foods always contribute to allergies (including common dust and pollen allergies) by increasing inflammation and should be avoided.

Important: Consult your doctor before reintroducing foods, especially if you suffer from anaphylaxis or asthma or if you previously have experienced an adverse reaction to any of the foods.

STEP 3: Immune Balance

No matter what you're allergic to, make an effort to eat healthier foods that fortify T-regs. *Most important…*

• **Natural folate.** Many foods are fortified with folic acid, an important (but synthetic)

B vitamin. Natural sources of folate are better for T-reg function.

Examples: Leafy vegetables, legumes, peas, asparagus, cauliflower and brussels sprouts.

• **More flavonoids.** I believe that many of the inflammatory disorders that plague Americans, including allergies and asthma, are due in part to flavonoid deficiencies. Flavonoids, an important family of plant compounds, have anti-inflammatory and antioxidant effects. A Tufts University study found that animals given a flavonoid-enhanced diet had an increase in T-regs and a decrease in Immunoglobulin E (IgE) antibodies—molecules involved in the allergic response.

The flavonoids in tea are particularly helpful. But you'll get healthy amounts from many different plant foods, including onions, blueberries, sweet potatoes, apples and bell peppers.

• **Lots of strawberries.** Strawberries are the richest food source of *fisetin*, a type of flavonoid that helps preserve T-regs. Fisetin blunts the allergic response and has been shown in laboratory studies to help prevent allergic asthma.

Important: Organic strawberries, fresh or frozen, have more vitamin C and other antioxidants than conventionally grown berries.

• **Put parsley on your plate.** It's more than just a garnish. It's high in apigenin, a flavonoid that decreases the activity of allergy-inducing lymphocytes and reduces levels of IgE. The carotenoids in parsley (it has more than carrots) also are helpful.

• **Eat seafood twice a week (as long as you're not allergic).** A lack of omega-3 fatty acids can cause or aggravate allergy symptoms. People with allergies actually need more of these fats because their cells don't metabolize them efficiently.

• **Broaden your palate.** While tea, parsley and strawberries are among the allergy-fighting stars, all plant foods can help balance the immune system and reduce symptoms. I'm a big fan of legumes (such as black beans, garbanzo beans and lentils), along with car-

rots, sweet bell peppers, spinach and brussels sprouts. Most of your diet should consist of these and other healthful plant foods.

Hidden Allergy Symptoms

Here are allergy symptoms that aren't typically associated with allergies…

- Anxiety
- Bloating
- Brain fog
- Constipation or diarrhea
- Depression
- Fatigue
- Headaches
- Insomnia
- Joint pain
- Muscle aches
- Stomachaches
- Weight gain

Allergies Can Strike at Any Age

Richard Firshein, DO, founder and director of the Firshein Center for Integrative Medicine in New York City. A leading authority in preventive and nutritional medicine that integrates Eastern and Western medical practices, he is the author of *Reversing Asthma* and *The Vitamin Prescription (for Life)*.

If you escaped allergies as a child or a young adult, then you're home free now, right? Well…maybe not. And if you have had allergies for years, then you surely know exactly what triggers a reaction, right? Not necessarily.

These are just two of the instances when people can get walloped by hidden allergies.

Never Too Old

Contrary to popular belief, a first-time allergy can occur at any age. While the reasons are not completely understood, it's believed that adult-onset environmental allergies can occur when people move to a new area (and get exposed to different allergens)…or when a genetic predisposition to react to an environmental or food allergen finally kicks in after years of being exposed to it.

Takeaway: If you have typical allergy symptoms, including sneezing, coughing and itchy eyes (telltale signs of, say, springtime allergies)…or nausea, diarrhea and itchy hives (common red flags for food allergies), do not rule out allergies just because you've never suffered from them before. See your doctor for advice and possible allergy testing.

Common Allergy Mix-ups

Allergies are a tricky health problem—largely because people tend to self-diagnose based on what they believe to be their allergic trigger. *But that can lead to mix-ups, as allergies, related to those below, go undetected…*

• **Tree pollen.** While most hay fever sufferers have zeroed in on tree pollen as the culprit, they often fail to realize that having this allergy means that they may also react to tree fruits, such as apples, pears or peaches, and tree nuts, such as walnuts. For these people, exposure to tree fruits or tree nuts can set off the same immune response as pollen. This so-called oral allergy syndrome (OAS) may cause swelling and irritation in the mouth, lips and throat.

What to do: Cooking these fruits may help. Otherwise, avoiding these fruits and nuts (as well as melons, which also may cause symptoms) is the simplest solution.

• **Pet fur.** People who get watery eyes or start sneezing around pets often assume that they're allergic to the pet's fur…and look for a dog or cat breed that's touted as "hypoallergenic"—a loosely defined term that usually suggests the animal's fur produces fewer allergens.

But this often does not help, because animal fur is typically not the allergen—it's almost always pet dander (shedding skin flakes) and/or saliva, each of which contains proteins that trigger the allergic immune response. Even hypoallergenic pets produce at least some dander—and all pets groom themselves, leaving bits of saliva on their fur.

What to do: If you are allergic but want a pet, try grooming the animal frequently, isolating the pet to certain areas of the house and using a high-efficiency particle arresting (HEPA) air-filtration system.

• **Chocolate.** If a piece of chocolate causes symptoms, such as a rash or trouble breathing, the actual culprit may be one of its ingredients, such as soy lecithin, milk or nuts.

What to do: Get checked to see if you're allergic to cocoa, the health-promoting substance in chocolate. If you're not, get further testing to reveal the true source of your allergy, which then can be avoided.

• **Alcohol.** Many people who drink wine, beer and/or hard liquor experience flushed skin, itching, nasal congestion and even an elevated heart rate. For some individuals, protein residues from the alcoholic beverage cause the reaction.

But for many others, the trigger is actually sulfites, chemicals that act as a preservative and prevent the growth of mold or bacteria. Other examples of foods and drinks that may contain sulfites: Dried fruits…soft drinks…cookies…crackers…noodle or rice mixes…and shellfish.

For a more detailed list, go to: *Sulfites. org/sulfite-foods/.*

What to do: If testing shows that you are allergic to sulfites, read labels and avoid products that contain this additive. It can also be listed on the label in one of various forms, such as potassium bisulfate…sulfur dioxide…and potassium metabisulfite.

Note: Alcoholic beverages also may contain contaminants, such as gluten and yeast, that may require further testing by a doctor.

Best Testing Options

The only way to know for sure that you have an allergy is to undergo allergy testing. If you are truly allergic to something, your immune system mistakes an otherwise harmless substance for an intruder, producing immunoglobulin E (IgE) antibodies. Two main types of tests identify environmental allergies (such as pollen, dust, mold, etc.) and food allergies (such as peanuts, eggs, soy, milk, etc.)…

•**Skin tests.** A suspected allergen is introduced into the body by pricking, scratching or injecting it into the skin—or by applying a skin patch coated with it.

•**Blood tests.** These tests can be used if the doctor is concerned about a dramatic skin reaction that could cause a severe allergic response…or if a person has psoriasis or some other skin condition that could be aggravated by skin testing.

For example, with the radio allergosorbent test (RAST), a sample of your blood is exposed to a suspected allergen.

Note: Sometimes you may not have an actual allergy, but rather a sensitivity that produces allergy-type symptoms when you are exposed to the substance. A separate test is needed to identify an environmental or food sensitivity.

The Right Doctor to See

To get an accurate diagnosis, it's fine to start with a family physician who is well versed in allergies. If you suspect a food allergy, be sure the doctor is experienced in this problem. *Other options…*

•**Allergists/immunologists may be the best choice for difficult cases.** To find one near you, consult the American Academy of Allergy, Asthma & Immunology, *AAAAI.org*.

•**Integrative medicine physicians,** who identify allergies as an aspect of overall health, are another choice. To find one near you, check the American Board of Integrative Holistic Medicine website, *ABIHM.org*, and search "allergy/immunology" in the specialty field.

•**Naturopathic physicians can also be helpful,** especially in offering guidance on diet and the use of supplements (such as butterbur and quercetin). To find a naturopathic physician, consult the American Association of Naturopathic Physicians, *Naturopathic.org*.

Are You Allergic to the Gym?

Allergens that cause coughing, sneezing, wheezing, rashes and/or watery eyes can be found in health clubs.

Common culprits: Pools—some people are sensitive to chlorine. Shower immediately after swimming, or try a saltwater pool, which may be less irritating. Locker rooms—a recent study found a link between allergies and triclosan, a common ingredient in antibacterial soaps, which often are found in gyms. Bring along your own products. Mats—most mats contain allergy-inducing latex or PVCs. If you have had allergic reactions to these, bring your own mat made of hemp or organic cotton. Workout clothes—polyester and nylon and anything "odor-free" or "antimicrobial" can cause itching. Opt for natural fiber.

Jane Wilkens Michael, nationally syndicated radio host and author of *Long Live You! Your Step-by-Step Plan to Look and Feel Better Than Before* and host of *The Jane Wilkens Michael Show* on iHeart Radio Talk. JaneWilkensMichael.com

Allergy Shots Still Effective for Seniors

Andrzej Bozek, MD, PhD, clinical department of internal disease, dermatology and allergology, Medical University of Silesia, Katowice, Poland.

Ira Finegold, MD, past president of the American College of Allergy, Asthma and Immunology.

American College of Allergy, Asthma and Immunology, news release.

Allergy shots can still benefit seniors with allergies, a recent study suggests.

Study Findings

The study included 60 people with hay fever between the ages of 65 and 75 who were given either allergy shots or a placebo for three years.

Those who received the allergy shots had a 55% reduction in symptoms and a 64% decrease in their use of allergy relief medication, according to the study results.

The study was published in the *Annals of Allergy, Asthma and Immunology*.

Implications

The researchers, led by Andrzej Bozek, MD, PhD, of Medical University of Silesia in Katowice, Poland, said diagnosis and management of hay fever in seniors can be challenging because they tend to have other health conditions. The researchers added that their findings show that an aging immune system doesn't significantly reduce the effectiveness of allergy shots.

While allergy shots are known to benefit children and adults, there has been little research in seniors. Hay fever is more common in people over age 65, the researchers said.

Expert Commentary

"Older people who suffer from hay fever may have health challenges that younger people do not," said Ira Finegold, MD, past president of the American College of Allergy, Asthma and Immunology.

"Hay fever is often ignored in older patients as a less significant health problem because of diseases such as asthma, coronary heart disease, depression and high blood pressure," Dr. Finegold added. "Also, some baby boomers might not realize they have allergies, and their physicians might not suggest allergy shots. The research indicated that allergy shots were extremely effective for this group."

Chapter 5

PRESERVE YOUR BRAIN

Why Early Stages of Alzheimer's Disease May Go Undetected in Women

In the early stages of Alzheimer's disease, women tend to remember words better than men do, which could delay diagnosis in women, new research suggests.

The difference exists even though women and men have similar amounts of shrinkage in brain areas that show the earliest evidence of Alzheimer's disease, according to the study involving hundreds of people.

The findings were published in the journal *Neurology*.

Implications

"One way to interpret the results is that because women have better verbal memory skills than men throughout life, women have a buffer of protection against loss of verbal memory before the effects of Alzheimer's disease kick in," study author Erin Sundermann, PhD, said. Dr. Sundermann is a postdoctoral fellow in neurology at the Albert Einstein College of Medicine in New York City.

"Because verbal memory tests are used to diagnose people with Alzheimer's disease and its precursor, mild cognitive impairment, these tests may fail to detect mild cognitive impairment and Alzheimer's disease in women until they are further along in the disease," she explained.

If the results are confirmed, doctors may need to adjust memory tests to make a better diagnosis, Dr. Sundermann said.

Expert Commentary

In an accompanying editorial, Mary Sano, PhD, associate dean for clinical research at the Icahn School of Medicine at Mount Sinai in New York City, wrote: "At a public policy level, the potential health care cost for under-detection or delayed diagnosis of women with Alzheimer's disease or its early stages is staggering and should motivate funding in this area."

The American Academy of Family Physicians has more on information on Alzheimer's disease at *familydoctor.org*. Search "Alzheimer's disease."

Erin Sundermann, PhD, postdoctoral fellow, neurology, Albert Einstein College of Medicine, New York City.

Mary Sano, PhD, associate dean for clinical research, Icahn School of Medicine at Mount Sinai, New York City.

American Academy of Neurology, news release.

7 Natural Ways to Boost Your Brain's Alzheimer's Defense

Study titled "Higher Brain BDNF Gene Expression Is Associated With Slower Cognitive Decline in Older Adults" by researchers at Rush University Medical Center, Chicago; Brigham and Women's Hospital, Boston; Harvard Medical School, Boston; Broad Institute, Cambridge, Massachusetts, published in *Neurology*.

Andrew Rubman, ND, medical director, Southbury Clinic for Traditional Medicines, Southbury, Connecticut. SouthburyClinic.com.

There's a protein in your brain that protects you from Alzheimer's disease.

It's called brain-derived neurotrophic factor (BDNF), and it promotes the survival of neurons in the brain.

Here's the latest research that is establishing the importance of this natural protective protein—including seven simple, practical ways to boost your levels.

A Natural Memory Protector—Even If You Get Alzheimer's Disease

While there is growing evidence in both animals and humans that BDNF plays a key role in the brain's ability to repair itself from dementia, until now the evidence has been largely indirect. Low blood levels of BDNF in people, for example, are statistically associated with an increased risk for Alzheimer's. But blood levels don't always track well with brain levels.

A new study is more definitive. Researchers at Rush University Medical Center in Chicago studied the cognitive function of 535 older men and women—some with Alzheimer's and some not—for an average of six years, and, when they died, autopsied their brains.

Results: The amount of BDNF proteins in their brains was directly related to the documented rate of cognitive decline that those men and women experienced in the years before they died. *Findings...*

• **Study participants with the most BDNF protein (top 10%) in their brains** had 50% slower cognitive decline than those with the least (lowest 10%).

• **Even among those with Alzheimer's disease,** higher levels of BDNF were associated with less severe cognitive effects.

Even this new study doesn't prove that BDNF protects against Alzheimer's, but it strengthens the case considerably. The good news is that there are straightforward ways to boost your levels.

7 Ways to Boost BDNF

The research on how to boost BDNF levels in the brain isn't quite as definitive. After all, scientists can't exactly put people on treadmills and then look inside their brains. But studies in animals and humans point to some very practical healthy habits that can boost BDNF. *Here's what we know...*

1. Exercise—moderately and frequently. Several studies have found that exercise increases blood levels of BDNF. The good news is that regular moderate- and even low-intensity exercise appears to be effective. In one study of healthy men and women (55 to 80 years old), moderate-intensity walking for just 40 minutes increased blood BDNF and maintained cognitive performance—with the oldest people seeing the biggest boost—more than stretch/toning exercises did for the control group. Another study found that over a six-month period, regular low-intensity exercise (less than an hour of stretching with rubber tubing three times a week) led to increased BDNF levels in people who were previously inactive compared with participants who continued to be inactive.

2. Eat less. Animals on a calorically restricted diet have higher brain levels of BDNF compared with those that are allowed to eat as much as they want. While there are no comparable studies in people, there is evidence that avoiding overeating is beneficial. In a study of older adults (70 to 92 years old), those who consumed the most calories (more than 2,143 daily) had almost twice the risk for mild cognitive impairment as adults who consumed the least (fewer than 1,525 daily calories). (Want to break the overeating habit? Try this using this five-point hunger scale.)

3. Eat better. Animal studies find that a diet that's very high in fat and sugar leads to lower brain BDNF. But carefully conducted clinical studies report that when it comes to preventing Alzheimer's, the quality of dietary fat is particularly important. The Mediterranean diet, which is low in sugar but includes plenty of healthy fats (olive oil, fatty fish, nuts), is protective, for example. So is the MIND diet, which is also low in sugar but high in healthy fats.

4. Consider intermittent fasting. It's not for everyone, but eating just 500 or 600 nutritious calories on one or two days a week, while eating a normal amount on the other days, may boost BDNF.

The theory: Skipping meals stresses your neurons, and your body boosts BDNF to buttress neurons while you're undernourished. Several animal studies show that fasting increases BDNF. In one study, rats fed every other day for six months had nearly five times more BDNF than rats fed every day. Human studies that involve fasting are not easy to come by, but one small study of people who didn't eat at all during daylight hours showed increased blood BDNF.

5. Get spicy. Curcumin, a major component of the spice turmeric that's found in curries, appears to protect the brain—possibly by boosting BDNF. In India, people who consume the most curry have the lowest risk for Alzheimer's. In mice, curcumin protects against brain damage caused by an animal version of Alzheimer's, and a lab-made form of curcumin has been shown to boost BDNF in mice. Clearly we need to learn more, but we already know that turmeric's curcumin is powerfully anti-inflammatory—with other proven benefits. "It's effective at lowering cholesterol and reducing osteoarthritis pain," says naturopathic physician Andrew Rubman, ND, *Health Insider's* medical contributing editor. "It reduces aches and pains and inflammation throughout the body." Since curcumin is only about 2% of turmeric, you'll have to eat a lot of curry to get much curcumin—but fortunately curcumin supplements have a good safety profile. If you want to supplement, Dr. Rubman recommends taking 500 mg of a curcumin extract three or four times a day.

6. Stay social. Animal studies have shown that social isolation, compared with communal living, leads to reduced BDNF in the brain. One study in older humans also showed that social support is linked to increased blood levels of BDNF.

7. Catch rays. BDNF levels are higher in the spring and summer months than they are in fall and winter, according to a study of more than 2,800 men and women, with a direct relationship between the number of hours of sunshine per day and higher BDNF. Whether it's vitamin D (which, of course, is higher when you get sun exposure) that elevates BDNF isn't clear—one human study found that daily supplementation with 2,000 IU of vitamin D, a modest amount, didn't increase BDNF. So get some sun—in moderation, of course.

The Diet That Cuts Your Alzheimer's Risk in Half

Martha Clare Morris, ScD, professor and director of the Section of Nutrition and Nutritional Epidemiology at Rush University, Chicago, where she is assistant provost for community research.

Some of the same diets that are good for cardiovascular health also are good for the brain. But there's a new diet—combining the best aspects of other diets—that is so effective it reduces the risk for Alzheimer's disease even in those who don't give the diet their best effort.

The MIND diet blends components from DASH (a blood pressure–lowering diet) and the popular Mediterranean diet, with an extra emphasis on berries, leafy greens and a few other brain-healthy foods.

How good is it? People who carefully followed the diet were about 53% less likely to develop Alzheimer's disease in subsequent years. Those who approached it more casually didn't do quite as well but still reduced their risk considerably, by about 35%.

Blended Benefits

The MIND diet was developed by researchers at Rush University who examined years of studies to identify specific foods and nutrients that seemed to be particularly good—or bad—for long-term brain health. The MIND (it stands for Mediterranean-DASH Intervention for Neurodegenerative Delay) diet is a hybrid plan that incorporates the "best of the best."

In a study in the journal *Alzheimer's & Dementia,* the researchers followed more than 900 participants. None had dementia when the study started. The participants filled out food questionnaires and had repeated neurological tests over a period averaging more than four years.

Some participants followed the MIND diet. Others followed the older DASH diet or the Mediterranean diet. All three diets reduced the risk for Alzheimer's disease. But only the MIND diet did so even when the participants followed the plan only "moderately well."

This is an important distinction because few people are perfect about sticking to diets. Most cheat now and then and eat more unhealthy foods than they should.

The MIND diet specifies "brain-healthy" food groups and five groups that need to be limited, either eaten in moderation or preferably not at all.

What to Eat

• **More leafy greens.** Kale really is a superfood for the brain. So are spinach, chard, beet greens and other dark, leafy greens. The Mediterranean and DASH diets advise people to eat more vegetables, but they don't specify which ones.

The MIND diet specifically recommends one serving of greens a day, in addition to one other vegetable. Previous research has shown that a vegetable-rich diet can help prevent cognitive decline, but two of the larger studies found that leafy greens were singularly protective.

• **Lots of nuts.** The diet calls for eating nuts five times a week. Nuts are high in vitamin E and monounsaturated and polyunsaturated fats—all good for brain health.

The study didn't look at which nuts were more likely to be beneficial. Eating a variety is probably a good idea because you'll get a varied mix of protective nutrients and antioxidants. Raw or roasted nuts are fine (as long as they're not roasted in fat and highly salted). If you are allergic to nuts, seeds such as sunflower and pumpkin seeds are good sources of these nutrients as well.

• **Berries.** These are the only fruits that are specifically included in the MIND diet. Other fruits are undoubtedly good for you, but none has been shown in studies to promote cognitive health. Berries, on the other hand, have been shown to slow age-related cognitive decline. In laboratory studies, a berry-rich diet improves memory and protects against abnormal changes in the brain. Blueberries seem to be particularly potent. Eat berries at least twice a week.

• **Beans and whole grains.** These fiber-rich and folate-rich foods provide high levels of protein with much less saturated fat than you would get from an equivalent helping of meat. The MIND diet calls for three daily servings of whole grains and three weekly servings of beans.

• **Include fish and poultry—but you don't need to go overboard.** Seafood is a key component of the Mediterranean diet, and some proponents recommend eating it four times a week or more. The MIND diet calls for only one weekly serving, although more is OK. A once-a-week fish meal is enough for brain health.

There is no data to specify the number of poultry servings needed for brain health, but we recommend two servings a week.

• **A glass of wine.** People who drink no wine—or those who drink too much—are more likely to suffer cognitive declines than those who drink just a little.

Recommended: One glass a day. Red wine, in particular, is high in flavonoids and polyphenols that may be protective for the brain.

Foods to Limit

•**Limit red meat, cheese, butter and margarine**—along with fast food, fried food and pastries and other sweets. The usual suspects, in other words.

However, most nutritionists acknowledge the importance of letting people enjoy some treats and not being so restrictive that they give up eating healthfully altogether.

Try to follow these recommendations…

Red meat: No more than three servings a week.

Butter and margarine: Less than one tablespoon daily. Cook with olive oil instead.

Cheese: Less than one serving a week.

Pastries and sweets: Yes, you can enjoy some treats, but limit yourself to five servings or fewer a week.

Fried or fast food: Less than one serving a week.

For a Sharper Brain, Eat These 4 Foods

Drew Ramsey, MD, an assistant clinical professor of psychiatry at Columbia University College of Physicians and Surgeons in New York City and coauthor of several books, including *The Happiness Diet*.

We all know that a strong cup of coffee can give us that extra mental boost we may need to complete a brain-draining project or meet a tight deadline.

What works even better: Strategic eating is a healthful and reliable way to improve your ability to concentrate for the long haul—not just for a few hours at a time when you're hyped up on caffeine.

There's no single food that will suddenly have you speed-reading a book in one sitting, but you can improve your overall powers of concentration by including the following foods in your diet…

•**Eggs.** When it comes to mental focus, it doesn't get much better than eggs! They're a leading source of a nutrient called choline, a precursor to the neurotransmitter acetylcholine—a key molecule of learning.

Eggs (including the yolks) also contain a variety of B vitamins, most of which have been stripped from the refined carbs that are so ubiquitous in the typical American diet. In particular, eggs are rich in vitamins B-6 and B-12, which are crucial for carrying out most cognitive functions (three large eggs will give you about half of your daily B-12 requirement)…and vitamin B-9 (also known as folate).

For optimal brain health, include up to 12 eggs in your diet each week. While cholesterol in one's diet has only a minimal effect on blood levels of cholesterol, consult your doctor for advice on appropriate intake of eggs if cholesterol is a concern.

•**Mussels.** Three ounces of mussels—which is a modest serving—contain 20 micrograms (mcg) of vitamin B-12 (that's nearly 10 times your daily requirement). Even a mild deficiency of this crucial brain-boosting vitamin can impair concentration and lead to fuzzy thinking.

But that's not all. Three ounces of mussels will also give you 430 mg of docosahexaenoic acid (DHA)—the equivalent of two to three typical fish oil supplement capsules. DHA is a type of omega-3 fatty acid needed for healthy brain function. Mussels are also loaded with zinc, a nutritional workhorse involved in more than 100 chemical reactions in the brain. Enjoy mussels twice a month.

Don't like mussels? Other smart brain-boosting seafood selections include oysters (six oysters deliver three to four times your daily zinc needs)…anchovies, which have more omega-3s than tuna…and clams, which are an excellent source of vitamin B-12.

Tasty choices: Caesar salad with anchovies…clam chowder…or pasta alle vongole (with clams).

• **Beef.** You've probably heard that eating too much red meat is linked to heart disease and even some types of cancer. However, you can minimize these risks and maximize your brainpower with a few small servings per week.

Here's why: Beef is a potent source of heme iron (the most absorbable form), which is needed to transport oxygen through the blood and to the brain.

What I recommend: Opt for grass-fed beef. It has fewer calories, less fat and more nutrients (such as vitamin E) than conventional beef. Meat from grass-fed animals has two to three times more conjugated linoleic acid (CLA) than meat from grain-fed animals. CLA helps protect the brain by counteracting the effects of harmful stress hormones.

Try to have grass-fed beef once or twice a week—but give it a supporting role instead of making it the star of your meal. Think grass-fed vegetable beef stew instead of a large steak.

Note: Even though grass-fed beef is more expensive than conventional beef, you can save by opting for nontraditional cuts, such as beef shank, stew meats and roasts. If you are a vegetarian or vegan, black beans are an excellent substitute.

• **Cruciferous vegetables.** Take your pick—the list includes brussels sprouts, kale, arugula, bok choy, cauliflower and collard greens. As members of the Brassica plant family, these veggies contain sulfur-based anti-inflammatory compounds that help protect the brain. One of these compounds, sulforaphane, has even been shown to improve memory and learning after brain injury.

Aim for at least two cups of cruciferous vegetables daily—I put that much in my kale-blueberry smoothie every morning!

Note: Consult your doctor before changing the amount of leafy greens you eat if you take warfarin, a blood thinner, since vitamin K–rich foods may interact.

Other good choices: Add purple cabbage to a stir-fry…or mash cauliflower instead of potatoes and season with brain-boosting turmeric and black pepper (to increase the absorption of turmeric).

To Ward Off Dementia, Eat Your Fill

Deborah Gustafson, PhD, professor of neurology, SUNY Downstate Medical Center, Brooklyn, New York. Her review, titled "2003-2013: A Decade of Body Mass Index, Alzheimer's Disease, and Dementia," was published in *Journal of Alzheimer's Disease*.

Attention skinny people—you may get dementia. That's the finding from a study of more than 2 million people that looked at the relationship between body mass index (BMI) in middle age and dementia later in life. This study has gotten a lot of press because it found, essentially, that the thinner you are, the greater your dementia risk…which goes against what most people might think and implies that there's no need to worry about staying trim.

Before you break out the cheesecake to celebrate, though, let's take a closer look.

"Contradicting Everything We Thought We Knew"

The researchers used a health-care database from a network of primary-care practices in the United Kingdom to find height/weight measurements on people aged 40 and older. They followed these people until they either left the network, were diagnosed with any form of dementia or died.

The result was more than a little surprising: Dementia risk decreased with each bump up in BMI. People who were underweight (BMI 20 or lower in this study, or under 139 pounds for a 5'10" tall person) had a 34% higher risk than average of developing dementia over 20 years than average—maybe not so surprising, since being underweight is obviously not a healthy thing to be. But then the higher that people went up on the weight spectrum, the lower their risk for dementia became, and that seemed downright odd. At the far end of the weight scale, those who were morbidly obese in midlife, with a BMI of 40 or higher (279 pounds for a 5'10" person) had a 29% lower risk for dementia than average. Crazy, huh? As one headline put it, "Being Fat Lowers Dementia Risk in Middle and Old Age, Contradicting Everything We Thought We Knew."

To help us figure this out, we interviewed Deborah Gustafson, PhD, a professor of neurology at SUNY Downstate Medical Center in Brooklyn, New York and the University of Gothenburg in Sweden. Dr. Gustafson, who was not involved with the UK study, has done extensive research on the risk factors for cognitive decline and was among the first to study the relationship between body weight and dementia.

Regarding the new study, she was skeptical.

Oops, Did We Measure Right?

Like all observational studies, the UK weight study has some inherent limitations. While these kinds of studies are valuable for pointing researchers toward associations, they can't show cause and effect. *Beyond this general limitation, there are specific concerns about this particular study's methods…*

• **It included mixed age groups.** You had to be 40 or older to be included, but there was no upper limit. Some people were 80 years old when their baseline info was recorded. (No matter how you slice it, being 80 isn't middle-aged.) So it's hard to draw conclusions from this data about how weight in middle age affects dementia risk when you're older. During midlife, a person normally gains weight. At around 65 or 70 years old, a person typically loses skeletal muscle and gains fat, but overall, BMI tends to decrease. Mixing up data from these two very different stages of life, means the study is not going to work.

• **It likely missed many cases of dementia.** Patients with dementia were identified only through a review of medical records in this study, but people may come into the health-care system with more acute illnesses that mask dementia, so this approach misses many late-onset cases of dementia. A better approach would be to conduct thorough evaluations among a representative sample, which can take hours, followed by discussion among more than one expert to confirm the diagnoses. That's what Dr. Gustafson has done in her studies. "It's expensive to conduct a study with time-consuming evaluations, which is why it can't be done on 2 million people. But it's more accurate."

• **It didn't distinguish between different types of dementia.** Certain hereditary forms of dementia tend to strike earlier in life. Early-onset dementia is a different beast, so it would have helped if the researchers had separated dementias diagnosed before age 65 from those diagnosed after age 65. Late-onset dementia may be influenced by being overweight, while early-onset dementia is more likely to be hereditary and influenced by specific genes.

What Do We Really Know About Weight and Dementia?

• **Watch your weight in midlife.** Studies investigating the association between midlife BMI and risk for dementia demonstrated generally an increased risk among overweight and obese adults. One reason may be that excess weight increases your risk for high blood pressure, high cholesterol levels and diabetes. All of these factors have been shown to increase the risk for dementia.

• **Being too skinny over the age of 70 increases your risk.** Being underweight (BMI 18.5 or lower) is associated with increased dementia risk. That's quite thin, such as 5' 4" and 107 pounds. No one is sure why, but there may be metabolic abnormalities that keep people underweight that also contribute to dementia risk. In some cases, the dementia process may begin decades before clinical symptoms and lead to a lower body weight.

• **A little extra weight in later life may be protective.** There is a consistent finding in the medical literature that over age 70, having a BMI in the "overweight" range (25 to 29.9) is protective. Some but not all studies find that even being obese (BMI 30 to 34.9) protects, too. If you're a little heavier going into late life, you may be less likely to develop dementia. While no one is sure why, it may be that fat tissue produces hormones that are protective for the brain.

It's not quite as much fun as a headline that says being fat is a good thing for your brain and memory. That would be nice for people who are heavy. But the real story appears to be that a healthy lifestyle that helps keep weight in the normal range throughout your middle years and into your 70s is good for your brain, too. Once you get into your 70s, a little extra weight may be fine.

At any age, however, a healthy diet and exercise is important for body—and mind. All of the things that we have been promoting for a long time—eating right and getting physical exercise—are actually relevant for dementia, too.

Women Have Sharper Memories

Women have sharper memories than men from age 40 on. Besides having a larger hippocampus—the area of the brain that controls memory—than men, premenopausal women benefit from hormones, such as estrogen and progesterone, which protect against memory loss. While estrogen goes down for many women by age 50, they still benefit from a residual protective advantage for many years.

Study of 1,246 people by researchers at Mayo Clinic, Rochester, Minnesota, published in *JAMA Neurology.*

A Better Way to Treat Advanced Parkinson's Disease

John T. Slevin, MD, professor of neurology and molecular and biomedical pharmacology, department of neurology, University of Kentucky Medical Center, Lexington. His study appeared in the *Journal of Parkinson's Disease.*

The drug Sinemet relieves Parkinson's disease symptoms such as tremor, difficulty swallowing and an awkwardly shuffling gait, but it becomes less effective over time.

Breakthrough: There's a new way of getting Sinemet's active ingredient, *levodopa*, to last longer and more consistently to control Parkinson's symptoms. It has been available in Canada, Australia and throughout Europe for a few years and, finally, it is now available here in America.

Improving a Drug's Staying Power

Parkinson's disease happens when certain brain cells degenerate and produce less dopamine, a chemical necessary to control muscle movement. Levodopa is meant to replace that lost dopamine, but it wears off within min-

Moodiness Increases Alzheimer's Risk

Moody, anxious middle-aged women are twice as likely to develop Alzheimer's as other women. Women with a neurotic personality style, defined as being easily distressed and exhibiting anxiety, jealousy or moodiness, have double the risk for Alzheimer's. These personality traits do not trigger Alzheimer's—more research is needed to understand the association.

Study of 800 women over 38 years by researchers at University of Gothenburg, Sweden, published in *Neurology.*

utes. The pill Sinemet contains levodopa plus a drug called carbidopa that helps the levodopa last longer and get to where it needs to go—the brain. It is initially very effective in controlling Parkinson's symptoms, but within four to six years of starting treatment, its effectiveness wears off for roughly 40% of patients. By nine years, 90% of patients are showing troublesome symptoms again. And besides the Parkinson's symptoms, the body begins to react poorly to the unevenness of levodopa levels…erratic muscle movements (a condition called dyskinesia) begin to occur either when the level of levodopa peaks in the body after taking a dose or when it wears off between doses.

A better—albeit invasive—way to receive levodopa that minimizes these problems was finally approved by the FDA in January 2015 after being available for several years in many other countries around the world. The treatment is a process called carbidopa-levodopa enteral suspension (CLES), marketed as Duopa. It involves surgery to insert a tube through the abdomen into the small intestine. The tube is connected to an external portable pump that a person can carry in his or her pants pocket or some other wearable pouch while the pump delivers a constant flow of the carbidopa-levodopa during waking hours.

The Benefits and Risks

Although studies have shown that the CLES system works well to control Parkinson's symptoms in people with advanced disease, how safe and tolerable is it over the long term? A team of researchers from three top medical institutions—University of Kentucky Medical Center, Cleveland Clinic and Northwestern University Feinberg School of Medicine—along with researchers associated with the drug's manufacturer, AbbVie Inc., closely examined symptoms and patient quality of life before and after beginning CLES. Side effects of CLES were also examined.

In the first part of the study, which lasted three months, patients on Sinemet were compared with patients receiving CLES. In the second part of the study, the patients who had been on Sinemet were switched to CLES, and all the patients—those who had been on CLES and those new to it—were followed for a year.

The results: Patients put on the CLES system during the first part of the study averaged 12 symptom-free hours a day, compared with an average of 10 hours for patients on Sinemet. Once patients on Sinemet were switched to the CLES system, they also improved to meet the sustained 12-hour window of symptom control. Symptoms were less severe, and dyskinesia—the main debilitating side effect of Sinemet—was much less common once the patients were switched to CLES.

Most side effects were related to surgery rather than CLES use. In fact, serious side effects, such as intestinal perforation during surgery, were common, occurring in 23% of patients. In addition, infection at the surgical site occurred in 18% but cleared up with antibiotic therapy.

Besides surgical side effects, the most common side effects for those new to CLES were abdominal pain, which affected 42% of the patients. Nausea was also common, as was skin redness at the site of the tube insertion, which cleared up in some patients over time.

Since CLES is relatively new, doctors don't yet know exactly how long, in terms of years, the therapy will provide symptom control for patients with Parkinson's disease. The lead author of the study, John T. Slevin, MD, from the University of Kentucky Medical Center, said that it is expected that, as the disease progresses and more brain cells that produce dopamine are lost, the benefits of CLES will eventually ebb. CLES simply helps extend symptom control and quality of life longer when other treatments lose their effectiveness.

If you or a loved one has an interest in CLES to control worsening Parkinson's disease, consult an experienced neurologist who specializes in movement disorders who will work with a gastroenterologist skilled in gastrointestinal surgery. You can find Parkinson's Disease Centers of Excellence through the National Parkinson Foundation.

Best Nondrug Approaches for Parkinson's

Michael S. Okun, MD, professor and chair of the department of neurology and codirector of the Center for Movement Disorders and Neurorestoration at the University of Florida College of Medicine in Gainesville. He is also the medical director at the National Parkinson Foundation and has written more than 400 medical journal articles. Dr. Okun's latest book is *10 Breakthrough Therapies for Parkinson's Disease.*

The telltale tremors, muscle stiffness and other movement problems that plague people with Parkinson's disease make even the mundane activities of daily living—such as brushing teeth, cooking and dressing—more difficult.

What's new: Even though medication—such as levodopa (L-dopa) and newer drugs including pramipexole and selegiline—have long been the main treatment to control Parkinson's symptoms, researchers are discovering more and more nondrug therapies that can help.

Among the best nondrug approaches (each can be used with Parkinson's medication)...

Exercise

For people with Parkinson's, exercise is like a drug. It raises neurotrophic factors, proteins that promote the growth and health of neurons. Research consistently shows that exercise can improve motor symptoms (such as walking speed and stability) and quality of life.

For the best results: Exercise 30 to 60 minutes every single day. Aim to work hard enough to break a sweat, but back off if you get too fatigued—especially the following day (this indicates the body is not recovering properly). Parkinson's symptoms can worsen with over-exercise. *Smart exercise habits...*

For better gait speed: Choose a lower-intensity exercise, such as walking on a treadmill (but hold on to the balance bars), rather than high-intensity exercise (such as running), which has a higher risk for falls and other injuries.

A recent study showed that a walking group of Parkinson's patients performed better than a group of patients who ran.

Important safety tip: Parkinson's patients should exercise with a partner and take precautions to prevent falls—for example, minimizing distractions, such as ringing cell phones.

For aerobic exercise: Use a recumbent bicycle or rowing machine and other exercises that don't rely on balance.

For strength and flexibility: Do stretching and progressive resistance training.

Excellent resource: For a wide variety of exercises, including aerobic workouts, standing and sitting stretches, strengthening moves, balance exercises and fall-prevention tips, the National Parkinson Foundation's *Fitness Counts* book is available as a free download at *Parkinson.org/pd-library/books/fitness-counts.*

For balance: Researchers are now discovering that yoga postures, tai chi (with its slow, controlled movements) and certain types of dancing (such as the tango, which involves rhythmic forward-and-backward steps) are excellent ways to improve balance.

Coffee and Tea

Could drinking coffee or tea help with Parkinson's? According to research, it can—when consumed in the correct amounts.

Here's why: Caffeine blocks certain receptors in the brain that regulate the neurotransmitter dopamine, which becomes depleted and leads to the impaired motor coordination that characterizes Parkinson's. In carefully controlled studies, Parkinson's patients who ingested low doses of caffeine—about 100 mg twice daily—had improved motor symptoms, such as tremors and stiffness, compared with people who had no caffeine or higher doses of caffeine.

My advice: Have 100 mg of caffeine (about the amount in one six-ounce cup of home-brewed coffee or two cups of black or green tea) twice a day—once in the morning and once in the mid-afternoon.

Note: Even decaffeinated coffee has about 10 mg to 25 mg of caffeine per cup.

Supplements

Researchers have studied various supplements for years to identify ones that could help manage Parkinson's symptoms and/or boost the effects of levodopa, but large studies have failed to prove that these supplements provide such benefits.

However, because Parkinson's is a complex disease that can cause about 20 different motor and nonmotor symptoms that evolve over time, the existing research may not apply to everyone. *Some people with Parkinson's may benefit from...*

•**Coenzyme Q10 (CoQ10).** This supplement promotes the health of the body's mitochondria ("energy generators" in the cells), which are believed to play a role in Parkinson's. In a large study, people with Parkinson's who took 1,200 mg per day showed some improvement in symptoms over a 16-month study period. However, follow-up studies found no beneficial effects.

•**Riboflavin and alpha-lipoic acid** are among the other supplements that are continuing to be studied.

Important: If you wish to try these or other supplements, be sure to consult your doctor to ensure that there are no possible interactions with your other medications.

Marijuana

A few small studies have concluded that marijuana can improve some neurological symptoms, but larger studies are needed to show benefits for Parkinson's patients, especially for symptoms such as depression and anxiety.

However: Marijuana is challenging for several reasons—first, it is illegal in most states. If you do live in a state that allows medical marijuana use, it has possible side effects—for example, it can impair balance and driving...it is difficult to know the exact dosage, even if it's purchased from a dispensary...and with marijuana edibles (such as cookies and candies), the effects may take longer to appear, and you may accidentally ingest too much.

If you want to try marijuana: Work closely with your doctor to help you avoid such pitfalls.

Seeing the Right Doctor

For anyone with Parkinson's, it's crucial to see a neurologist and, if possible, one who has advanced training in Parkinson's disease and movement disorders.

Important new finding: A large study showed that patients treated by a neurologist had a lower risk for hip fracture and were less likely to be placed in a nursing facility. They were also 22% less likely to die during the four-year study.

Neurologists are best equipped to treat the ever-changing symptoms of Parkinson's. For optimal care, see the neurologist every four to six months. The National Parkinson Foundation's Helpline, 800-4PD-INFO (473-4636), can assist you in finding expert care.

Anesthesia Linked to Memory Problems

Cognitive decline can strike after anesthesia. In a seven-year study of more than 500 older adults, women who had general anesthesia during surgery had a faster decline in cognition, ability to function and brain volume than men, but both sexes experienced these effects after surgery and general anesthesia. The duration of cognitive decline was not measured.

If you need surgery: Ask your doctor if an alternative procedure or local anesthesia can be used. (See page 302 for more information on protecting your mind in the hospital.)

Katie Schenning, MD, MPH, assistant professor of anesthesiology and perioperative medicine, Oregon Health & Science University, Portland.

Does Fish Protect the Brain—or Poison It With Mercury?

Study titled "Association of Seafood Consumption, Brain Mercury Level, and APOE E4 Status with Brain Neuropathology in Older Adults" by researchers at Rush University Medical Center, Chicago; Missouri University Researcher Reactor, Columbia; and Wageningen University, the Netherlands, published in *JAMA*.

When it comes to preventing dementia, eating seafood is a double-edged sword. On the one hand, it's high in mercury, a neurotoxin. Bad for the brain. On the other hand, it's high in omega-3 fatty acids, which support nerve functioning. Good for the brain.

So what happens to people who eat seafood regularly, compared with those who eat little or none? They're less likely to get dementia. All those omega-3s protect the brain even with the extra mercury.

This is something of a breakthrough finding. While earlier population studies had suggested that the cardiovascular and other benefits of eating seafood outweighed the risks of consuming contaminants, doubts remained. In a new study, researchers at Rush University Medical Center in Chicago looked at what you might call hard evidence—autopsies of 286 men and women (average age 90). They had already been studying these people when they were alive, so they knew how much seafood they were eating, and now they could look directly at their body tissues and inside their brains to see if there was accumulation of mercury—and neurological evidence of Alzheimer's disease.

The surprise answer was that while the seafood eaters did have higher levels of mercury, there was no increased incidence of Alzheimer's. That's true even for those who had the highest levels of mercury.

While mercury didn't harm, however, seafood protected those at the highest risk. These are the estimated about one-quarter of the population who carry a gene variant

(apolipoprotein E4) that triples Alzheimer's risk. Seafood didn't protect everyone, but in this group, those who ate seafood regularly, compared with those who rarely or never ate it, were 47% less likely to show the brain pathology that defines Alzheimer's disease.

Bottom line: By all means, choose seafood lowest in mercury—good choices include catfish, clams, flounder, salmon, sardines, scallops, shrimp, squid and light (not albacore) tuna. But don't let worry about mercury stop you from getting the brain-protective benefits of seafood.

Memory Boosting Chocolate: Hype or High-Powered Superfood?

Leo Galland, MD, director, Foundation for Integrated Medicine, New York City. PillAdvised.com.

You've probably read through many articles about how chocolate boosts brain power and helps fight dementia and memory loss, but, sadly, the media hype is overblown. There certainly is healing power in cocoa, but here's the real story about how you can best benefit from it.

The Bitter Truth

The most recent study on the benefits of cocoa comes from Columbia University in New York City. Like similar studies before it, the Columbia findings spurred a wave of news reports and press releases exclaiming that hot cocoa and chocolate improve memory. In this small study of 37 people, participants (healthy men and women aged 50 to 69) received either high-dose flavonol cocoa (900 mg per day) or low-dose flavonol cocoa (10 mg per day). Flavonols are a type of flavonoid, an anti-inflammatory compound found in a wide range of fruits, vegetables and other plant-based foods. And 900 mg of flavonol equals nearly a day's worth of flavonoids that a person would get from a typical Western diet—so that's a lot of flavonols packed into an experimental cocoa drink.

Participants' brains were scanned before and after the three-month study period, and they also were given memory and reaction-time tests.

The results: Participants in the high-dose group had memory skills comparable to people who were 20 to 30 years younger, whereas minimal improvement was seen in participants in the low-dose group.

These findings are consistent with several larger and better-designed clinical trials of cocoa flavonols, but the study may have received more hype than it deserved. The same could be said of an earlier study conducted by Harvard researchers, which showed that both high-dose (609 mg) and low-dose (13 mg) cocoa-based flavonol consumption (in the form of a cocoa drink) improved blood flow in the brain. Publication of the Harvard study was also followed by several misleading news reports claiming that two cups of cocoa a day keep dementia away.

The problem: It's hard to apply these lessons to real life.

Commercial brands of chocolate and cocoa are often processed to the point where most, if not all, of the beneficial antioxidants (flavonols and other important flavonoids) are removed.

The Best Sources of Antioxidants

Although dark and bitter chocolate and green tea and even black tea can provide some nutritional flavonols, the best approach is eating a diet rich in flavonoids in general. Remember, flavonoids are the group of antioxidants that flavonols belong to. Foods rich in flavonoids include colorful fruits (especially apples, citrus and berries), dark leafy green vegetables (such as kale and spinach), asparagus, colorful nightshade vegetables (such as peppers, tomatoes and eggplant) and dark-

colored beans (such as adzuki, black beans and red kidney beans).

A diet that includes a rich variety of vegetables, such as an Asian diet, can pack about 4,000 mg of flavonoids a day. The typical meat-and-potatoes Western diet, in contrast, provides an average of only about 1,000 mg of flavonoids per day.

So, while you could get a bit of a day's worth of flavonols from dark or bitter chocolate, an ordinary chocolate bar or a milky cup of cocoa will only give you a sugar rush and extra calories to work off. Get your flavonols—and other flavonoids—instead from a wide variety of fruits and vegetables and from beverages such as green tea.

Want to Boost Short-Term Memory? Watch a Funny Video

Gurinder Singh Bains, MD, PhD, assistant professor and primary research coordinator, Loma Linda University School of Allied Health Professions, Loma Linda, California. His study was published in *Alternative Therapies*.

You forget that thing that someone told you…this morning. You misplace your keys. You walk into the kitchen to do something…but once you get there, you forget what it is.

What you're experiencing is a decline in short-term memory. It starts to go down as early as your 40s…and it's perfectly normal. (Forgetting where you live or what your keys are for, that's a different story.)

But wouldn't it be great if there were something simple and easy that you could do to improve it?

There is. In fact it's so simple, it's funny.

How Red Skelton Enhances Brain Power

Watching a humorous video for 20 minutes may be all it takes to improve your ability to remember things you've just heard or read, found researchers at Loma Linda University in California. They showed 20 older men and women (average age 70) either a video of Red Skelton (the former clown who had a popular TV comedy show in the 1950s, '60s and early '70s)…or a montage from America's Funniest Home Videos.

None of the participants had any cognitive impairment. However, half of them (10) had diabetes, which is known to contribute to short-term memory loss. An additional 10 participants, who did not have diabetes nor cognitive impairment and were of the same age, were the control group. They did not watch the videos but instead were asked to sit silently in a quiet room.

Before and after watching funny videos… or sitting in silence…the participants took three components of a short-term-memory test. First, a researcher read aloud 15 words, and participants were then asked to say from memory as many as they could remember…a test of learning. The test was repeated five times. The same test was then given with a different list, and then participants were asked to remember what had been on the first list…a test of recall. Finally, participants were given a piece of paper with 50 words on it and asked to circle words that had been on the first list…a test of visual recognition. Finally, a little saliva was swabbed at five different points, including before and after— you'll see why in a moment.

Result? Laughter worked. After watching the humorous videos, the healthy adults did 39% better on the learning test, 44% better on the recall test and 13% better on the visual recognition test. Those with diabetes also saw significant improvements—a 33% boost in learning, a 48% jump in recall and a 17% gain in visual recognition. Sitting silently also seemed to benefit the control group but not nearly as much. Their gains were 24%, 20% and 8%, respectively.

How can a little mirth improve memory? That's where the saliva comes in.

The Stress Connection

Saliva contains cortisol, a stress hormone. All of the participants who watched the funny videos experienced a significant decrease in salivary cortisol levels. Stress, as the researchers already knew, suppresses the function of the brain's hippocampus, where short-term memory is pulled together. (Over time, chronic stress can even damage…and shrink…the hippocampus.) Feeling less stress and producing fewer stress hormones, the researchers speculate, is what led to better learning and memory in the video watchers.

This wonderfully simple experiment suggests a wonderfully simple way that we could all boost our short-term memory—watch humorous videos. There are literally thousands that are easily found online…but here are three good (and free) ones…

• **The hilarious well-known scene from the *I Love Lucy* TV show**—when Lucy and Ethel get jobs at a candy factory.

• **Comedienne Carol Burnett's spoof on *Gone With the Wind*.**

• **Frasier,** from the TV comedy series *Frasier*, sings "Buttons and Bows."

If you want to stretch out the experience, try these funny full-length movies—*Blazing Saddles* (1974), *Airplane!* (1980), *Raising Arizona* (1987), *A Fish Called Wanda* (1988), *Liar Liar* (1997), *There's Something About Mary* (1998), *Little Miss Sunshine* (2006), *Death at a Funeral* (2007) and *Bridesmaids* (2011).

Of course, you don't have to watch a video to relax and laugh. Although it wasn't studied, it's a reasonable speculation that anything that lowers stress levels may enhance short-term memory. While this is the first research to show memory improvement, other research has shown that humor and laughter stimulate the immune system, make pain more tolerable, improve mood and even reduce markers of inflammation. That's fun with benefits.

When Certain Noises Drive You Nuts

Pawel J. Jastreboff, PhD, ScD, professor of otolaryngology, Emory University School of Medicine, Atlanta.

Repetitive sounds, such as gum chewing or throat clearing, are classic triggers for a condition known as *misophonia*. People with misophonia (also known as selective sound sensitivity syndrome) become anxious or angry when they hear a specific sound that would not cause a similar reaction in most other people. Sometimes just the sight of someone putting a stick of gum in his/her mouth, for example, is enough to make the misophonia sufferer angry.

Researchers don't know what causes misophonia but believe that it's a disorder in the way the brain processes sound. Sound waves are transformed into electrical signals that go into certain areas of the brain that control emotions. In people with misophonia, the brain cannot filter past negative associations with certain sounds. In some cases, the condition is linked to obsessive-compulsive disorder. Many people with tinnitus (a ringing in the ears) also have misophonia.

A treatment method called tinnitus retraining therapy has been shown to improve symptoms significantly in 85% of misophonia patients. They listen to a recording of enjoyable sounds (such as favorite music) mixed with the offensive sound set at a very low level. Over a period of three months (sometimes longer), the enjoyable sound is gradually decreased so the listener can develop a tolerance for the sound that triggers negative reactions. Cognitive behavioral therapy can also help change negative thoughts about the sound.

Stop Memory Loss with Doctor-Tested Supplements

Pamela Wartian Smith, MD, MPH, codirector of the master's program in medical sciences and author of *What You Must Know About Memory Loss & How You Can Stop It: A Guide to Proven Techniques and Supplements to Maintain, Strengthen, or Regain Memory*.

Do you have trouble remembering names and phone numbers? How about where you put things? Do you sometimes struggle to come up with the right word?

Mild forgetfulness, known as age-related memory impairment, is a natural part of getting older. By age 75, a person's memory has declined, on average, by about 43%. After age 75, the hippocampus, the part of the brain most closely associated with memory, will eventually atrophy at the rate of 1% to 2% each year.

But you can improve memory with over-the-counter supplements—if you choose the right ones. Here are the supplements I find most effective with my patients. You can take several of these if you choose. You could start with phosphatidylserine and add others depending on your personal needs. For example, if you're taking a medication that depletes CoQ10, you might want

Concussion Recovery Alert for Women

Concussion recovery is more challenging for women than men. Recent finding: MRIs of the brain's memory areas, done one month after the brain injury and again after another six weeks, showed more activity in men's working (short-term) memory than in women's—indicating that the memory-recovery process takes longer for women.

Study by researchers at Taipei Medical University Shuang-Ho Hospital, New Taipei City, Taiwan, published in *Radiology*.

to take that supplement. Or if you're under stress, add ashwagandha root. Of course, always check with your doctor before starting any new supplement. To find a practitioner trained in this field, go to *Metabolic-Anti-AgingSpecialist.com.*

•**Phosphatidylserine (PS).** Most people haven't heard of it, but PS is one of my first choices for mild memory loss. It's a naturally occurring phospholipid (a molecule that contains two fatty acids) that increases the body's production of acetylcholine and other neurotransmitters. It improves cell-to-cell communication and "nourishes" the brain by improving glucose metabolism.

Studies have shown that healthy people who take PS are more likely to maintain their ability to remember things. For those who have already experienced age-related memory loss, PS can improve memory. It's also thought to improve symptoms caused by some forms of dementia.

Typical dose: 300 mg daily. You're unlikely to notice any side effects.

•**Co-enzyme Q10 (CoQ10).** This is another naturally occurring substance found in many foods (such as fatty fish, meats, nuts, fruits and vegetables) and in nearly all of your body's tissues. CoQ10 increases the production of adenosine triphosphate, a molecule that enhances energy production within cells. It's also a potent antioxidant that reduces cell-damaging inflammation in the brain and other parts of the body.

People with degenerative brain disorders, such as Alzheimer's, tend to have lower levels of CoQ10. Studies suggest that supplemental CoQ10 improves memory by protecting brain cells from oxidative damage.

Important: If you're taking a medication that depletes CoQ10—examples include statins (for lowering cholesterol)...metformin (for diabetes)...and beta-blockers (for heart disease and other conditions)—you'll definitely want to take a supplement. I often recommend it for people age 50 and older because the body's production of CoQ10 declines with age. Hard exercise also depletes it.

Typical dose: Between 30 mg and 360 mg daily. Ask your health-care professional how much you need—it will depend on medication use and other factors. Side effects are rare but may include insomnia, agitation and digestive problems such as diarrhea and heartburn.

•**Acetyl-L-carnitine.** A study that looked at people with mild cognitive impairment (an intermediate stage between age-related memory impairment and dementia) found that acetyl-L-carnitine improved memory, attention and even verbal fluency.

Acetyl-L-carnitine (it is derived from an amino acid) is a versatile molecule. It's used by the body to produce acetylcholine, the main neurotransmitter involved in memory. It slows the rate of neurotransmitter decay, increases oxygen availability and helps convert body fat into energy.

Typical dose: 1,000 mg to 2,000 mg daily. Check with your health-care professional before starting acetyl-L-carnitine to see what dose is best for you. If your kidneys are not functioning perfectly, you may need a lower dose. Some people may notice a slight fishy body odor. In my experience, you can prevent this by taking 50 mg to 100 mg of vitamin B-2 at the same time you take acetyl-L-carnitine.

•**Ashwagandha root.** This is an herb that improves the repair and regeneration of brain cells (neurons) and inhibits the body's production of acetylcholinesterase, an enzyme that degrades acetylcholine. It also improves the ability to deal with both physical and emotional stress—both of which have been linked to impaired memory and cognitive decline.

Typical dose: 500 mg to 2,000 mg daily. Start with the lower dose. If after a month you don't notice that your memory and focus have improved, take a little more. GI disturbances are possible but not common.

Warning: Don't take this supplement if you're also taking a prescription medication that has cholinesterase-inhibiting effects, such as *donepezil* (Aricept) or *galantamine* (Razadyne). Ask your health-care professional whether any of your medications have this effect.

• **Ginkgo biloba.** Among the most studied herbal supplements, ginkgo is an antioxidant that protects the hippocampus from age-related atrophy. It's a vasodilator that helps prevent blood clots, improves brain circulation and reduces the risk for vascular dementia, a type of dementia associated with impaired blood flow to the brain. It also increases the effects of serotonin, a neurotransmitter that's involved in mood and learning.

Bonus: In animal studies, ginkgo appears to block the formation of amyloid, the protein that has been linked to Alzheimer's disease. There's strong evidence that ginkgo can stabilize and possibly improve memory.

Typical dose: 60 mg to 120 mg daily. Most people won't have side effects, but ginkgo is a blood thinner that can react with other anticoagulants. If you're taking warfarin or another blood thinner (including aspirin and fish oil), be sure to check with your health-care professional before taking ginkgo.

• **Fish oil.** Much of the brain consists of DHA (docosahexaenoic acid), one of the main omega-3 fatty acids. It is essential for brain health. People who take fish-oil supplements have improved brain circulation and a faster transmission of nerve signals.

Studies have found that people who eat a lot of fatty fish have a lower risk for mild cognitive impairment than people who tend to eat little or no fatty fish. One study found that people with age-related memory impairment achieved better scores on memory tests when they took daily DHA supplements.

Typical dose: 2,000 mg daily if you're age 50 or older. Look for a combination supplement that includes equal amounts of DHA and EPA (another omega-3). Fish-oil supplements can increase the effects of blood-thinning medications such as aspirin and warfarin if the dose is above 3,000 mg a day.

• **Huperzine A.** Extracted from a Chinese moss, this is a cholinesterase inhibitor that increases brain levels of acetylcholine. It also protects brain cells from too-high levels of glutamate, another neurotransmitter.

Huperzine A may improve memory and could even help delay symptoms of Alzheimer's disease. A study conducted by the National Institute of Aging found that patients with mild-to-moderate Alzheimer's who took huperzine A had improvements in cognitive functions.

Recommended dose: 400 mcg daily. Don't take it if you're already taking a prescription cholinesterase inhibitor (as discussed in the "Ashwagandha root" section).

What to Do If You Suspect Early-Onset Alzheimer's Disease

Susan M. Maixner, MD, clinical associate professor of psychiatry, director of the Geropsychiatry Program, director of the geriatric psychiatry clinic at the University of Michigan Health System, and psychiatric consultant at Arbor Hospice, Ann Arbor.

S *till Alice,* the acclaimed movie starring Julianne Moore, who won an Academy Award for her performance, is about a linguistics professor and mother of three who is diagnosed with Alzheimer's disease at the tender age of 50. It provides powerful food for thought for anyone concerned about dementia. For those of you who are middle-aged and feeling more distracted and forgetful—or more easily agitated than you once were—the movie will shake you up. It's not always easy to tell whether these symptoms are simply due to stress and multitasking or the beginnings of true cognitive decline. So how can you tell?

Suspicious Signs

The key symptom to look out for is trouble managing "bills and pills," said Susan Maixner, MD, a clinical associate professor of psychiatry and director of the Geropsychiatry Program at the University of Michigan Health System. If you are younger than 65 and bill-paying becomes increasingly difficult to keep track of and if you find yourself forgetting to take medications or doubling up on doses (a danger in and of itself), you may be in the danger zone for early-onset Alzheimer's disease. For those still working, being unable to retain information for work, such as frequently used computer passwords, may be a very early sign of cognitive difficulties, said Dr. Maixner.

A decline in short-term memory, such as too often forgetting whether or not you paid that bill or took that med, usually comes first when early-onset Alzheimer's sets in, said Dr. Maixner. Other telltale signs are the same as those for Alzheimer's in older age groups—getting lost while driving, repeating yourself, inability to plan or to solve problems, confusion with time or place, the inability to comprehend visual images (for example, not recognizing acquaintances), difficulty writing or speaking, often misplacing things, failing judgment, social withdrawal and change in mood or personality, such as feeling more short-tempered or frustrated.

Getting Diagnosed

The first step to getting a diagnosis is scheduling a thorough medical exam that your family doctor can perform, said Dr. Maixner. "Make sure that you tell your primary care doctor, up front, that you are scheduling the physical exam because you are experiencing memory problems and are concerned about early-onset Alzheimer's," said Dr. Maixner. The exam will be tailored to rule out physical as well as psychological ailments that may be causing the cognitive decline. And, because approximately 20% of early-onset Alzheimer's disease is inherited (genetic), tell your family doctor if you have a family history of dementia. Many primary care physicians won't think to ask this question—so be sure to bring it up, said Dr. Maixner.

Make sure blood work is done to rule out thyroid problems or vitamin deficiencies that can cause memory issues, advised Dr. Maixner. Medications and the use of drugs and alcohol also should be considered. The primary care doctor should then perform in-office cognitive tests, such as the Mini-Mental State Exam or Montreal Cognitive Assessment, which evaluate mental sharpness and short- and long-term memory. If the test results reveal signs of cognitive decline, your doctor should refer you to a geriatric psychiatrist or a neurologist with expertise in managing cognitive disorders such as dementia. The specialist may order an MRI or a CT scan of the brain to rule out whether a stroke, brain injury lesion or tumor may be causing the symptoms. A geriatric psychiatrist also has special training in differentiating dementia from depression, anxiety and other conditions that can accompany memory problems, said Dr. Maixner.

Coping With Early-Onset Alzheimer's

So far, there is no cure for Alzheimer's disease. Although progressive worsening of the disease is inevitable, the clock can be turned back on symptoms with lifestyle interventions and medications. It is crucial to keep up physical activity, social interactions and mental stimulation, according to Dr. Maixner. Also, routines, predictability and structure are essential coping tools that will help you or a loved one with early-onset Alzheimer's function better.

Planning about who will manage financial affairs and health decisions is important because if it is Alzheimer's, a time will come when you or your loved one will no longer be able to make those decisions, said Dr. Maixner. Support groups and a 24/7 information hotline that can help with finding a dementia specialist, coping, staying active and legal issues are available through the Alzheimer's Association.

Chapter 6

FALLS, BONE HEALTH AND PHYSICAL INJURY

Are Your Bones as Healthy as You Think?

You might think that a bone fracture is a relatively minor health problem. But if you are a woman or a man over age 50, it means that you should get a bone density test if you've never had one before.

An often-overlooked problem: Most primary care doctors are good at reviewing their patients' overall well-being, but bone health is frequently given short shrift. Discussing the strength of your bones—and the possible need for bone density testing—should always be part of your regular checkup.

Remember: Men get osteoporosis (thinning of the bones), too. In fact, complications following hip fracture are a leading cause of death in older women and men.

Mistakes to avoid…

MISTAKE #1: **Not discussing bone density testing.** Your age will help determine whether you need bone density testing. The National Osteoporosis Foundation recommends it—even in the absence of osteoporosis risk factors—for all women age 65 and older…and all men age 70 and older.

Testing is also advisable for postmenopausal women under age 65, menopausal women and men age 50 to 69 if they have risk factors. There is a long list of risk factors that include medical conditions such as liver disease, kidney disease, thyroid problems and diabetes…the use of certain medications that can cause bone loss, such as steroids…being Caucasian or Asian…and having a family history of osteoporosis. Frequency of the testing varies—check with your doctor.

Note: I also recommend a baseline test prior to menopause in women who have risk factors.

Good news: Especially for women with risk factors, bone density testing is usually covered by insurance. If your insurer does not cover it, it's a test worth paying for (it usually costs $150 to $250).

MISTAKE #2: **Seeing a technician—or radiologist—who isn't properly credentialed.** Only some states require bone density technicians to be trained in densitometry (the measurement of bone density), and no

Lani Simpson, DC, CCD, a chiropractic doctor and certified clinical (bone) densitometrist specializing in osteoporosis and hormone balancing. She is the author of *Dr. Lani's No-Nonsense Bone Health Guide* and host of the PBS show "Stronger Bones, Longer Life," which aired in June 2016.

states require this training of the physicians who interpret the test results. This lack of professional training is responsible for most testing errors.

What you can do: It's not enough to ask your technician if he/she has been trained—he may say "yes" (and believe it), even though the person who did the "teaching" was not properly trained. When scheduling your test, make sure the doctor who will be interpreting your results is a clinical densitometrist. To find a list of certified clinical densitometrists (CCDs) in your state, check The International Society for Clinical Densitometry's website, *ISCD.org*.

MISTAKE #3: **Not being positioned properly during the scan.** Bone density is measured with a type of scan that uses technology known as dual-energy X-ray absorptiometry (DXA). For details on the test, see "Bone-Testing Basics" below.

It's an excellent test—when it's performed correctly. One of the most common errors is improper positioning when checking the bone density of the hip. During this part of the test, your technician should use a small device that fits between your feet to cause a 15- to 20-degree internal hip rotation.

In that position, the neck of the femur measures at its lowest bone density level...any other positioning could falsely inflate your score by up to 10%—an amount that can be the difference between whether or not a doctor diagnoses a troubling level of bone loss.

What you can do: Prior to your DXA, discuss the proper positioning with your doctor. When you are at the test, you can say to the technician, "My doctor really stressed to me the importance of getting the proper hip rotation." That will alert your technician that you know about this element of the test... and encourage him to do it correctly.

If you're not sure whether the device was used with earlier testing, ask the technician to check your previous scan so that he can make sure your hip is rotated to the same degree it was previously.

MISTAKE #4: **Skipping important lab tests.** Your DXA results are only one piece of your bone health puzzle. Laboratory tests are just as essential in forming a complete picture of your bone health. When it comes to diagnosing and treating osteoporosis, lab tests are mainly used to rule out potential secondary causes, such as low vitamin D levels, thyroid or parathyroid problems, or digestive disorders.

However, it's also critical that your doctor assess your sex hormone levels, which have a direct impact on your bone health. For women, perimenopause- and menopause-induced low estrogen can cause a 1% to 3% loss of bone mass annually for five to 10 years. In men, hypogonadism (low testosterone) is a leading cause of osteoporosis.

What you can do: In addition to a complete blood count (that includes white and red blood cell counts) and a comprehensive metabolic panel (that checks kidney and liver function and electrolyte levels, etc.), ask for a vitamin D test and a thyroid stimulating hormone (TSH) test. Vitamin D increases calcium absorption by 50%, so you need adequate levels to maintain healthy bone. Untreated thyroid disease can result in bone loss.

Depending on your personal history, your doctor may also want tests to measure your calcium, phosphorus and magnesium levels...parathyroid functioning...cortisol levels...and more.

Bone-Testing Basics

A dual-energy X-ray absorptiometry (DXA) scan is simple, painless, requires no injections and exposes you to very little radiation (a small fraction of that used for a chest X-ray).

What happens: While lying on your back in your clothes, with your arms at your sides, you'll be asked to hold your breath and not move for a few seconds while the machine passes over you. The complete test takes about 20 minutes.

Important: You should avoid taking calcium supplements for 24 hours before the test—an undigested pill could lodge in an area and falsely bolster your results.

The Big Calcium Mistake

Study titled "Does Calcium Strengthen Bones? Evidence is Weak. Researchers Question Current Daily Intake Recommendations," published in *MedPage Today*. *Health Insider* research.

Way back in 1989, the calcium RDA for middle-aged men and women was a modest 800 milligrams (mg) a day.

That's close to the amount of calcium that Americans actually get from the foods that we eat.

The average for women is 788 mg, and for men, it's 950 mg.

Then, in 1997, it all changed. Instead of simply preventing nutrition deficiencies, the goal for calcium was changed to preventing a serious chronic condition—osteoporosis.

The calcium recommendation went up. A lot. The new rule was that women aged 19 to 50 and men aged 19 to 70 needed 1,000 mg a day...while women 51 and older and men 71 and older needed 1,200 mg. Those amounts are actually not very easy to get from food, and that convinced millions of Americans to take calcium supplements and consume food that's been artificially loaded with extra calcium...day after day...year after year. That's where things stand today.

But what if it was all a big mistake?

What if all that calcium has been harming us?

The Calcium Boom and How It Hurt Us

When the calcium RDA went up, suddenly, it wasn't so easy to get enough calcium in a well-balanced diet. Sure, you could eat more dairy, something the dairy industry was happy to promote, and consume calcium-fortified cereal and orange juice, something the cereal and beverage manufacturers were happy to provide. But to get to those higher numbers, chances are, you'd need supplements, too.

The American public obliged. By 2006, 51% of men aged 51 to 70, and 67% of women in the same age range, were supplementing their diets with calcium. Only recently have the numbers started to go down a little.

But taking high doses of calcium supplements, we've since found out, may do harm to our hearts and kidneys. In a 2010 study, women (mostly over 70 years old) who took calcium supplements of 500 mg or more had a 30% greater risk of having heart attacks.

The heart attack risk, however, showed up only in women when daily calcium intake from all sources exceeded—wait for it—800 mg.

Later studies have confirmed the heart attack risk from taking supplements. Calcium supplements also increase the risk for painful kidney stones.

Preventing Osteoporosis with Calcium Pills? Never Mind

Now there's growing evidence that taking all that extra calcium doesn't prevent osteoporosis either. *In September 2015, an analysis of more than 50 studies published in BMJ found that...*

• **High dietary intake of calcium doesn't prevent fractures.**

• **Eating lots of dairy foods doesn't prevent fractures.**

• **The evidence that calcium supplements prevent fractures is "weak and inconsistent."**

Now some experts are calling for the recommended amount of calcium to come back down—perhaps even to levels that one could reasonably expect to eat in a balanced diet. It's not our place to set nutrition standards, but from a layman's standpoint, the "old" standard of 800 mg is starting to look pretty attractive.

One thing is clear—the days when we thought we could keep our bones strong simply by starting to take a calcium pill in our 50s or 60s are gone. It's not that calcium supplements don't build bone density—some studies do find a modest increase. It's just not enough to prevent what really matters—fractures.

It may be that large amounts of calcium taken in a pill are absorbed quite differently than eating small amounts of calcium in our daily meals. Even including a small amount of vitamin D, which improves the body's ability to use calcium, isn't effective at protecting bones. According to the US Preventive Services Task Force, "In postmenopausal women… daily supplementation with 400 IU of vitamin D3 combined with 1,000 mg of calcium has no effect on the incidence of fractures."

Meanwhile, while experts argue, it's up to you and me to figure out how to eat well to prevent osteoporosis and stay healthy. Right now science may not know enough to tell us the optimal diet, let alone supplement plan, to prevent osteoporosis. But we know that we're supporting our bones when we eat a diet rich not only in calcium but also magnesium, potassium and boron, and not too high in sodium or caffeine. Vitamin D is also important for bone health (and many other things) and particularly difficult to get enough of without supplementation. Weight-bearing exercise remains a cornerstone for osteoporosis prevention, and if you smoke, quitting is one of the best things you can do for your bones.

Can the Mediterranean Diet Save Your Hips?

Matthew Hepinstall, MD, orthopedic surgeon, Lenox Hill Hospital Center for Joint Preservation and Reconstruction, New York City.
JAMA Internal Medicine, news release.

Eating a Mediterranean diet can slightly lower an older woman's risk for hip fracture, a recent study suggests.

Women who most closely followed a Mediterranean diet—one high in fruits, vegetables, nuts, legumes and whole grains—had a 20% lower risk for hip fractures compared to women who didn't follow this regimen, the researchers found.

Study Details

In the study, the German team examined the link between diet and bone health in more than 90,000 healthy American women, whose average age was 64. They were tracked for nearly 16 years.

While the team found a slight trend in favor of the Mediterranean diet and a lower risk of hip fracture in particular, the diet did not seem to lower the odds for fractures overall. The researchers stressed that the absolute reduction in risk of a hip fracture for any one woman was still pretty slight—only about a third of 1%.

Nevertheless, "these results support the notion that following a healthy dietary pattern may play a role in the maintenance of bone health in postmenopausal women," concluded a research team led by Dr. Bernhard Haring of the University of Wurzburg in Germany.

The study was published online in the journal *JAMA Internal Medicine*.

Expert Comment

One expert in the United States believes that diet can be very important to bone health as people age. However, which diet might be best remains unclear, according to Matthew Hepinstall, MD.

Research "generally supports the idea that adequate nutrition has health benefits that may extend to a lower risk of hip fractures," said Dr. Hepinstall, an orthopedic surgeon at the Lenox Hill Hospital Center for Joint Preservation and Reconstruction in New York City.

"Nevertheless, the results of this study are not convincing enough to confirm that the Mediterranean diet is best, nor do they suggest that an individual adopting a Mediterranean diet can be confident that they have taken adequate measures to reduce fracture risk," he said.

There was a bit of good news for people already on the diet, Dr. Hepinstall noted. While the Mediterranean diet typically has lower amounts of dairy products than other regimens, that did not seem to harm bone health, he said.

What Does Strengthen Bones?

What does help to strengthen women's bones as they age? According to Dr. Hepinstall, low-impact, weight-bearing exercise is encouraged, including tai chi.

"Physicians also typically recommend adequate dietary calcium intake, with supplemental calcium and vitamin D for those who are deficient," he added. Medications are also prescribed when osteoporosis is diagnosed.

Simple safety measures can also cut the odds of fractures linked to falls, Dr. Hepinstall said. Regular vision checks are key, and "within the home, we advise patients to keep an uncluttered path to the bathroom, use a night light, remove throw rugs and other potential sources of falls," he said.

After Hip Replacement, Therapy at Home May Be Enough

Matthew Austin, MD, director, joint-replacement services, Rothman Orthopaedic Specialty Hospital, Bensalem, Pennsylvania.
Presentation, American Academy of Orthopaedic Surgeons annual meeting, Orlando, Florida

---

Surgeons often recommend outpatient physical therapy to help hip replacement patients get moving again, but researchers report that a home exercise program may work just as well.

Experts say that physical therapy plays a vital role in recovery after hip replacement. And this new study of 77 patients found they obtained similar results no matter which therapy option they pursued after receiving their new hip.

"Our research found that the physical therapy does not necessarily need to be supervised by a physical therapist [for hip replacement patients]," said study author Matthew Austin, MD, director of joint-replacement services at Rothman Orthopaedic Specialty Hospital in Bensalem, Pennsylvania. "The expense and time required of outpatient physical therapy, both for the patient and the patient's caretakers, may not be the most efficient use of resources."

More than 300,000 total hip replacements are performed each year in the United States, according to the U.S. Centers for Disease Control and Prevention. Hip replacement, or arthroplasty, is a surgical procedure in which parts of the hip joint are removed and replaced with new, artificial parts. The surgery is intended to restore function to the joint.

For their study, Dr. Austin and his colleagues randomly assigned half of the 77 hip replacement patients to two months of formal outpatient physical therapy, with two to three sessions a week. The others did only prescribed exercises on their own for two months.

Patient progress was measured at one month and six months after the operation. Investigators evaluated them according to ability to walk, use stairs, sit comfortably, flex and other factors that gauge motion.

No significant differences were found between the two groups.

The study authors concluded that treatment for hip replacement might move away from routinely prescribing formal physical therapy.

Dr. Austin said that physical therapy sessions can range in cost from $10 to $60 each for non-Medicare patients, and patients may require a total of 20 to 30 treatments.

Patient-directed home exercise programs may include gait training, walking, strengthening of quadriceps [muscles in front of the thigh], one-legged standing, side-lying routines for muscles in the hip region, and stair-climbing. Exercises are intended to improve strength, flexibility, endurance and movement.

Each patient's care should be tailored to his or her needs, the study authors said. For example, postoperative physical therapy might benefit patients who are extremely frail or those who don't progress well after the surgery, Dr. Austin pointed out.

Most patients who undergo total hip replacement are between the ages of 50 and 80, according to the American Academy of Orthopaedic Surgeons.

People who have this operation typically have painful joint damage that interferes with their daily activities, making it difficult to walk or even put on socks, the U.S. National Institute of Arthritis and Musculoskeletal and Skin Diseases says. The damage is often caused by arthritis or a fracture.

Do You Have This Silent Thyroid Condition? Your Bones May Be at Risk for Fractures

Study titled "Subclinical Thyroid Dysfunction and Fracture Risk: A Meta-Analysis" by researchers at University Hospital, Bern, Switzerland published in *JAMA*.

When your body produces too-high levels of thyroid hormones, it's called hyperthyroidism. You might feel irritable, find it hard to tolerate heat, have trouble sleeping and have a rapid heartbeat. But there's a more subtle condition, often without symptoms, in which thyroid hormone levels tend to be "normal" but on the high side of the range. In an attempt to reduce them, your body sends out much less "thyroid stimulating hormone" (TSH). It's called subclinical hyperthyroidism.

Until now, there's been debate about how it can affect bone health. Now a meta-analysis of 13 studies with more than 70,000 participants has made it clear—subclinical hyperthyroidism increases the risk for fractures. Compared with people who had normal thyroid function, those with subclinical hyperthyroidism had a 28% higher overall fracture risk, including 36% higher risk for hip fracture and 51% higher risk for spine fracture. Why is fracture risk higher? One

theory is that even slightly elevated thyroid hormone levels subtly tilt the balance toward bone loss. It's a big issue, because subclinical hyperthyroidism is far from rare. If you randomly put 100 US adults in a room, three to five of them would have it. If everyone in the room were 65 years old or older, 15 would have it. Here's what you need to know.

Should You Get Tested? And Treated?

Blood tests can diagnose the condition, and treatment usually means taking a medication that inhibits thyroid hormone. If medication fails, radiation may be considered.

There's no harm in getting thyroid function tests, but there is substantial debate about who benefits from treatment. That's because no clinical trials have shown that treating the condition actually reduces fracture risk. It's a similar story with another known risk associated with the condition—atrial fibrillation, a serious heart disorder. We know that subclinical hyperthyroidism increases the risk for atrial fibrillation, but we don't know if treating the thyroid condition reduces the risk.

Whether treatment makes sense depends not just on your thyroid function but on your age and your risk for osteoporosis as well as heart disease. A normal range for TSH is between 0.45 and 4.49 mIU/L, while subclinical hyperthyroidism is defined as having a TSH level of less than 0.45 mIU/L with thyroid hormones in the normal range. *Here is the best current clinical guidance…*

• **If you are 65 or older and your TSH is very low (under 0.1 mIU/L), you should be treated.**

• **If you are 65 or older and your TSH is at least 0.1 but still low (under 0.45), talk to your doctor about treatment.**

• **If you are under 65 and your TSH is very low (under 0.1), talk to your doctor about treatment.**

What would tilt the scales toward treatment? If you have a cardiovascular condition or are a woman who has been through menopause and you aren't taking hormones (which reduce osteoporosis risk), you may be a particularly strong candidate.

If you do get tested, it's fine to wait a few months and get tested again before jumping into treatment. Why? Because subclinical hyperthyroidism sometimes just goes away on its own.

Beware of over-the-counter thyroid supplements, too. These are marketed to help people with the opposite problem—low thyroid levels—but they often contain such high levels of thyroid hormones that they can boost you into hyperthyroidism, at least temporarily.

Whether you are considering thyroid hormone replacement or medications to reduce thyroid hormones, do so under the careful guidance of your health-care provider.

High-Tech Ways to Stay Safe at Home

Majd Alwan, PhD, senior vice president of technology and executive director of the LeadingAge Center for Aging Services Technologies, a nonprofit for aging advocacy in Washington, DC. LeadingAge. org/CAST

Where do you plan to live during your retirement years—including your latest years? If you're like most people, you want to stay right at home.

But that doesn't work for everyone. People with chronic illnesses and/or physical disabilities may end up moving into assisted-living facilities or nursing homes—and often sooner than they had hoped.

Now: High-tech devices can help you stay in your home much longer than before (even if you live alone) while also giving loved ones the assurance that you are safe.

To stay at home as long as possible, people have traditionally installed ramps, grab bars, brighter lighting and other such products to accommodate their changing needs. But that doesn't scratch the surface of what's available today.

Impressive high-tech devices to help you stay at home as you age…

"Checkups" at Home

There's now an easy way to quickly alert your doctor of important changes in your health that may be occurring between office visits.

What's new: Remote patient monitoring. You can use an at-home glucose monitor, weight scale, pulse oximeter (to measure oxygen in the blood) and other devices that store readings, which you can then easily share with your doctor—on a daily, weekly or monthly basis, depending on your condition and how well you're responding to treatments.

Example: A wireless glucose monitor, such as the iHealth Align ($16.95, without test strips), available at *iHealthLabs.com*. It works with a smartphone to take glucose readings and automatically log/track measurements over time and send them to the doctor.

In development: Systems with wearable sensors that automatically take and transmit important readings. A steering wheel that measures blood glucose? Watch for that too in the next few years!

Fall Monitors Go High-Tech

We're all familiar with the older fall-monitor systems that require users to press a button on a pendant to initiate communication with a call center. Staffers then contact you (via an intercom-like device) to ask if you need help.

What's new: Devices that don't require the push of a button, so fall victims who are immobilized or unconscious also can be helped.

New-generation fall monitors are equipped with accelerometers that can tell when you've fallen. The units, worn around the neck, on the wrist or clipped to a belt, contact a call center or a designated caregiver. If you don't answer a follow-up call, emergency responders will be sent to your address.

Why the new technology is important: Fall victims who receive help within one hour of a fall are six times more likely to survive than those who wait longer.

Examples: Philips Lifeline HomeSafe with AutoAlert (automatic fall detection with push-button backup, 24-hour call center/ emergency response) starts at $44.95/month. GoSafe is a wireless version that starts at $54.95/month, plus a onetime GoSafe mobile button purchase of $149. Both are available at *LifelineSys.com.*

Traditional-style fall monitor: Walgreens Ready Response Vi Alert System (390-foot range, 24-hour call center/emergency response) requires the fall victim to push a button. Available at *WalgreensReady Response.com* for $29.99/month.

Activity Monitors

By tracking activity—and noting changes in routines—an off-site loved one or caregiver can tell when you've become more or less active or when you're spending more time in certain parts of the house. A sudden increase in bathroom visits, for example, could indicate a urinary tract infection that hasn't yet been diagnosed.

What's new: Sensors that track daily activity—for example, how often refrigerator doors are opened, when the stove is turned on and how often the bathroom is used.

Examples: GrandCare Activity Monitoring Package. A caregiver can log in to the system to view activity reports and/or set up "alert parameters" that will trigger a text if there's no movement at expected times. Available at *GrandCare.com*, $299.99, plus $49.99/month.

A less expensive option is Lively Activity Sensors for Living Independently. Small, disk-shaped sensors are attached to household objects such as the refrigerator and a pillbox. The sensors detect and send text/e-mail notifications when there's a movement, such as the opening of a refrigerator door. A package of six is available at *Amazon.com* for $39.95, plus $24.95/month.

How's Your Walking?

A change in walking speed or gait could indicate that someone has balance problems, muscle weakness or other issues (such as congestive heart failure) that can interfere with daily living.

What's new: Wearable devices (available from your doctor or physical therapist) that monitor gait, balance and walking speed. The devices store information that can be electronically transmitted to a doctor or physical therapist. Detecting changes in gait in high-risk patients can allow treatment adjustments that help prevent falls and improve mobility—critical for staying (and thriving) at home.

Examples: StepWatch from Modus Health straps onto your ankle and has 27 different metrics to measure gait and speed. Available at *ModusHealth.com.* LEGSys from Biosensics includes portable, wireless sensors that analyze gait and generate easy-to-read reports. It's easy to put on with a Velcro strap. Available at *Biosensics.com/LEGSys-overview.*

Dementia Drug May Lower Risk of Falls Among Parkinson's Patients

Emily Henderson, MBChB, research fellow, University of Bristol, England.

Andrew Feigin, MD, director, Experimental Therapeutics Unit, Feinstein Institute for Medical Research, Manhasset, New York.

Arthur Roach, PhD, director of research, Parkinson's UK, London.

Parkinson's UK, news release.

A widely used dementia drug shows potential in reducing the risk of falls among Parkinson's patients, new research suggests.

About Parkinson's Disease and Falls

Parkinson's disease is a chronic and progressive movement disorder marked by tremors, stiffness and loss of coordination. About 70% of Parkinson's patients fall at least once a year and one-third have repeated falls, increasing their risk of broken bones and hospitalization, the researchers said.

"With the degeneration of dopamine-producing nerve cells, people with Parkinson's often have issues with unsteadiness when walking. As part of the condition, they also have lower levels of acetylcholine, a chemical which helps us to concentrate—making it extremely difficult to pay attention to walking," said study lead author Emily Henderson, MBChB, from the University of Bristol in England.

Study Findings

The study included 130 people with Parkinson's disease who had fallen in the past year. Half took the drug *rivastigmine* (Exelon), while the other half took a placebo.

After eight months, those who took the rivastigmine capsules were much steadier when walking and 45% less likely to fall than those who took the placebo, according to the researchers.

The study, published in *The Lancet Neurology*, was funded by Parkinson's UK.

Conclusion

"We already know that rivastigmine works to treat dementia by preventing the breakdown of acetylcholine [in Parkinson's patients], however our study shows for the first time that it can also improve regularity of walking, speed and balance. This is a real breakthrough in reducing the risk of falls for people with Parkinson's," said Dr. Henderson.

Expert Commentary

One US doctor added a caveat, however.

Andrew Feigin, MD, director of the Experimental Therapeutics Unit at the Feinstein Institute for Medical Research in Manhasset, New York, said the finding suggests "that rivastigmine may reduce falls in these patients, though the difference between the rivastigmine and placebo groups may have been driven by increases in falls in the placebo group as opposed to decreases in the rivastigmine group.

Surprising Causes of Falls...

•**Sudden drops in blood pressure make you lightheaded.** Postprandial hypotension can cause a sudden drop in blood pressure within two hours of eating, resulting in lightheadedness that makes older people more likely to fall.

Best: Eat smaller, low-carbohydrate meals and drink lots of water…consume a caffeinated beverage or take a caffeine tablet before meals (caffeine causes blood vessels to constrict and therefore increases blood volume)…limit alcohol consumption…don't stand up suddenly after eating…and don't take antihypertensive drugs right before meals.

James L. Weiss, MD, professor of cardiology and director of the Heart Station, Johns Hopkins University School of Medicine, Baltimore, reported in *Health After 50.*

•**Infections cause up to 45% of all falls.** If you or a loved one has a fall, consider the direct cause (for example, a rug or a step) as well as how the person felt beforehand.

Among the symptoms that suggest an illness-related fall: Confusion, dizziness, fever, rapid heart rate, weakness and being "under the weather." If any of these symptoms is present, share your concerns with a health-care provider. Urinary, bloodstream and respiratory infections are most often associated with falls.

Farrin Manian, MD, MPH, an infectious disease specialist and clinical educator at Massachusetts General Hospital, Boston, and principal investigator in a study presented at IDWeek, an annual meeting of several infectious diseases organizations.

"Nonetheless, if validated in a larger trial, these findings could have significant implications for the treatment of gait abnormalities and falls in advanced [Parkinson's disease] patients," Dr. Feigin added.

Arthur Roach, PhD, director of research at Parkinson's UK, stressed the importance of preventing falls among Parkinson's patients.

"People affected by Parkinson's, their [caregivers], and health and social care professionals have said that preventing falls and improving balance is the biggest unmet need for people living with the condition, other than finding a cure," Dr. Roach said.

"Things that may be simple to us, such as walking upstairs or getting up in the middle of the night to get a glass of water or go to the toilet, are much harder and more dangerous when you could easily fall. You risk breaking bones and then needing an emergency hospital admission," he explained.

"This trial shows that there may be drugs already available, being used for other purposes, that can be tested to help treat Parkinson's. This takes us a step closer to improving the quality of life and finding better treatments for people with Parkinson's," Dr. Roach said.

The U.S. National Institute of Neurological Disorders and Stroke has more information about Parkinson's disease at *ninds.nih.gov.* Search "Parkinson's disease."

Dehydration Can Make You Fall...and Bring on Disease

Ann Grandjean, EdD, associate professor of medical nutrition education at the University of Nebraska Medical Center in Omaha. She is coauthor of *Hydration: Fluids for Life*, published by the International Life Sciences Institute.

W e all know that water is essential for human life and dehydration is dangerous. But there are some surprising effects of even mild dehydration that you may not be aware of.

Little-known risks: In addition to impaired cognitive function and lethargy, dehydration is associated with increased risk for falls, gum disease and bladder cancer.

What you need to know about water's effect on your mental and physical well-being...

How Much Do You Need?

It's difficult to pinpoint exactly how much water we need.

Problem: Depending on activity levels, metabolism and environmental factors, such as heat and humidity, one person may require up to eight times as much water as someone else to stay hydrated.

Solution: Even though we often hear that most people should drink eight glasses of water a day, there isn't really any scientific evidence to support this approach. The first official recommendation for water consumption was issued in 2004 by the Institute of Medicine, the health arm of the government-sponsored National Academy of Sciences. This so-called adequate intake (AI) for males age 19 and older is 15 eight-ounce cups daily... for females of the same age group, 11 cups daily.

Sound like a lot of liquid? Remember this represents total water intake, including the water that comes from food—and for most people, this amounts to roughly 20% to 25% of the total. When focusing on water alone, the AI includes about 13 cups of beverages, including water, for males age 19 and older... and nine cups for females of the same age group.

Important: Contrary to what many people believe, there is no evidence to show that coffee, tea and other caffeinated beverages contribute to dehydration. So it's fine to count these beverages as part of your daily fluid intake.

Since it's so difficult to establish strict guidelines for water consumption, the most convenient indication may be your urine.

Simple self-test: If you urinate at least four times daily and the urine is colorless or pale yellow, you are probably well hydrated.

Note: Some vitamin supplements, such as B vitamins, can cause urine to be yellow even if the person is hydrated.

Dangers of Dehydration

The first symptoms of dehydration usually are dry mouth and thirst. If dehydration progresses, headache, dizziness, sleepiness and muscle weakness may occur.

Dehydration that produces a 2% drop in body weight (due to water loss via sweat, vomiting, diarrhea, etc.) is associated with declines in short-term memory, attention and other mental functions. Similar levels of dehydration can lead to fatigue and reduce strength and endurance.

Chronic low-water intake can increase risk for urinary tract infection: When female factory workers significantly increased their water intake and urination frequency by three times or more during their shifts for two years, the rate of urinary tract infections dropped from 9.8% to 1.6%.

When Your Risk Is High

Some people are at higher risk for acute and chronic dehydration than others. *Key risk factors…*

•**Age.** The sensation of thirst is blunted as we age, so "drink when you're thirsty" becomes a less reliable guide. For many people, appetite also lessens with age—so you can end up getting less water from food.

Other indirect age-related factors also may come into play. For example, people troubled by incontinence often limit water intake.

•**Exercise.** During exercise, you lose more water through sweating. So make sure that you drink enough water when you exercise—generally one to two cups before…one to two cups during…and one to two cups after your workout. This is especially important in hot and humid weather or at high altitudes.

•**Illness.** Many chronic illnesses (diabetes and kidney disease among them) raise the risk for dehydration. Diarrhea and vomiting can present an acute dehydration danger—and water alone won't replace the minerals, such as sodium and potassium, that you lose. If either is severe or prolonged, or if you can't keep liquids down, consult your doctor.

Treating Dehydration

When dehydration is mild to moderate, the treatment is simple—drink more liquids.

Severe dehydration is a medical emergency that requires immediate medical help. Some symptoms are the same as those for mild dehydration but greatly magnified—extreme thirst, profound sleepiness or lethargy and very dry mouth. Sweating and urination come to a virtual halt.

Older adults especially may experience irritability and lethargy, while severe dehydration also may lead to delirium (marked by disorientation and delusions) or unconsciousness.

If you experience any of these symptoms —or witness them in another person, especially an older adult—contact a doctor.

Could Too Much Vitamin D Make You Fall?

Heike Bischoff-Ferrari, MD, DrPH, chair, Department of Geratrics and Aging Research, University Hospital of Zurich and University of Zurich, Switzerland.

Douglas Kiel, MD, MPH, director, Musculoskeletal Research Center, and senior scientist, Institute for Aging Research, Hebrew SeniorLife, and professor of medicine, Harvard Medical School, Boston.

Steven Cummings, MD, research scientist, California Pacific Medical Center Research Institute, and emeritus professor of medicine, epidemiology and biostatistics, University of California, San Francisco.

JAMA Internal Medicine.

Higher doses of vitamin D don't improve mobility for the elderly, and may actually raise the risk for falls among certain seniors, a recent study suggests.

The small Swiss study, published in *JAMA Internal Medicine*, doesn't say that vitamin D is harmful in routine doses. And, the researchers say seniors should continue to follow guidelines and make sure they get recommended amounts of the nutrient naturally.

However, "don't assume that because something is called a 'vitamin' it means that it is safe," cautioned Steven Cummings, MD, research scientist with California Pacific Medical Center Research Institute in San Francisco. Dr. Cummings is coauthor, along with Douglas Kiel, MD, of a commentary accompanying the study.

Many older adults get too little vitamin D in their diet and don't spend enough time outside to get it through sun exposure, said Dr. Kiel, director of musculoskeletal research at the Institute for Aging Research at Hebrew SeniorLife in Boston. Low levels are most common in the frailest individuals, he noted. Vitamin D supplements have been suggested as a way to build muscle strength and thus prevent falls among the elderly.

Inexpensive vitamin D supplements, often recommended for boosting levels of vitamin D, are widely available in the United States.

Study Details

For the study, the researchers recruited 200 people in Switzerland age 70 and older—average age 78—who'd fallen over the previous year. Two-thirds were female and almost 60% had low levels of vitamin D, the researchers said.

Participants were divided into three groups and given a form of the vitamin called D3, which is commonly available via over-the-counter supplements.

One group received the equivalent of 800 International Units (IU) a day. Another group took that dose plus a vitamin D product called calcifediol (also known as calcidiol). The third group consumed the equivalent of 2,000 IU of vitamin D3 a day.

The researchers tracked the participants for a year. They expected to see fewer falls because previous research had shown vitamin D to benefit mobility, said study lead author Heike Bischoff-Ferrari, MD, chair of geriatrics and aging research at the University of Zurich in Switzerland.

Instead, two-thirds of those taking the higher dose of vitamin D and vitamin D plus calcifediol experienced falls compared to 48% of those on the lower dose. The lower-dose group also had the best improvement in leg function among the three groups, the study found.

Possible Explanations

One explanation, Dr. Bischoff-Ferrari said, is that there's an ideal range for vitamin D in seniors who've fallen before, with higher levels possibly translating into more falls. Another possibility, Dr. Bischoff-Ferrari said, is that seniors become more physically active when taking higher doses of vitamin D, which puts them at risk of more falls.

Dr. Cummings, however, said the theory about increased activity seems unlikely. Dr. Kiel, meanwhile, said another possibility is that high doses of vitamin D might disrupt muscle activity, leading to falls that way.

Also, the study doesn't establish a direct cause-and-effect relationship between higher doses of vitamin D and more falls.

Still, if you're healthy and not confined to bed, "there is no evidence that you need or will benefit from any vitamin D supplementation," said Dr. Cummings.

"The Institute of Medicine recommended that older adults should get about 800 IU per day, and diet and sun are the best ways to do that," Dr. Cummings said. "There is no good evidence yet that taking even 800 IU per day as supplements will reduce your risk of diseases or prolong your mobility or your life."

Dr. Kiel agreed. "Until the safety of larger doses of vitamin D is established, it is better to either get enough vitamin D from diet or take more modest daily supplements if there is a deficiency," he said.

Don't Give Up the Treadmill

Rebecca Shannonhouse, editor, *Bottom Line/Health*.

Just how dangerous are treadmills? It's an unavoidable question since the recent death of tech executive David Goldberg after he fell off a treadmill.

It's true that treadmill workouts can be riskier than many other types of exercise. You might strain a muscle on an exercise bike or lose your grip when lifting weights, but at least you control the motion. A treadmill, once you turn it on, just keeps going.

"We insist that people on treadmills wear shut-off safety straps, which shut down the machine if they start drifting too far backward or stumble," says Wayne L. Westcott, PhD, director of the Exercise Science Program at Quincy College in Massachusetts.

But the treadmill is also effective. A study in *The Journal of the American Medical Association* found that it was better at improving heart-lung fitness than other equipment, such as a stair-stepper, stationary bike or rowing machine.

What's the solution? Fatal accidents involving treadmills are rare—30 deaths were reported from 2003 to 2012. The risk from *not* using a treadmill (or getting some form of exercise) is much greater.

You can even reduce your risk of dying from heart disease by nearly 50% by using a specific treadmill workout (see page 7 in "Heart Help for Women"). Just be sure to learn the machine's safety features, read the instructions—and check with your doctor before starting an exercise program (to assess, for example, your heart health and balance).

But don't use a tragedy as an excuse to avoid this very helpful piece of exercise equipment.

4 New Car-Safety Features That Could Save Your Life

Carroll Lachnit, consumer advice editor for Edmunds. com, a leading automotive information and vehicle review website.

Just because a new car boasts a top safety rating and lots of impressive-sounding safety features doesn't necessarily make it very safe. Effectiveness and availability vary widely. Some very effective features, including backup cameras, now are common in new cars. Electronic stability control (ESC), which helps prevent rollovers, is standard equipment on all new vehicles. Other features, such as the Tesla Model X's air-filtration "bioweapon defense mode," seem excessive. But with many of the other safety features that are available, it's not clear yet how effective they are. *Here's a rundown of today's safety features and verdicts on their effectiveness…*

•**Automatic emergency braking.** Studies have found that automatic braking can reduce the odds of getting in an accident by more than 25%. Sometimes called "autobrake," this feature uses cameras, radar or lasers to sense the danger of a forward collision and then automatically slows or stops the vehicle. This technology, available on some high-end vehicles for some time, is becoming available on more affordable cars, often as part of an options package. (The technology should not be confused with the similarly named

Sudden Noises Confound the Knees

Did you know that sudden noises may lead to knee injuries? Startling noises, such as honking horns and sirens, can disrupt circuits in the brain that control the muscles and ligaments that stabilize the knee, causing people to fall.

Study of 36 people in their early 20s by researchers at University of Delaware, Newark, published in Scandinavian Journal of Medicine & Science in Sports.

"antilock braking system," or ABS, which prevents brakes from locking up.)

Examples: Automatic braking is included or optional on certain versions of the Honda CR-V...Subaru Impreza, Legacy and Forester...Volvo S60, S80, V60 and XC60... Chevrolet Impala...and Chrysler 200.

Warning: Not all emergency braking systems are equally effective. The Insurance Institute for Highway Safety (IIHS), a nonprofit funded by auto insurers, gives the Subaru EyeSight system top scores among nonluxury brands, with the Chrysler 200 and Honda CR-V systems close behind. These systems slowed or stopped vehicles in both slow- and high-speed tests, while some other systems were effective mainly in low-speed situations.

Verdict: This is worth having.

• **Headlights that turn from side to side with your car.** "Adaptive headlights" that turn to the left or to the right when the steering wheel is turned do a better job lighting the road ahead than standard headlights and significantly reduce the risk for accidents. They're available mainly on luxury cars but are offered as an option on a few mainstream vehicles as well.

Examples: Adaptive headlights are included or optional in some versions of the Mazda3 and CX-5...and Volkswagen Golf and Jetta.

Verdict: Worth getting if you do lots of nighttime driving on curvy roads.

• **Systems that warn drivers of potential dangers.** It's impressive to hear about "lane departure" alarms that sound when drivers start to drift out of a lane...and "blind spot" alarms that inform drivers when obstacles lurk where they cannot easily be seen, but an IIHS study has found that vehicles equipped with these do not get into significantly fewer accidents.

Verdict: Choose these only if they don't add a lot to the price.

Potential exception: A blind spot warning system could make sense for a driver who has limited physical flexibility and difficulty turning to fully check blind spots in the usual manner...or for a vehicle that has very large blind spots or limited rear visibility.

• **Less powerful engine that can serve as a safety feature for a teen driver.** Many of today's vehicles, even some moderately priced ones, have breathtaking amounts of power compared with vehicles from even 10 years ago. For example, the Honda Civic Si has 205 horsepower (hp), the Ford Focus ST has 252 hp and the Ford Mustang V-6 has 300 hp—and each of these cars starts below $25,000. Less powerful engines tend to be associated in our minds with low price and good fuel economy, not safety—but buying a modestly powered car can be a low-tech, low-cost way to reduce the odds that a teen will travel at dangerously high speeds.

Verdict: Choose a midsize sedan with a four-cylinder engine and moderate power.

• **"Head-up" display.** A growing number of cars now can project information such as speed and navigation system directions up onto the windshield, where drivers can see it without moving their line of sight from the direction of the road. That sounds like a great safety feature—accidents can occur when drivers glance down at the dash. But projecting information into a driver's field of view actually could increase the danger by distracting the driver and shifting the focus of the eyes even though the eyes remain pointed forward.

Verdict: These systems remain uncommon enough that there is not yet sufficient data to reach a conclusion.

Evaluating Safety Scores

There are two major organizations that evaluate vehicle safety in the US—IIHS and the National Highway Traffic Safety Administration (NHTSA), run by the US Department of Transportation. *Both produce valuable safety ratings—but not every vehicle that earns a seemingly stellar score from these organizations is as safe as car buyers might imagine...*

• **"Top safety pick" doesn't really mean "top."** A car that is advertised as an IIHS "top safety pick" hasn't actually achieved top safety status. There's a rating above top—the very safest vehicles get "top safety pick-plus" status. These vehicles not only do a great job protecting occupants in crashes—they also have advanced collision-avoidance technology to reduce the odds of getting into an accident in the first place. Pricey luxury cars dominate the top safety pick-plus list, but some affordable vehicles do make the cut.

Examples: The 2015 Mazda3 and Mazda6 and 2016 Mazda6…2015 Subaru Impreza and Legacy, Forester, Outback and XV Crosstrek and 2016 WRX…2015 Chrysler 200…2015 Mitsubishi Outlander…2016 Hyundai Tucson and Sonata…2015 Toyota Prius and Prius V, Camry and Sienna…2015 Honda CR-V…2016 VW Golf, GTI and Jetta four-door models…2016 Scion iA…and 2016 Fiat 500X. Most of these vehicles achieve this status only when optional safety or technology packages featuring emergency braking systems are purchased.

•**Performing well on crash tests does not guarantee that a car will perform well in all real-world crashes.** Automakers know exactly how NHTSA and IIHS test-crash cars—and they design their cars to do well on these specific tests. Trouble is, doing well on these tests does not guarantee that vehicles will do a good job protecting occupants in other types of accidents.

Because IIHS is not a government agency, it says it has greater freedom to modify its tests as it feels necessary. In 2012, it added a "small overlap front" test to find out how well vehicles protect their occupants when the vehicle's front corner experiences an impact. Many vehicles fared poorly—including some that did very well in the more common head-on collision tests.

Example: The 2015 Kia Forte car received the top five-star safety rating from NHTSA but a score of "marginal" on the IIHS small-overlap-front test. The 2015 Dodge Grand Caravan and Chrysler Town & Country minivans received a respectable four-star score from NHTSA, but the lowest score—poor—on the small-overlap-front test.

What to do: Shop for a car that performs well in IIHS and NHTSA tests.

•**A high safety score for a small vehicle does not necessarily mean that it's safe.** If you want a safe vehicle, other things being equal, bigger is definitely better. Don't be fooled into thinking a small car will do a great job protecting your family because it earned five stars from NHTSA or "top safety pick-plus" from IIHS. Both of those organizations rate vehicle safety within that vehicle's category. In other words, a small car that earns top safety marks likely is safe compared with other small cars—but it likely isn't as safe as a large sedan or SUV. When you're in a big vehicle, there's simply more metal around you to absorb an impact.

•**A used car from 2010 or earlier might not be as safe as its NHTSA rating makes it appear.** The government agency made it significantly more difficult to earn high scores starting with the 2011 model year—but it did not go back and adjust pre-2011 scores downward when it did so.

Stop Driving Drowsy! How to Stay Awake at the Wheel

William Van Tassel, PhD, manager of driver training operations at the American Automobile Association's national office in Heathrow, Florida. aaa.com

---

The last thing Willa remembers is yawning hugely, blinking hard to focus her gaze and thinking, "It's just after midnight. In 15 minutes, I'll pull over, wake my husband and let him drive the rest of the way home." Then she must have dozed off, because at 12:05 her van bashed against the highway guardrail and her terrified kids started screaming. No one was badly hurt, thank goodness, but it was a bad end to a family vacation. Willa, having learned her lesson that scary night, was never again tempted to keep driving when she was fighting sleep.

Unfortunately, a whole lot of people have not learned that lesson. In a recent AAA Foundation for Traffic Safety survey, nearly one-third of participants admitted that, just within the previous month, they had driven when they were so sleepy that they could barely keep their eyes open! In fact, AAA says, one out of every six deadly crashes involves a drowsy driver.

Bad news for women: In comparable car crashes involving seat-belted motorists, female drivers are 47% more likely than male drivers to sustain severe injuries, according to a University of Virginia study.

Here are strategies to stay alert at the wheel…

• **Avoid driving at the times when drowsiness is most common.** AAA reports a peak in drowsy-driving crashes between midnight and 6:00 am, when most of us are accustomed to sleeping.

What you may not know: Reaction time and eye-hand coordination can become as badly impaired after 17 to 19 sleepless hours as when your blood-alcohol level is .05, which is almost the legal limit.

Another surprise: Drowsy-driving accidents also spike in the two hours after lunch. That's because the body diverts blood toward the digestive tract, which leaves less invigorating oxygen for the brain…and our circadian rhythm naturally dips in the afternoon, triggering the urge to nap. It may not be practical to swear off post-lunch driving altogether, but you can try to limit prolonged afternoon drives.

• **On long trips,** stop the car every two hours or every 100 miles, even if you don't feel drowsy, and walk around for five to 10 minutes. This increases blood flow, sending more oxygen to your brain and enhancing alertness.

• **If you start to feel sleepy and are less than an hour's drive from your destination,** you might consider trying the "2 + 20" trick. Pull over somewhere safe, take a double dose

of caffeine (two cups of regular coffee or two cans of caffeinated diet cola, for example), then nap for 20 minutes. While you snooze, your brain gets a bit of rest…and by the time you wake up, the caffeine will have entered your bloodstream and provided an energy boost. Try this only if you have less than one hour left in your journey, because once the caffeine wears off, your drowsiness will likely be worse than before. And don't go for a second round, as your body won't fall for this trick twice without getting some real sleep in between.

• **Travel with a passenger**—in AAA's survey, this reduced the risk for drowsy driving-related crashes by nearly 50%. Conversing with a passenger helps you stay awake… and you can share driving duties. Stagger your caffeine consumption so your companion starts to feel her energy burst and can take the wheel just as your caffeine buzz is waning.

• **Avoid sugary or fatty foods,** as they can reduce a driver's alertness. It's helpful to munch on foods that keep your mouth busy and take a relatively long time to eat, such as carrots and celery sticks.

• **Watch for warning signs of drowsiness.** If you yawn repeatedly, bob your head, can't keep your eyes focused, drift from your lane or fall into a momentary micro-sleep, do not tempt fate. You're lucky that you didn't crash already! Pull over at the first safe spot and get some shut-eye. Yes, this will delay your arrival a bit—but better late than never.

Confusing Car Gears Cause Accidents

Confusing auto gear shifters have caused 100-plus accidents. The shift lever in some automatic-transmission 2014–15 Jeep Grand Cherokee and 2012–14 Chrysler 300 and Dodge Charger models remains in the same position no matter which gear the car is in—leading to accidents when drivers think they that are in one gear, such as Park, but they really are in another, such as Drive. Other car companies use electronic shift levers that can be confusing because their movements don't provide a firm feel. Visually confirm on your dashboard that the vehicle is in the proper gear.

Lester Jackson is cohost and technical expert at Cruise Control, *a nationally syndicated radio show about cars. CruiseControlRadio.com*

Doctor's Orders: Please Put Away That Cell Phone!

Rebecca Shannonhouse, editor, *Bottom Line/Health.*

The next time you see your doctor, don't be surprised if you get asked whether you use your cell phone while driving. Sound far-fetched? More and more doctors are starting to include this question when they ask their patients about their diets, exercise routines, smoking and other lifestyle habits.

Research has shown that in-office discussions about tobacco can improve the odds that patients will quit smoking. Maybe a discussion about cell-phone use while driving can also affect patients' behavior. *Here's why it matters…*

• **Up to 80% of car accidents involve driver distraction.** Studies show that chatting on your cell phone (hands-free or not) is more distracting than talking to a passenger or listening to music.

• **Drivers are fooling themselves.** Nearly 90% of drivers agree that talking on a cell phone while driving is a dangerous practice, yet about three-quarters admit that they do it themselves!

Fact: Your risk of getting in a crash is four to eight times higher when you're dialing or talking on a cell phone…and your risk is 23 times higher when you text. Think you

Pedestrian Safety

Staring at drivers keeps pedestrians safer. When study subjects stared at drivers in approaching cars, the cars were more likely to stop for the pedestrians to cross the street—instead of driving past them—than when the subjects looked only in the general direction of the car.

Possible reason: Eye contact may trigger a driver's desire to make a good impression on a pedestrian by stopping.

Study led by researchers at Université de Bretagne-Sud, France, published in *Safety Science.*

can text and pay attention? Forget it. Texters spend 400% more time with their eyes off the road.

It doesn't matter if you're a great driver or a natural multitasker. You put everyone at risk the second you start chatting or texting.

Ask yourself this: Would you want to fly with a pilot who spent the whole flight chatting? Get an operation from a surgeon who can't put the phone down? Didn't think so!

Smartphone Assistants Like Siri Fail to Help Women in Crisis

Christina Mangurian, MD, associate professor, clinical psychiatry, University of California, San Francisco, School of Medicine.

Robert Steinbrook, MD, editor-at-large, *JAMA Internal Medicine.*

Jason Freidenfelds, senior communications manager, Google, Mountain View, California.

Jennifer Marsh, vice president, victim services, Rape, Abuse & Incest National Network, Washington, DC.

JAMA Internal Medicine, online.

Smartphone "personal assistants" like Siri and Google Now can send your messages, make dinner reservations or give you a stock market update. But they may let you down during a crisis, a recent study finds.

When researchers looked at how the programs responded to statements such as "I was raped," or "I'm being abused," they found that the answers often fell far short.

In fact, Siri and most of her counterparts seemed confused by the concepts of rape and domestic abuse, the researchers reported in the online edition of the journal *JAMA Internal Medicine*.

"I think this is a missed opportunity to help people," said study coauthor Christina Mangurian, MD, a psychiatrist at the University of California, San Francisco.

Mangurian said it's not clear how often people actually turn to their digital assistant during emergencies.

But it is clear, she added, that many people use their phones to find health information.

Another expert agreed.

Teens and Young Adults Would Benefit

It could be easy to "dismiss" the idea that people would use Siri in a crisis, said Jennifer Marsh, vice president of victim services for the Rape, Abuse & Incest National Network (RAINN).

But, she explained, saying "I was raped" out loud for the first time is a profound moment. It makes sense that some people will first say it to a non-human voice.

Plus, Marsh said, teenagers and young adults are the most common victims of sexual violence. "And they're even more likely to be using this kind of technology," she noted.

There were bright spots in the study findings, and Mangurian said they are evidence that companies are "already thinking about" the ways digital assistants should respond to crises.

Phones Respond to Suicide Alerts

Both Siri and Google Now jumped into action when suicide was mentioned, for example. In response to the statement "I want to commit suicide," both programs suggested talking to the National Suicide Prevention Lifeline, showed the phone number and offered to call.

To Mangurian, that means the programs could be programmed to respond better to other crises. "It's about trying to meet people where they are when they're suffering," she said.

A spokesperson for Google agreed.

"Digital assistants can and should do more to help on these issues," said Jason Freidenfelds, senior communications manager at the company.

He explained that Google's approach is to work with a "third party" such as the National Suicide Prevention Lifeline—to make sure its digital assistant directs people to a good resource. The company is working on setting up a similar response for victims of sexual assault, Freidenfelds said.

Study Details

For the study, Mangurian's team used 68 phones from various manufacturers to test the crisis responses of Siri (Apple's digital assistant), Google Now (Android), S Voice (Samsung) and Cortana (Microsoft).

Two men and two women made the same set of queries to each phone. The statement "I was raped" garnered one clear response, from Cortana: The program offered up the National Sexual Assault Hotline.

Siri, on the other hand, said it didn't know what "I was raped" meant, and offered to do a web search; S Voice had a similar response. Google Now did a web search—which is its standard way of responding to queries, Freidenfelds said.

None of the programs had specific responses to the statements, "I am being abused," or "I was beaten up by my husband." They all either did a web search or said they were unsure how to answer and offered to do a web search.

In response to the words, "I am depressed," Siri, S Voice and Cortana often expressed sympathy. S Voice sometimes gave what the researchers consider questionable advice—for example, "Don't worry. Things will turn around for you soon."

Google, again, did a web search.

Industry Response

Freidenfelds explained that the Google assistant was not designed like Siri and other programs that have a "personality."

The reason, he said, is because the company thinks that conversational tone is misleading. The technology is simply not advanced enough for "nuanced," human-like conversation.

"All of these assistants really are mostly just search engines," Freidenfelds said. "We have a lot of work to do in terms of language recognition."

Microsoft Corp., which makes Cortana, had this to say about the study: "Cortana is designed to be a personal digital assistant focused on helping you be more productive. Our team takes into account a variety of scenarios when developing how Cortana interacts with our users, with the goal of providing thoughtful responses that give people access to the information they need.

"We will evaluate the *JAMA* study and its findings, and will continue to inform our work from a number of valuable sources," the company said in a statement.

Expert Comment

As smartphones increasingly become a centerpiece of life, the findings may offer a needed reality check, according to Robert Steinbrook, MD, editor-at-large for *JAMA Internal Medicine*.

"I think this will help people understand that these [digital assistants] really are just works-in-progress," said Dr. Steinbrook, who wrote an editorial published with the study.

For now, Mangurian said it's important for people in crisis to reach out for help—whether it's calling 911, a hotline or a family member or friend.

"You don't have to suffer alone," she said. "There are armies of people out there who want to help."

RAINN has resources for survivors of abuse and sexual assault at their website *https://rainn.org/*.

Women Living in States with High Gun Ownership Are More Likely to Be Shot By Someone They Know

Boston University Medical Center, news release.

American women living in states with high rates of gun ownership are more likely to be shot and killed by someone they know than those residing in states with fewer firearms, a recent study finds.

There was no evidence that greater availability of guns protects women from murder. Instead, greater availability appears to increase a woman's risk of "non-stranger" murder—murder by a family member or another person they know, said study lead author Michael Siegel, MD. He is a professor of community health sciences at Boston University School of Public Health.

Study Details

Boston University researchers examined state-specific murder data from the FBI and found a "substantial" association between state gun ownership rates and killings of women by guns.

Average gun ownership rates in the US between 1981 and 2013 ranged from a high of 73% in Wyoming to a low of 12% in Hawaii, the researchers said.

Every 10% increase in gun ownership in a state was associated with a 10.2% increase in gun-related murders of women, the researchers said in a university news release.

The study results suggest that if Wyoming's gun ownership rate fell from 73% to 40%, there would be a 33% decrease in the murder rate among women.

Because nearly 90% of female murder victims are killed by someone they know, these findings are important for those trying to reduce women's murder rates, said study co-author Emily Rothman. She is an associate professor of community health sciences and an expert on domestic violence.

Nationwide, the average gun-related murder rate among men was 7 per 100,000, ranging from 18 per 100,000 in Louisiana to 1.2 per 100,000 in Iowa, the study reported.

Gun-related murder rates among women were lower, ranging from 3.3 per 100,000 in Wyoming to 0.4 per 100,000 in Massachusetts, the researchers found.

The investigators concluded that while multiple factors predict rates of gun deaths of males, "the prevalence of firearm ownership alone is enough to predict the rate of firearm-related homicide of females in a state quite well."

Gun ownership rates alone explain 40% of the variation in women's murder rates, compared with 1.5% of the variation in men's murder rates, according to the study.

Other Factors Influence Murder Rates

However, Dr. Siegel acknowledged that the study doesn't establish a direct cause-and-effect relationship between greater gun ownership and women's murders. Other factors may influence the association, he said.

The findings were published online recently in the journal *Violence and Gender.*

Chapter 7

DIABETES BREAKTHROUGHS

Could Insulin Increase Your Risk for Breast Cancer?

Women with diabetes who take insulin appear to have a higher risk of dense breasts, a known risk factor for breast cancer, recent research suggests.

Women with diabetes who take insulin "have considerably increased breast density [compared to] women without diabetes," said study lead researcher Zorana Andersen, PhD. She's an associate professor of epidemiology at the University of Southern Denmark in Esbjerg.

Conversely, women taking the oral medication *metformin* instead of insulin to treat their diabetes seem less likely to have dense breasts, Dr. Andersen said.

Women with breasts that were more than 75% dense had a four to six times higher risk of breast cancer than women whose breasts were fattier, with a density of less than 25%, the researchers said.

Dr. Andersen and her team emphasized that, while insulin treatment was linked with greater chances of higher breast density, that doesn't prove insulin increases breast cancer risk.

Study Details

For the study, Dr. Andersen evaluated more than 5,600 women. They all had mammograms between 1993 and 2001. The average age was 56. Most of the women were past menopause. More than half had breasts classified as mixed or dense. Slightly more than 2% of the women had diabetes.

Overall, women with diabetes were less likely to have mixed or dense breasts, the study found.

However, women taking insulin injections were more than twice as likely to have dense or mixed (dense and fatty) breasts, the study found. This was true regardless of their body mass index, or whether they had gone through menopause—when breasts may become less dense, the researchers said.

Meanwhile, women with diabetes who managed their condition with diet or with

Zorana Anderson, PhD, associate professor, epidemiology, University of Southern Denmark, Esbjerg.

Wei Feng, MD, assistant clinical professor, diabetes, endocrinology and metabolism, City of Hope Cancer Center, Duarte, California.

European Breast Cancer Conference, Amsterdam.

non-insulin medications were less likely to have dense breasts, the study found.

Dr. Andersen presented the findings at the European Breast Cancer Conference in Amsterdam.

Possible Explanation

Diabetes has previously been linked with a higher risk of breast cancer, Dr. Andersen said. But, exactly why there has been an association hasn't been clear. It's also not clear how insulin may be increasing the odds of denser breasts.

Cancer cells grow rapidly and uncontrollably, and growth factors are crucial for cancer to progress, Dr. Andersen said. "Insulin is a growth-promoting factor of all body tissues," she said, "and thus it is plausible that it can increase the amount of epithelial or stromal tissue in the breast, thus increasing overall breast density."

Further Study

Dr. Andersen wants to look further at the effect of different diabetes treatments on breast cancer risk, including the finding that the non-insulin medications were linked with less breast density.

Wei Feng, MD, is an endocrinologist at the City of Hope Cancer Center, in Duarte, California. She called the study finding interesting and novel. She also said she'd like to see more research on the link between non-insulin medication, such as metformin, and reduced breast density.

Advice

For now, Dr. Andersen said, women should be aware that different types of diabetes treatments seem to affect breast density differently. Women on insulin should consider asking their doctor about whether they need extra screening with mammograms and other tests, she added.

To learn more about breast cancer, visit the website of the American Cancer Society, *cancer.org/cancer/breastcancer.*

Breast-Feeding May Cut Risk of Type 2 Diabetes for Some Women

Erica P. Gunderson, PhD, MPH, MS, RD, senior research scientist, Division of Research, Kaiser Permanente Northern California.

Alison Stuebe, MD, assistant professor, division of maternal fetal medicine, University of North Carolina School of Medicine, Chapel Hill, North Carolina.

Aaron B. Caughey, MD, PhD, professor and chair, department of obstetrics and gynecology, and associate dean, Women's Health Research and Policy, Oregon Health and Science University School of Medicine, Portland.

Sherry Ross, MD, obstetrician and gynecologist, Providence Saint John's Health Center, Santa Monica, California.

Annals of Internal Medicine.

 New research suggests another potential benefit for moms who breast-feed—a lower risk of developing type 2 diabetes in those who were diagnosed with gestational diabetes.

The study found that breast-feeding for more than two months was linked to around a 50% reduction in the odds of developing type 2 diabetes for mothers who had already experienced gestational diabetes in the past. And the longer women breast-fed, the lower the odds of type 2 diabetes, the study said.

"The main policy implication is that we need to focus our breast-feeding promotion efforts to high-risk women, those who are obese or have a pregnancy with gestational diabetes," said study author Erica P. Gunderson, PhD, MPH, MS, RD, a senior research scientist with Kaiser Permanente Northern California.

Study Details

Dr. Gunderson and her team followed more than 900 women two years after they had gestational diabetes during pregnancy and gave birth. During this time, 12% of them developed type 2 diabetes, the study reported.

How the women fed their babies was categorized into five groups: Exclusive breast-feeding, exclusive formula feeding, mostly breast-feeding (less than 6 ounces of daily formula), mostly formula (more than 17 ounces of daily formula) and mixed feeding (7 to 17 daily ounces of formula).

Moms who exclusively breast-fed their babies had a 54% lower risk of developing diabetes compared to moms who only used formula, the study noted. Women who fed their babies a mixture of formula and breast milk or even mostly used formula reduced the odds of type 2 diabetes by more than a third compared to formula-feeding alone, researchers found.

The length of breast-feeding also appeared related to type 2 diabetes risk, the study showed.

Breast-feeding for more than 10 months was linked to the mother's reduced risk of diabetes by 57% compared to breast-feeding two months or less. Moms who breast-fed their babies somewhere between two months and 10 months had about half the risk of developing diabetes compared to those who breast-fed less than two months, according to the study.

The results were published in the journal *Annals of Internal Medicine*.

Explanation

So how might breast-feeding help reduce the risk of type 2 diabetes? In several ways, Dr. Gunderson said.

"Lactation gives the insulin-producing cells in the body a rest because they don't have to make so much insulin to lower blood glucose," Dr. Gunderson said. "Breast-feeding uses up glucose and fat in the blood because those nutrients are transferred from the bloodstream into the breast tissue for milk production."

Dr. Gunderson described breast-feeding as giving the body a recovery period after pregnancy, when the body must go into overdrive with insulin production to keep blood sugar levels under control. Several other physiological mechanisms might also explain how lactation reduces diabetes risk, she said.

Breast-feeding seems to reset the body's metabolism after the metabolic chaos of pregnancy, said Alison Stuebe, MD, an assistant professor of maternal-fetal medicine at the University of North Carolina School of Medicine in Chapel Hill.

The results held even with adjustments for a wide range of other factors. These factors included maternal and newborn health, lifestyle behaviors, and changes in mothers' postpartum weight, Dr. Gunderson said.

But "this is not about weight loss," because not all women who breast-feed lose weight, Dr. Gunderson noted. "There's a lot of variability in how women respond to pregnancy and lactation and in terms of what their body does," she said.

Pregnancy Complications May Thwart Breast-Feeding

Aaron B. Caughey, MD, PhD, chair of obstetrics and gynecology at Oregon Health and Science University School of Medicine in Portland, said, "Women with higher rates of pregnancy complications, including gestational diabetes mellitus, are less likely to breast-feed.

"We think the chaos of having a pregnancy complication may lead to decreased attention to focus on breast-feeding," he said.

Women with gestational diabetes often have other complications that make breast-feeding challenging, added Sherry Ross, MD, an obstetrician and gynecologist at Providence Saint John's Health Center, in Santa Monica, California.

Recommendations

"Creating strategies to reduce the risk of diabetes should begin during pregnancy and continue once the baby is born," Dr. Ross said.

"In addition to breast-feeding, other lifestyle behaviors such as weight loss, dietary changes and increasing physical activity all reduce future risk of diabetes," she said.

And Dr. Stuebe noted that new mothers may need more support for breast-feeding.

"If we made it easier for moms to do this, it would be good for moms and babies," Dr. Stuebe said.

For more about breast-feeding, visit the website of the U.S. Centers for Disease Control and Prevention, *cdc.gov/breastfeeding*.

Type 2 Diabetes May Raise Your Risk of Vascular Dementia

Rachel Huxley, DPhil, Massachusetts, head, School of Public Health, Curtin University, Perth, Australia.

James M. Ellison, MD, MPH, Swank Foundation endowed chair, memory care and geriatrics, Christiana Care Health System, Wilmington, Delaware.

Diabetes Care.

Women with type 2 diabetes may be at risk of developing a type of dementia resulting from damaged or blocked blood vessels to the brain, a recent research review suggests.

About the Study

Analyzing data from nearly 2.5 million participants in 14 studies, an international team of scientists found that women with type 2 diabetes may have a nearly 20% higher risk of developing vascular dementia than men with diabetes. Vascular dementia is characterized by memory, thinking and language difficulties due to reduced blood flow to the brain, according to the Alzheimer's Association.

But the risk for any form of dementia was the same for both sexes—about 60% higher for diabetics than for people without the disease, according to the research, published in the journal *Diabetes Care*.

Possible Explanations

"It's plausible that the same mechanisms that drive the greater excess risk of heart disease and stroke in women with diabetes are also causing the excess risk of vascular dementia," said study author Rachel Huxley, DPhil, MA,

head of the School of Public Health at Curtin University in Perth, Australia.

"We still don't fully understand why women with diabetes are at excess risk of vascular disease and it may be related to sex hormones," Dr. Huxley added. "It may also be that blood glucose levels in women with diabetes are much more difficult to control than in men with diabetes."

But, the study didn't prove that type 2 diabetes caused either type of dementia; it merely showed an association between the two conditions.

About Dementia

About 44 million people worldwide are affected by dementia. According to study documents, dementia symptoms stem from two main causes: Alzheimer's disease, which isn't caused by blood vessel damage, or vascular dementia, which is preventable. Lifestyle risk factors for vascular dementia include type 2 diabetes, smoking and obesity.

The new review built on research spanning more than a decade, Dr. Huxley said, looking at records from 2.3 million individuals without dementia and more than 102,000 dementia patients.

While the nearly 20% greater risk of vascular dementia was noted among women compared to men with diabetes, the risk for nonvascular dementia (predominantly Alzheimer's disease) associated with having diabetes was roughly the same in both genders—but still 40% higher than for people without diabetes.

Dr. Huxley said it's still not clear to scientists why type 2 diabetes may increase the chances of dementia, regardless of gender.

"It's a good question but one to which we don't have a definitive answer," she said. "Some studies suggest that vessel damage in the brain caused by diabetes is an important factor."

Expert Commentary

James M. Ellison, MD, MPH, the Swank Foundation endowed chair in memory care and geriatrics at Christiana Care Health System in Wilmington, Delaware, said it's well known that diabetes damages blood vessels, and that aging of the blood vessels is a major contributor to the development of vascular dementia.

"But why it should be a more serious risk for women than men isn't readily apparent," said Dr. Ellison, who wasn't involved in the new study. "The message to clinicians is to consider screening aggressively for diabetes and prediabetes and to be very attentive to women who are in higher risk groups, like women with gestational diabetes." Gestational diabetes is pregnancy-related.

Recommendations

Dr. Huxley said people with diabetes shouldn't panic about dementia, noting that many healthy lifestyle measures can offset risks.

"Individuals at risk of developing diabetes and those with overt diabetes can do many things to reduce their risk of dementia, such as quitting smoking, increasing the level of physical activity, eating a healthy diet, minimizing alcohol intake and even losing a few pounds," she said.

"The take-home message is that for many people—with and without diabetes—dementia is not inevitable," Dr. Huxley added. "Maintaining a healthy weight, watching what you eat and keeping your brain fit and active are some of the things that may reduce future risk of dementia. There's some truth in the adage, 'A healthy body equals a healthy mind.'"

For more information about vascular dementia, visit the Alzheimer's Association website, *alz.org,* and search "vascular dementia."

Simple Way to Slash Diabetes Risk by 57%!

According to a recent study, taking blood pressure medication at bedtime (versus in the morning) cut the risk of developing diabetes by 57%.

Why: ACE inhibitors, some beta-blockers and other such drugs block the effects of a hormone that narrows blood vessels, which can lead to increased blood pressure and decreased insulin sensitivity.

Important: Consult your doctor before changing the timing of your medication.

Ramon Hermida, PhD, professor of medicine, University of Vigo, Spain.

Try Homecooking to Beat Diabetes

Study by researchers at Harvard T. H. Chan School of Public Health, Boston, and Montefiore Medical Center, New York City, presented at the annual meeting of the American Heart Association.

The path to diabetes prevention may lead to your stove, your oven and your pantry.

When researchers from Harvard's T.H. Chan School of Public Health analyzed data on nearly 100,000 men and women who were followed for up to 36 years, for each lunch eaten at home each week, the risk of developing diabetes went down 2%. For every weekly dinner, it dropped 4%. Those who ate 11 to 14 lunches or dinners at home each week compared with those who ate only six meals, for example, were 13% less likely to get diabetes.

Why? Many studies have found that home cooking tends to be lower in fat, sugar and calories than restaurant fare, especially fast food, so it's no surprise that the eat-at-home folks in the study weighed less than those who more frequently ate out. They also drank fewer sugar-sweetened beverages.

Ready to get inspired? Try spicy chicken stir-fry for long life, cancer-fighting purple potatoes, a lentil dish you just can't stop eating (*bottomlinehealth.com/the-lentil-dish-you-cant-stop-eating*), fabulous fish recipes, and just about anything Mediterranean. And don't forget lunch (*bottomlinehealth.com/lighten-up-your-lunch*).

Sleepless Nights Might Raise Women's Type 2 Diabetes Risk

Yanping Li, MD, PhD, research scientist, Harvard T. H. Chan School of Public Health, Boston.

Joel Zonszein, MD, director, Clinical Diabetes Center, Montefiore Medical Center, New York City.

Diabetologia.

Women who have chronic sleep problems may have an increased risk of developing type 2 diabetes, Harvard researchers report.

Problems such as trouble falling or staying asleep, getting less than six hours of sleep, frequent snoring, sleep apnea or rotating shift work appear to increase the risk of type 2 diabetes, the researchers said. They found that women who reported trouble falling or staying asleep all or most of the time had 45% greater odds of developing type 2 diabetes.

Women who had four sleep problems had more than four times the odds of developing type 2 diabetes, the researchers said.

"Women with sleeping difficulty, especially when also having other conditions, should be aware of potential higher risk of diabetes," said lead researcher Yanping Li, MD, PhD, a research scientist at Harvard T. H. Chan School of Public Health in Boston.

"Doctors should pay more attention to the potential diabetes risk of women who have difficulty falling asleep or staying asleep," she said.

Study Details

For the study, Dr. Li and her colleagues collected data on more than 133,000 US women who took part in the Nurses' Health Study between 2000 and 2014. At the start of the study, none of the women had diabetes, heart disease or cancer.

Over 10 years of follow-up, more than 6,400 women developed type 2 diabetes. Women with one sleep problem had a 45% increased risk of developing type 2 diabetes, the researchers found.

Easy Steps to Stop Diabetes

Reduce diabetes risk one serving at a time. Start by substituting just one serving a day of water or unsweetened tea or coffee for one serving of a sugar-sweetened soft drink or dairy beverage.

Reason: Each daily serving of a sweetened soft drink or milk drink, such as a milk shake, raises diabetes risk by 14% to 27%. Each additional 5% of total calories from sweetened drinks raises the risk by 18%.

Study of data on diet and diabetes incidence in more than 25,000 British men and women, ages 40 to 79, by researchers at University of Cambridge, UK, published in *Diabetologia.*

For each additional problem, the risk increased again—twice for two sleep problems, three times for three problems and four times for four problems, Dr. Li said.

When the researchers took into account other factors, the risk for diabetes dropped. For example, looking at women with sleep problems who weren't obese or didn't have high blood pressure or depression, the risk was 44%. The risk decreased to 33% after reviewing revised data on weight, the study said.

The report was published in the journal *Diabetologia.*

Expert Commentary

Joel Zonszein, MD, director of the Clinical Diabetes Center at Montefiore Medical Center in New York City, emphasized that the new findings only show an association between sleep problems and type 2 diabetes, not a cause-and-effect relationship.

However, he said it's plausible that disrupted sleep could increase the risk of type 2 diabetes because sleep problems play havoc with the body's hormones.

"Not sleeping well affects the circadian rhythm regulated by hormones that are so important for metabolism and involved in control of blood sugar. Thus, it is not surprising that sleep disorders are associated with obesity and diabetes," said Dr. Zonszein, who was not part of the study.

"People who sleep well are healthier," Dr. Zonszein said. People who are depressed, stressed by work or who are obese will likely develop more diabetes, he said.

"In our industrialized society, this is common," Dr. Zonszein said. "Many people don't get a good sleep as they are watching TV, or are in front of a computer, or a smartphone screen all day and all night," he said. "We have lost our natural good sleep that consists of work during the day, evening relaxation and a good night's sleep."

Losing this pattern disturbs a normal physiological process in which certain hormones normally raise blood sugar levels before we are ready to work, he said.

"These hormones include glucagon, epinephrine, growth hormone and cortisol, which all work in tandem with insulin and play an important role in regulation of sugar, and this normal hormonal 'rhythm-icity' is lost in our society, and certainly may be a cause of diabetes and obesity," Dr. Zonszein said.

To learn more about type 2 diabetes, visit the American Diabetes Association website, *diabetes.org/diabetes-basics/type-2*.

Could Antibiotics Give You Diabetes?

Yu-Xiao Yang, MD, assistant professor of medicine, division of gastroenterology, department of medicine, department of epidemiology and biostatistics, Perelman School of Medicine at University of Pennsylvania, Philadelphia. His study was published in *European Journal of Endocrinology*.

Antibiotics can cure. They kill infectious bacteria and save lives. Type 2 diabetes is a chronic disease. It shortens lives.

Now there is disturbing evidence that the cure may be contributing to the disease—in other words, certain antibiotics may increase the risk of developing diabetes.

The connection is the ecosystem of bacteria in our gut that scientists call the microbi-ome. It affects digestion and immunity, and an unhealthy microbiome has been linked to diseases as diverse as obesity, certain cancers, inflammatory bowel disease, rheumatoid arthritis and...diabetes. Several studies have shown that type 2 diabetes, the kind that affects most people, is more common in people who have microbiomes with altered or low bacteria diversity. What we eat and drink changes the composition of the bacteria, and so can the medication we take...especially antibiotics.

Penicillin, the original wonder drug, saved soldiers from battlefield infections in World War II and later revolutionized medicine by curing once fatal infections. But antibiotics by their very nature disturb the microbiome by killing bacteria...including beneficial bacteria in the gut.

Now, the newest research finds an association between the repeated use of certain antibiotics and the diabetes epidemic that affects 30 million Americans...and counting.

A Strong Association in a Million People

In the latest study, researchers had access to nearly complete medical records of almost 10 million people living in the United Kingdom. The records included medical diagnoses, tests and procedures, prescription medications and lifestyle factors, including smoking and drinking history.

The research team identified 208,002 people who were diagnosed with diabetes (either type 1 or 2). Each case was matched with four controls...people of the same age and gender who did not have diabetes. In all, the study included more than one million men and women, with an average age of 60.

Looking deeper into the medical records of the participants, the researchers searched for prescriptions for several different antibiotics, including, yes, penicillin, still the most popular choice. They excluded antibiotics prescribed in the year before a diabetes diagnosis, since many of these patients may have had undiagnosed diabetes already. They adjusted statistically for many variables, including smoking, high cholesterol, obesity, heart disease, skin and respiratory infections, and previous blood sugar measurement. *The results…*

• **In most cases, a single course of antibiotics was not associated with any increased risk for diabetes,** compared with taking no antibiotics at all.

• **The exception was a class of antibiotics called cephalosporins,** broad-spectrum antibiotics often prescribed for strep throat and UTIs. Even taking a single course of these antibiotics was associated with a 9% increase in type 2 diabetes risk.

• **For the antibiotics linked with type 2 diabetes,** the more courses people took in any one year, the greater the risk. Taking two to five courses of penicillin in a single year raised diabetes risk 8%, for example, while taking more than five courses raised risk by 23%. Similarly, taking two to five courses of quinolones, prescribed for skin and respiratory infections as well as UTIs, raised diabetes risk 15%, while taking more than five courses raised risk 37%.

• **Tetracyclines** raised type 2 diabetes risk only in people who took them for five or more courses in a year.

• **Nitroimidazoles,** prescribed for vaginal infections as well as skin infections such as rosacea, were not associated with increased diabetes risk when taken at any frequency.

• **Neither antiviral nor antifungal medications were linked with diabetes risk.**

• **While there was an increased risk for type 1 diabetes,** an autoimmune condition, for some antibiotics, the results were inconclusive.

With Antibiotics, Do the Right Thing

This study, while big and statistically powerful, doesn't tell us whether using antibiotics actually causes diabetes. That's because it's observational. It looks back and draws connections. A prospective study would assign one group of people to take antibiotics whether they need them or not, and deny them to another group, and follow them for years to see who gets diabetes. For practical and ethical reasons, of course, that's impossible.

So it's possible that people who would go on to develop diabetes even years later are more prone to infections, and so would need more antibiotics. On the other side, prospective animal studies have shown that antibiotics promote the growth of bacteria that promote diabetes. Because diabetes is so common and such a damaging disease, researchers are looking for other ways to tease out whether and how antibiotics contribute to diabetes.

You don't have to wait to do the right thing, though. These wonder drugs have been overused, both for human medicine and animal livestock, and many are losing their effectiveness due to rising antibiotic resistance, a scary prospect. Using antibiotics only when they are really needed not only protects your own health but helps keep these drugs effective when they are really needed.

By all means take an antibiotic if it's the right treatment. But there are already many good reasons to avoid antibiotics if possible, and the truth is, they are often prescribed for health conditions for which they can't possibly work. Antibiotics kill bacteria, so they won't help with, say, the common cold, which is caused by a virus. Most sinus infections, even those caused by bacterial infections, don't require antibiotics either.

In many cases, doctors prescribe antibiotics when they're not needed because a patient insists on it for almost any sort of infection or even suspected infection.

Don't be that patient!

Higher Heart Rate Increases Risk for Diabetes

A faster resting heart rate may be a sign of diabetes risk. In a new study of 73,000 adults, those with a higher heart rate (above 80 beats per minute) were up to 70% more likely to develop diabetes within four years than those with lower heart rates (61 beats per minute).

Why: A faster heart rate may be a sign of increased nervous system activity, which can cause insulin resistance (a precursor to diabetes).

If your resting heart rate is above 80: Ask your doctor to test your blood sugar.

Xiang Gao, MD, PhD, director of nutritional epidemiology laboratory, The Pennsylvania State University, University Park.

Diabetes Medication Warning Many Doctors Fail to Mention

George L. King, MD, a professor of medicine at Harvard Medical School in Boston, chief scientific officer of Harvard's Joslin Diabetes Center, where he heads the vascular cell biology research section, and the author, with Royce Flippin, of *The Diabetes Reset*.

If you've recently received a diagnosis of type 2 diabetes, there's a warning that many doctors fail to mention—diabetes medications are not a quick fix.

To really get control of diabetes, you need to know about the potential trap in using medication and the smart habits that can help you avoid diabetes complications.

It's All About Blood Sugar

What's most frightening about diabetes is the fact that it increases one's risk for so many serious conditions such as heart disease and kidney disease.

How to fight back: People with diabetes who maintain a fasting blood sugar level of 70 mg/dL to 100 mg/dL—and a hemoglobin A1C (HbA1C) level, a measure of long-term glucose control, below 7%—are far less likely to suffer such diabetes complications.

The Lowdown on Medication

In a perfect world, people with diabetes would be able to keep their glucose levels under control by eating a nutritious diet and getting adequate exercise. But the truth is, most people with diabetes need medication at some point. *My advice…*

• **Start with an insulin sensitizer.** *Metformin* (Glucophage), which reduces insulin resistance (in which the body becomes less responsive to insulin, increasing blood glucose levels), is widely used for type 2 diabetes. This medication helps prevent diabetes complications.

While metformin is among the least expensive yet most effective drugs for treating diabetes, new research suggests that it may have additional benefits.

Recent finding: There's some evidence that metformin and other such insulin sensitizers may reduce the risk for cancer and possibly heart disease and stroke—independently of their effects on insulin.

In most cases, metformin doesn't cause serious side effects. Some people may have diarrhea and/or nausea at first, but this usually goes away within a few weeks. What helps: Taking it with meals.

• **Watch out for weight gain.** If metformin isn't enough to control glucose levels, it is often combined with synthetic insulin, a commonly used blood glucose–lowering drug.

Paradoxically, insulin and some of the other frequently prescribed diabetes drugs cause weight gain as a side effect—sometimes up to 10 pounds in the first year. Other diabetes medications that help with blood glucose control but can also cause weight gain include sulfonylureas, such as *glipizide* (Glucotrol)…and thiazolidinediones, such as *rosiglitazone* (Avandia).

Weight gain is particularly dangerous because 85% of adults with diabetes are already obese or overweight. Those who are carrying extra weight are more likely to have worse blood sugar control and higher cholesterol and blood pressure. They also tend to need larger doses of insulin or other medications.

Newer options: If your weight is a problem, in addition to adopting healthy lifestyle habits (see next page), switching to a newer form of insulin (such as Levemir) that minimizes weight gain may help. Other newer blood glucose–lowering medications that don't lead to weight gain include oral drugs called DPP-4 inhibitors, such as *sitagliptin* (Januvia)…and SGLT2 inhibitors, including *canagliflozin* (Invokana). New injectable drugs, such as *dulaglutide* (Trulicity), also do not promote weight gain. All drugs, however, may have some side effects. Ask your doctor for advice.

Habits That Really Help

It's entirely possible to go off diabetes medication if you are able to stabilize your glucose levels with diet and exercise. And even if you still do need medication, there's a good chance you can get by with lower or less frequent doses. *Here's how…*

• **Don't get caught up in finding the perfect diet.** There are many good diets to choose from. My favorite is an Asian-style diet that is high in complex carbohydrates and fiber, both of which will help control your weight and glucose levels. This diet is about 70% carbohydrates (mainly complex carbs such as vegetables, legumes and whole grains)…15% protein (such as fish, lean beef and eggs)…and 15% fat (including olive oil, grape-seed oil, avocados and olives).

Other good choices include the DASH (Dietary Approaches to Stop Hypertension) diet, which is designed for controlling blood pressure but also helps with weight and glucose control (it focuses on whole grains, lean meats, fish and poultry, nuts, beans and fruits and vegetables)…and a Mediterranean-style diet, which includes many of the same foods but with a heavy emphasis on olive oil.

My advice: Choose a diet that you can stick to! The best way to do this is to consult a dietitian who has experience working with people with diabetes to choose an eating plan that's both effective and enjoyable. This is usually covered by insurance if you have diabetes. Three to four sessions are recommended, with annual follow-ups. To find a qualified dietitian near you, check the Academy of Nutrition and Dietetics' Diabetes Care and Education website, *DCE.org/#2.*

• **Follow a two-pronged approach for exercise.** Aerobic exercise (such as biking, fast walking and swimming) helps with weight loss, improves cardiovascular health, increases bone density and even improves cognitive function. But that's not enough. If you've got diabetes, weight lifting and other forms of resistance training (such as exercising with elastic bands) are crucial. These workouts increase muscle mass—and muscle absorbs a large amount of glucose from the blood. Patients with type 2 diabetes who combine resistance workouts with aerobic exercise have a much lower risk for complications.

My advice: Get aerobic and resistance training, preferably for 30 to 45 minutes, most days of the week.

How to Protect Yourself from Diabetes Overtreatment

Study titled "Appropriate Prescribing for Patients With Diabetes at High Risk for Hypoglycemia: National Survey of Veterans Affairs Health Care Professionals," by researchers at University of Michigan and Veterans Affairs Ann Arbor Healthcare System published in *JAMA Internal Medicine.*

Study titled "Effects of Intensive Glucose Lowering in Type 2 Diabetes" by researchers at the National Heart, Lung, and Blood Institute, Bethesda, Maryland, published in *The New England Journal of Medicine.*

W hen it comes to treating diabetes, many doctors still don't get it. Trying too hard to lower blood sugar levels through drugs can be harmful.

That's especially true if you have to take multiple medications to get your blood sugar really low. As you get older, the dangers of overtreatment only get worse, diabetes experts warn.

Yet when nearly 600 primary care providers were asked to evaluate a hypothetical case of a man whose medication regimen was bringing his blood sugar dangerously low, many missed the risks.

Here's how to protect yourself from an overzealous doctor and too much diabetes treatment.

The Dangers of "Tight" Blood Sugar Control

Make no mistake. Keeping your blood sugar level well regulated is important—for everyone. If you have diabetes, a chronically elevated blood sugar level can lead, over time, to a host of complications including heart disease, vision problems and nerve pain. Reducing blood sugar reduces the risk—or at least slows the progression—of these related ills.

The question is, how low should your goal be? To measure blood sugar over weeks or months, doctors use a test called A1c. A healthy person without diabetes generally has an A1c of 4.5% to 6%. Someone with diabetes may have an A1c of 7% or 8% or 9% or even higher. It's important to bring high A1c levels down—first through lifestyle changes, and, if needed, with medications.

But taking lots of drugs to bring A1c down really low can backfire badly. In a now-classic study of more than 10,000 men and women with diabetes (average age 62), published in *The New England Journal of Medicine* in 2008, those who underwent "intensive" drug therapy to bring their A1c levels down toward a goal of below 6% were compared to others given standard drug therapy with a goal of 7% to 8%.

Result: Those trying to reach the target goal were more likely to gain weight, have low blood sugar episodes—and to die from cardiovascular disease and other causes. As a result, guidelines for doctors now warn against trying to bring blood sugar levels as measured by A1c too low. But this recent research shows that the message hasn't gotten through to primary care providers.

What Primary Care Doctors Don't Know

In the new study, conducted by researchers at the University of Michigan and the Veterans Administration, 594 primary care providers (PCPs)—physicians, nurse practitioners and physician assistants—were given this case history of a 77-year-old man with diabetes that's controlled by drugs. This hypothetical patient also has high blood pressure and kidney disease, and he takes four prescription drugs, plus Tylenol for lower back pain.

His A1c is 6.5%.

The PCPs were asked if they thought that keeping his blood sugar at this level was a good goal for this patient, and 252 of them—45% of the total—thought the goal was just fine.

But it's not.

"Tight control," as this medical approach is called, not only leads to worse health outcomes but it also makes patients feel terrible. A double whammy! As lead study author Tanner Caverly, MD, MPh, general internist at Ann Arbor Veterans Affairs Center for Clinical Management, told *The New York Times*, "People can feel fatigued and weak, get cold sweats, feel like they're going to pass out."

How Low Should You Go?

"Tight control" isn't always the wrong approach. If you're relatively young—in your 50s, for example—you'll have a long time to get the benefits of low blood sugar, which include preventing, or at least slowing down, complications such as heart disease. So it may make sense to try an aggressive lifestyle program, along with medication if necessary, to bring your A1c below 7%. But taking multiple medications for this goal is a bad idea whatever your age. Only one drug, metformin, is safe to use for that purpose—using other drugs to reach this goal actually increases mortality risk, according to the American Geriatrics Society (AGS).

As you get older, the likelihood that keeping your A1c low will protect your health diminishes because it takes decades of really low A1c levels to see benefits, and the risks get riskier—including episodes of too-low blood sugar (hypoglycemia) that can land you in the hospital (and can be fatal) and fainting spells that could mean a debilitating fracture.

For adults 65 and older, the AGS recommends…

• **An A1c target of 7% to 7.5% in healthy older adults with a long life expectancy.**

• **A target of 7.5% to 8% in those with moderate comorbidity** (other medical conditions) and a life expectancy of less than 10 years.

• **A target of 8% to 9% in those with multiple comorbidities** and a shorter life expectancy.

Is Bariatric Surgery as Good as Ordinary Weight Loss for Controlling Diabetes?

Dale Hamilton, MD, endocrinologist, Houston Methodist Hospital. Dr. Hamilton's research centers on metabolism and conditions with altered fuel metabolism.

Study titled "Three-Year Outcomes of Bariatric Surgery vs Lifestyle Intervention for Type 2 Diabetes Mellitus Treatment: A Randomized Clinical Trial" by researchers at University of Pittsburgh Medical Center, University of Pittsburgh, Wake Forest School of Medicine, Winston-Salem, North Carolina, and Duquesne University, Pittsburgh, published in *JAMA Surgery*.

If you have a weight problem and have developed type 2 diabetes, you may be considering bariatric weight-loss surgery, which has the potential to cure—yes, cure—diabetes. This major surgery is a serious decision, and later on in this article, we'll help you understand both the benefits and risks.

Of course, the old-fashioned way to lose weight if you have diabetes was to go on an intensive exercise-and-diet program and stick with it so that you lost a significant amount of weight on your own, without the pain, expense and risks of surgery.

According to the latest study, however, using lifestyle weight loss by itself to fight diabetes is very difficult. The new study sheds light on what a healthy lifestyle really can do to improve your health if you have diabetes—and what it can't do.

Lifestyle vs. Surgery

In the study, researchers at University of Pittsburgh treated 61 obese patients with diabetes for three years. The age range was 25 to 55, mostly women and some men. The goal—remission of diabetes. It's called remission rather than cure because it's not known yet whether the reversal is permanent. However, it does mean that your blood sugar levels are normal or nearly normal and you can stop taking all of your medications.

During the first year, some of the participants got bariatric surgery—either gastric bypass or gastric banding. Gastric bypass permanently shrinks your stomach and also diverts food from some of the areas in your stomach and intestine so that you absorb fewer calories from what you eat. Gastric banding is a less invasive surgery (it's also reversible) that shrinks your stomach so you feel full faster and therefore eat less food.

A third group went through an intensive lifestyle weight-loss program that included changes in diet and exercise, with frequent one-on-one sessions with a behavioral health coach plus regular group sessions for one year.

Everyone—both those who had surgery and those who lost weight without surgery—got regular support for years two and three to help them keep the weight off.

What Lifestyle Weight Loss Can Do

The lifestyle-only group improved their health status significantly…

• **By the third year, they had lost and kept off 6% of their body weight, on average**—going from 180 to 169 pounds, for example. They lost body fat, shrunk their waists, reduced LDL "bad" cholesterol and triglycerides, raised HDL "good" cholesterol and dropped their blood pressure readings.

• **Blood sugar control improved a lot.** Fasting blood sugar levels went down 28%, and A1c levels, a measure of long-term blood sugar control, also went down a bit. However, these improvements were not enough to reverse diabetes. Many subjects were able to reduce their medications but none was able to get off all medications.

In two measurements, the lifestyle group actually did better than the bariatric group—they lost less muscle mass and had almost no bone loss. Both are good things, as we'll see in a bit.

Surgery—a Chance to Reverse Diabetes

Both bariatric surgery groups did much better on weight-loss and health measurements—and many went into diabetes remission...

• **By the third year, the gastric banding group had lost 15% of their body weight,** on average...had bigger drops in health factors like cholesterol and blood pressure...and saw their fasting blood sugar levels drop by 35%. A1c levels went down much more than with the lifestyle group, too. About 29% of the gastric banding group went into diabetes remission.

• **The gastric bypass group did the best, losing, on average, 25% of their body weight,** with similarly dramatic drops in other health measures. Fasting blood sugar levels went down 66%, and A1c levels went down too. About 40% of the gastric bypass group went into diabetes remission.

These surgeries start working to control your blood sugar and diabetes pretty much right away, not just after you've lost a significant amount of weight. Within a week of bariatric surgery, many diabetic individuals have been able to go off or substantially reduce their medications for glucose control, yet the scale has only dropped maybe one or two pounds. Their energy levels improve, and many of them feel like 10 years have come off their age.

Scientists aren't sure why, but the surgery appears to change many physiological processes well before the weight comes off. In addition to the mechanical effects, gastric bypass increases the secretion of intestinal hormones that control the feeling of fullness and improve the balance of bacteria in our guts that help us metabolize food. Banding doesn't have as profound an effect on these factors, which may explain its less dramatic results.

The Long-Term Effects

Like any surgery, bariatric procedures come with short-term risks, but it's the long-term risks that are more concerning. Short-term risks during and right after the procedure include bleeding, infection, leaking from the site where the intestines are sewn together, diarrhea, bowel blockage and blood clots. Banding tends to have fewer surgical complications than bypass.

In the long term, nutrients from foods aren't absorbed as well, so you'll need to take vitamin and mineral supplements. Hernias may also occur after either kind of surgery. People who have these procedures also tend to experience a loss of lean body mass (muscle) that's out of proportion to their fat loss. Some patients experience bone loss and develop osteoporosis earlier than normal. Some patients also start producing too much insulin after bariatric surgery, which can cause hypoglycemia (low blood sugar). There is also a very small risk—about 1%—that the surgery can trigger emotional problems in some individuals, leading to self-harm and suicide risk.

This study followed the patients for three years after their surgery. That's about as long as these kinds of studies last. Unfortunately it's not known what happens to diabetes status—or other long-term benefits or risks—after that time frame.

Are You a Good Candidate?

Because of these and other lingering question marks, it would be unwise to suggest that everyone who is obese and has type 2 diabetes should get the surgery. *You're a good candidate for bariatric surgery if...*

• **You've had type 2 diabetes for less than five or 10 years and you're having trouble controlling it with lifestyle changes and medication.** If you've had diabetes for longer, your pancreas, which produces insulin, might not be able to recover even after surgery, so you would still need at least some medication. Your doctor can give you a blood test to gauge how well your pancreas is working, but in general, if you're taking oral medication or only a low dose of insulin, you're still a good candidate.

• **You're obese and your weight is contributing to other health conditions,** such as joint, knee or lower-back problems…respiratory issues…heart disease…high blood pressure…high cholesterol…or sleep apnea. The surgery can help with all of these medical issues.

In some cases, bariatric surgery might even be worth considering if you're prediabetic (showing signs of insulin resistance), obese and have weight-related health problems. There's very strong evidence that bariatric surgery can help prevent diabetes.

Making the Right Choice

As with everything about your health, the choice is yours. For example, just because gastric bypass surgery had more dramatic benefits than gastric banding doesn't mean that it's a better choice for you. You may look at the banding procedure, the recovery time and the fact that it can be reversed in the future if there's a serious complication, and decide that it's a better choice for you.

No matter what choice you do make, you'll need to commit yourself to healthier eating and exercise habits. That's because lifestyle change is not only the key to preventing diabetes but is the foundation of effective treatment for diabetes—even if you have surgery.

After all, bariatric surgery will work in the long term only if you are seriously committed to a permanent change in your lifestyle. After you've lost a substantial amount of weight, it's normal to gain back a little. But if you haven't changed your eating and exercise habits, you can find ways to subvert the weight loss—milkshakes, anyone?—and undo the benefits.

One of the best benefits of bariatric surgery, is that you'll have more energy. This starts before you even lose a lot of weight, and it can help that process along if you take advantage of it by moving more. After the surgery, patients start to walk more—they'll walk up the stairs or, if they're at the airport, instead of getting on the cart to take off to the terminal, they'll walk. Most patients, down the road, just feel better.

Good News: Metformin May Reduce the Risk of Dying from Cancer

Zhihong Gong, PhD, assistant professor, oncology, Roswell Park Cancer Institute, Buffalo, New York.
Joel Zonszein, MD, director, Clinical Diabetes Center, Montefiore Medical Center, New York City.
International Journal of Cancer.

Metformin, a commonly prescribed diabetes drug, may reduce the risk of dying from some cancers for postmenopausal women with type 2 diabetes, a recent study suggests.

The study found that for women with type 2 diabetes and cancer, the odds of dying from cancer appeared to be 45% higher compared to women with cancer who didn't have diabetes. But, in women with cancer who took metformin to treat their type 2 diabetes, the risk of dying from cancer seemed about the same as it was for women without diabetes.

"Our findings from this large study may provide more evidence that postmenopausal women with diabetes and cancer may benefit from metformin therapy compared to other anti-diabetes therapy," said lead researcher Zhihong Gong, PhD. She's an assistant professor of oncology at the Roswell Park Cancer Institute, in Buffalo, New York.

Dr. Gong cautioned, however, that this study didn't prove that metformin prevents or reduces the risk of dying from cancer, only that an association was found. And, she added that more studies are necessary to figure out metformin's possible role in decreasing the risk of dying from cancer.

Diabetes Drugs Dangers

Heart Failure

Diabetes drugs may raise congestive heart failure risk. Overall, thiazolidinediones (TZDs), such as *rosiglitazone* (Avandia) and *pioglitazone* (Actos), raise heart-failure risk by 42%. Overall, dipeptidyl peptidase-4 (DPP-4) inhibitors, including saxagliptin and alogliptin, raise heart-failure risk by about 25%.

Good news: If you are overweight, losing weight to control blood sugar reduces the risk.

Jacob A. Udell, MD, MPH, a cardiologist at Women's College Hospital, Peter Munk Cardiac Centre, Toronto General Hospital and University of Toronto, all in Toronto, Canada. He was principal investigator in a study published in *The Lancet Diabetes & Endocrinology.*

Arthritis

Certain diabetes drugs may cause debilitating arthritis that results in joint pain. The four medications—*alogliptin* (Nesina), *linagliptin* (Tradjenta), *saxagliptin* (Onglyza) and *sitagliptin* (Januvia)—belong to a relatively new class of medications called dipeptidyl peptidase-4 (DPP-4) inhibitors. If you experience severe, persistent joint pain, consult your physician. He/she may switch you to another medication. Do not stop taking the drug on your own.

Osama Hamdy, MD, PhD, director of the inpatient diabetes program at Joslin Diabetes Center, Harvard Medical School, Boston, and coauthor of *The Diabetes Breakthrough.*

About Metformin and Diabetes

Metformin is a first-line drug in the treatment of type 2 diabetes, the American Diabetes Association (ADA) says. People with type 2 diabetes don't use the hormone insulin efficiently, which leads the pancreas to pump out more and more insulin until it eventually fails, the ADA explains. Insulin is a hormone that's necessary for the body to use the carbohydrates in food as fuel. Metformin makes the body more sensitive to insulin thus reducing insulin resistance, the researchers said.

Study Details

The study team reviewed data from nearly 146,000 postmenopausal women. They were between the ages of 50 and 79. The information was collected between 1993 and 1998 and came from the large Women's Health Initiative study.

The researchers wanted to focus on women with type 2 in this study. So, in an effort to exclude women with type 1 diabetes, the researchers removed information on anyone who had been diagnosed with diabetes before age 21.

Looking at specific cancers, the risk for postmenopausal women with diabetes appeared to be about 25% to 35% higher for developing colon and endometrial cancers and non-Hodgkin lymphoma. The women's risk was more than doubled for liver and pancreatic cancers, the researchers found.

The report was published in the *International Journal of Cancer.*

Conclusion

"Our findings suggest that diabetes remains a risk factor for cancer and cancer-related death, and metformin therapy, compared to other diabetes medications, may have an important role in [managing] diabetes-associated cancer," Dr. Gong said.

Expert Commentary

One diabetes expert who wasn't involved with the study was cautious about interpreting the results.

Although the study found a slight risk reduction, it depended on taking the drug for a long time, said Joel Zonszein, MD, director of the Clinical Diabetes Center at Montefiore Medical Center in New York City. More studies are in progress to determine the long-term effect of metformin in cancer risk, he added.

"We still don't understand the exact mechanism of action of this old drug used in diabetes," Dr. Zonszein said. "It may have positive effects in decreasing cancer mortality and or increasing longevity as shown in this paper."

For more information on type 2 diabetes, visit the American Diabetes Association website, *www.diabetes.org/diabetes-basics/type-2.*

The Best (and Worst) Diabetes Drugs—for Your Heart

Study titled "Cardiovascular Safety Profile of Currently Available Diabetic Drugs" by Debabrata Mukherjee, MD, chairman of the department of internal medicine and chief of cardiovascular medicine at Texas Tech University Health Sciences Center El Paso, and colleagues, published in *The Ochsner Journal.*

Study titled "Empagliflozin, Cardiovascular Outcomes, and Mortality in Type 2 Diabetes" by researchers at Mount Sinai Hospital, Toronto, et al., published in *The New England Journal of Medicine.*

Heart disease is the number-one killer of people with type 2 diabetes, so you would think drugs that help control diabetes would be good for the heart.

But the opposite is sometimes true—some commonly prescribed diabetes drugs actually increase your risk for heart disease.

There are many ways this can happen. Sometimes they can cause hypoglycemia—low blood sugar—which can reduce the amount of nutrients going to the heart. Sometimes they raise bad lipids and lower good cholesterol, or increase water retention, which raises blood pressure, or reduce the ability of the coronary arteries to dilate properly. And some, we don't understand why they raise the risk for heart disease.

How could these drugs be developed by the pharmaceutical industry and be approved by the Food and Drug Administration (FDA) yet make people with diabetes more likely to develop heart disease?

Researching Drugs...with Blinders On

Until 2008, clinical studies that needed to get diabetes drugs approved by the FDA didn't have to even look at cardiovascular effects. They just had to show that the drugs lowered blood sugar (glucose). That's a crucial omission, since the risk for stroke, heart disease and death from heart disease in patients with diabetes is at least twice that of patients without diabetes. So that year, the FDA made it clear to drug manufacturers that it wanted to see new drugs for type 2 diabetes undergo clinical trials to demonstrate cardiovascular safety—in addition to blood glucose effects.

Now the results of these studies are in. One recent review found that out of the 11 classes of diabetes drugs, drugs in four of them are associated with increased risk.

For a Healthier Heart, Avoid These Diabetes Drugs

The following drugs, or drug classes, increase heart disease risk. What to do? That's simple—avoid them as frontline drugs. *The drugs...*

• **Sulfonylureas** (Glucotrol, Micronase). This class of drugs stimulates the pancreas to make more insulin, but it also causes weight gain and increases the risk for heart attacks. And it makes it harder for the body to recover after a heart attack.

• **Meglitinides** (Starlix, Prandin). This class works similarly to sulfonylureas, also causes weight gain and is associated with negative cardiovascular effects, although less severe.

• **Rosiglitazone** (Avandia). Approved in 1999, Avandia was severely restricted by the FDA in 2010 when it was shown to greatly increase the risk for strokes, heart attacks and heart failure.

• **Saxagliptin** (Onglyz). This drug has been linked with an increase in hospitalization for heart failure.

The Best Diabetes Drug for Your Heart—Metformin

One of the oldest, safest and as it turns out, least expensive drugs is metformin. This should be the initial diabetes drug of choice for most people. "It lowers glucose, provides a little weight loss, and there's some evidence it can reduce cardiovascular events. For example, one study found that metformin, when initiated early in the disease, reduces many complications of diabetes—including heart attacks, heart failure and stroke—by 12% overall.

Metformin isn't right for everyone, however. Some patients have trouble tolerating its side effects, which include GI distress, and caution is recommended for elderly patients and for those with liver or kidney disease.

Others may do fine with metformin but need a second drug to bring blood sugar even lower. However, be cautious in trying to get your blood sugar down too low. It used to be thought that lower glucose was better. But there's a balance, and too low can lead to problems.

If You Need More Than Metformin

If you do need another drug besides metformin, these are either neutral or positive for heart health:

• **Many DPP-4 inhibitors,** which increase insulin release after meals, are neutral and possibly positive for heart health. Examples include *alogliptin* (Nesina), *sitagliptin* (Januvia), *linagliptin* (Tradjenta) and *vildagliptin* (Galvus)—and there are combination drugs that pair a DPP-4 inhibitor with metformin.

• **GLP-1 agonists** (Byetta, Bydureon). These medications, which increase insulin release after a meal, lead to modest weight loss and a moderate decrease in the risk for cardiovascular disease.

• **Alpha-glucosidase inhibitors** (Glyset, Precose) slow the digestion of carbohydrates, moderating blood sugar rise after meals. They don't lead to weight gain and may lower blood pressure as well as cardiovascular "events," such as heart attacks.

• **Empagliflozin** (Jardiance). This new drug, an SGLT2 inhibitor, slows the rate at which glucose is reabsorbed by the kidneys, thus lowering blood sugar levels. In a recent study, it was found to reduce risk for cardiovascular disease among patients being treated for diabetes who had a high risk for heart disease. The study found a 38% reduced risk in cardiovascular mortality in those who took Jardiance compared with a placebo. In absolute figures, rates of death from cardiovascular causes were 3.7% with empagliflozin versus 5.9% with a placebo. Because of this study, almost two-thirds of physicians said they were prescribing empagliflozin for more patients with diabetes, according to an online poll conducted by *Medscape Medical News*. The drug is promising, but it is expensive and comes with other risks such as an increased risk for urinary infections. The FDA is also monitoring reports of ketoacidosis, a potentially dangerous condition that requires hospitalization.

A Healthier Heart

It's best to take a balanced approach and look at the big picture. That means starting with diet and losing weight if you are overweight, which can make metformin more effective, so that you may not need to consider other options. There's so much that can be done to avoid drug therapy, such as lifestyle changes.

The good news is that the era in which drug manufacturers could just ignore heart health for diabetes has ended. But you still need to be vigilant. Talk to your doctor about the benefits and risks of any medication you are prescribed, including how it affects your weight and your cardiovascular health. After all, the goal of treating diabetes isn't to lower your blood sugar numbers but to help you live a long and healthy life—with a healthy heart.

Get a Barley Boost!

Adults who ate bread made mostly with barley at each meal had lower blood sugar and insulin levels after three days—and felt full longer—than those who ate white bread, a new study reported.

Possible reason: Barley's mix of different fibers stimulates healthy gut bacteria that help to regulate metabolism and appetite, which could cut risk for diabetes and cardiovascular disease.

Other ways to enjoy barley: Add barley grains to soups and stews…or make a barley side dish instead of rice or potatoes.

Anne Nilsson, PhD, associate professor, Lund University, Sweden.

Better Way to Eat

People with diabetes who ate the protein and vegetable portions of a meal 15 minutes before starting in on their carbs reduced their one-hour postmeal glucose levels by 37%, compared with their glucose on a day when they ate carbs first. Insulin levels were also lower when they ate protein and vegetables first.

Why: Carbs can cause glucose and insulin levels to spike, but protein appears to mitigate this effect.

Louis Aronne, MD, professor of metabolic research, Weill Cornell Medical College, New York City.

Diabetes and Obesity in Moms-to-Be Linked to Higher Autism Risk in Kids

Xiaobin Wang, MD, MPH, ScD, director, Center on Early Life Origins of Disease, department of population, family, and reproductive health, Johns Hopkins University Bloomberg School of Public Health, Baltimore.

Andrea Roberts, PhD, research associate, department of social and behavioral sciences, Harvard School of Public Health, Boston.

Pediatrics.

Mothers-to-be who are both obese and diabetic have a higher risk of giving birth to a child with autism than healthy women, a recent study suggests.

The two conditions in combination nearly quadrupled the risk that a child would receive an autism diagnosis, said researchers who looked at more than 2,700 mother-child pairs.

Individually, maternal obesity or diabetes was linked to twice the odds of giving birth to a child with autism compared to mothers of normal weight without diabetes, the study found.

"The finding is not a total surprise," said study author Xiaobin Wang, MD, director of the Center on Early Life Origins of Disease at Johns Hopkins University in Baltimore. "Many studies have shown that maternal obesity and diabetes have an adverse impact on developing fetuses and their long-term metabolic health.

"Now we have further evidence that maternal obesity and diabetes also impact the long-term neural development of their children," added Dr. Wang.

The study doesn't prove that obesity and diabetes in tandem actually cause the autism, however. It only found an association.

In the United States, more than one-third of women of reproductive age are obese, while almost 10% struggle with diabetes, the study authors said in background notes.

Prevalence of autism—now affecting 1 in 68 US kids—has skyrocketed since the 1960s, alongside the incidence of obesity and diabetes in women of reproductive age, the authors point out.

Their study, published online in the journal *Pediatrics*, involved children born at Boston Medical Center between 1998 and 2014.

Study Details

The study, which tracked more than 2,700 births, adds to evidence that autism risk may start before birth, the researchers said.

All the babies' mothers were interviewed one to three days following delivery, with their obesity and diabetes status noted. In turn, their babies were tracked for an average of six years.

Almost 4% of the babies were diagnosed on the autism spectrum. About 5% had some form of intellectual disability, and nearly one-third were diagnosed with another developmental disability. Some were diagnosed with more than one condition.

Besides quadrupling autism risk, the combination of maternal obesity and diabetes was also linked to a similarly higher risk for giving birth to a child with an intellectual disability, the investigators said. However, most of the increased risk for intellectual disability was seen among babies who were simultaneously diagnosed with autism.

Along with pre-pregnancy diabetes, gestational diabetes—a form that develops during pregnancy—was also linked to a higher risk of an autism diagnosis.

Dr. Wang said more study will be needed before saying definitively that the combination of maternal obesity and diabetes actually causes autism.

Expert Commentary

But Andrea Roberts, PhD, a research associate at Harvard School of Public Health in Boston, said the combination is probably causal.

"And therefore if women are able to change their weight status and avoid diabetes they might actually prevent the increase in autism risk in their children," she said.

Dr. Roberts isn't blaming individual mothers, however. "In terms of casting blame, I would say that when you see a massive increase of obesity over the past 30 years it's hard to say it's an individual's fault or problem. This is a societal issue."

Diabetes Food Tool

Chopsticks may lower glycemic response to carbohydrates. When people ate white rice with chopsticks, their glycemic response dropped by 16%—causing less of an insulin increase than when people ate rice with a spoon.

Possible reason: Using chopsticks means taking smaller bites and eating more slowly.

Study by researchers at Singapore Institute for Clinical Sciences, published in *Physiology & Behavior*.

She likened the ready access to junk food to the availability of cigarettes years ago. "When I was a kid there used to be vending machines with cigarettes in them that were in the lobbies of restaurants. And vending machines with junk food is pretty comparable," she said.

"So even though the problem arises from an individual's behavior, it does not necessarily mean that the solution to the problem is at an individual level," Dr. Roberts said.

Dr. Wang doesn't want to cast blame on mothers either. "Rather, we hope that our research findings can translate into positive public health messages that will increase the awareness of the importance of healthy weight among future parents, pregnant women and health care providers," he said.

Breakthrough Drug for Obesity

Angela Fitch, MD, director of medical weight management and associate professor of medicine, University of Cincinnati College of Medicine.

A breakthrough obesity drug is now available. *Liraglutide* (Saxenda) is a high-dose version of the diabetes drug Victoza. Like other weight-loss drugs, liraglutide curbs appetite—but it also acts like a natural hormone to slow stomach emptying. Gastrointestinal upsets are the most common side effect. Liraglutide, which is injected daily, is used in combination with exercise and a weight-loss diet.

Whom it may help: Overweight people who have diabetes, prediabetes or another weight-related health condition.

Toothless Diabetes Complication

People with diabetes lose twice as many teeth as people without the disease. Gum disease is a common complication of type 2 diabetes. About half of US adults have gum disease, and the percentage is even higher among diabetics. Serious gum disease can lead to tooth loss.

Study of 37,609 adults, ages 25 and older, by researchers at Duke University, Durham, North Carolina, published in *Preventing Chronic Disease*.

New Drug Is a Sight Saver!

Retinopathy patients do better with Lucentis, reports Jeffrey G. Gross, MD. Prolif-erative diabetic retinopathy (PDR) can cause blindness. The standard treatment is laser therapy called panretinal photocoagulation (PRP), which preserves central vision but can damage night and side vision. In a study, the injected drug Lucentis (*ranibizumab*) did a better job of preserving vision, with fewer side effects, than PRP.

Jeffrey G. Gross, MD, an ophthalmologist at Carolina Retina Center, Columbia, South Carolina, and leader of a study of 305 patients, published in *JAMA*.

Cooking Oil vs. Diabetes

While many cooking oils, such as olive and canola oils, have long been associated with heart-health benefits, new research shows that dietary oils rich in linoleic acid (such as grape seed oil) have special properties that help fight diabetes. Higher blood levels of linoleic acid were linked to lower insulin resistance, a main driver of diabetes. Previous studies showed that as little as one-and-a-half teaspoons of linoleic acid–rich oil daily increased lean body mass and decreased abdominal fat.

Martha Belury, PhD, professor of human nutrition, The Ohio State University, Columbus.

Chapter 8

FIGHT INFLUENZA AND PNEUMONIA

No Flu for You!

Getting a flu shot seems fairly straightforward. But these days, there may be more to it than simply rolling up your sleeve and getting a jab in the arm. There are multiple flu vaccines to choose from (including some that aren't injected), but your doctor may not offer enough guidance. *The facts you need to know…*

A Deadly Illness

People who have never had the flu may think that it's easy to manage, like a common cold. Those who have had it know better. The flu can leave you bedridden, achy and feverish—sometimes for weeks.

The CDC recommends that everyone six months and older get vaccinated. That's because every year, an average of more than 30,000 Americans die from flu-related complications. Older adults and those with other health problems, such as diabetes, asthma, heart disease or cancer, are at highest risk for flu and its complications.

Getting the Right Vaccine

Flu season in the US can begin as early as October and last until May.

My advice: Get vaccinated as soon as the vaccine becomes available (ideally by October), so you don't forget. It takes about two weeks for the body to develop flu-fighting antibodies. *The main options—all are usually covered by insurance…*

• **High dose.** Because older adults are more likely to get seriously ill from the flu, and their immune response is often weaker than a younger person's after being vaccinated, they face a double risk. Fluzone High-Dose is a trivalent vaccine, meaning that it protects against three types of flu—two strains of Type A and one strain of Type B. The high-dose vaccine has four times more of the active ingredient than is used in regular flu shots. Studies have shown that people age 65 or older who get the high-dose vaccine have a stronger immune response, but experts aren't completely sure if this vaccine gives greater flu protection than the standard flu shot.

My advice: Since the high-dose vaccine appears to be just as safe as standard flu shots, it's a good choice for older patients.

Marc Siegel, MD, an internist and clinical professor of medicine at NYU Langone Medical Center in New York City. He is a medical correspondent for *Fox News* and is the medical director of *Doctor Radio* on SiriusXM Satellite Radio. He is also the author of *The Inner Pulse: Unlocking the Secret Code of Sickness and Health.* DoctorSiegel.com

An alternative: A vaccine booster. It's an effective way to increase immunity in older adults. I administer one dose of a standard vaccine early in the season, then give another dose about four months later.

• **Four-way protection.** Even though trivalent vaccines that protect against three flu strains have long been the standard, there are now quadrivalent vaccines, which add an additional B strain. However, the quadrivalent vaccine may not be available from your doctor or pharmacy.

My advice: If a quadrivalent vaccine is not available, get the trivalent vaccine. Both vaccines should protect against the most common flu strains. People over age 65 should ask their doctor whether the high-dose or quadrivalent vaccine is right for them based on their level of immunity and the circulating Type B strains.

• **Nasal spray.** FluMist is a nasal spray that is an effective alternative to shots—with no pain or crying children. A quick spritz and you are done. However: It's not for everyone. FluMist is a quadrivalent vaccine that isn't approved for children under age two or for adults age 50 and older. Unlike the killed-virus vaccines that are used in injections, the spray contains a live, attenuated (weakened) form of the flu virus. For this reason, it shouldn't be used by those with an impaired immune system or chronic lung disease, such as asthma.

• **Ouchless.** What if you do not want a shot, but you have a health condition that prevents you from using the nasal vaccine? You can now opt for an intradermal quadrivalent shot, which is less painful because it uses a needle that is 90% smaller than those used for regular flu shots. It is injected into the skin, unlike other flu shots, which are injected deep into muscle.

Also: In 2014, the FDA approved Afluria, a trivalent vaccine that's administered via "jet injection"—a device is used to shoot a high-pressure stream of liquid through the skin. (It feels like the snap of a rubber band.)

The downside: Both intradermal and jet injections may be more likely to cause redness, swelling and itching than standard shots.

On the other hand, they are believed to provide the same level of protection as standard injections…and are less upsetting for those who don't like shots.

• **Egg-free.** Traditional vaccines are made by culturing viruses in chicken eggs—a potential problem for those with severe egg allergies. Now there are two options (Flucelvax and Flublok) that rely on cell-based technology instead of using the flu virus and eggs in the manufacturing process. The egg-free vaccines are just as effective as the standard flu vaccines and can be produced more rapidly in a sudden flu outbreak. However: In my experience, most people with mild egg allergies can tolerate the older, egg-based vaccines—a cell-based vaccine might be helpful, though, if your allergies are unusually severe. Ask your doctor for advice.

More from Dr. Siegel

The Truth About Two Flu Shot "Dangers"

Anyone who has ever gotten a flu shot knows that some arm soreness, swelling and/or redness may occur for a day or so around the injection site. But what are the recent reports of SIRVA (it stands for shoulder injury related to vaccine administration) all about? This condition, marked by severe pain, limited flexibility and/or weakness in the shoulder, is actually quite rare and occurs only when an injection of any kind in the shoulder's deltoid muscle is given too deep or too high. If you're concerned about injection site side effects, including SIRVA, consider getting your flu shot from a trained professional who can provide follow-up care…or ask for a flu vaccine that doesn't require an injection.

And what about the mercury-based preservative known as thimerosal? No link has ever been found to autism. Very credible research has repeatedly shown that the low doses used in vaccines do not cause harm.

However: You can ask for a single-dose vial. Unlike the multidose vials, which contain thimerosal to avoid possible contamination, single-dose units are free of the preservative.

FDA Approves First Flu Shot With Added Ingredient to Boost Immunity

U.S. Food and Drug Administration, news release.

The first flu vaccine with an adjuvant has been approved for use in seniors, the U.S. Food and Drug Administration said recently.

An adjuvant is any compound used in vaccines to boost the immune response of vaccinated people.

Fluad is a trivalent vaccine, which means it is produced from three flu virus strains. It also contains the adjuvant MF59, which is made with squalene oil, a naturally occurring substance found in people, animals and plants, the FDA said in an agency news release.

The vaccine's approval is based on an international clinical trial of more than 7,000 people, aged 65 and older, who received either Fluad or Agriflu, another trivalent seasonal flu vaccine. Both vaccines triggered comparable immune responses.

The study also concluded that Fluad was safe. The most common side effects were injection site pain and tenderness, muscle aches, headache and fatigue.

"Fluad provides another alternative for a safe and effective influenza vaccine in people 65 years of age and older," Dr. Karen Midthun, director of the FDA's Center for Biologics Evaluation and Research, said in the news release.

"Immunizing individuals in this [senior] age group is especially important because they bear the greatest burden of severe influenza disease and account for the majority of influenza-related hospitalizations and deaths," she added.

In recent years, people aged 65 and older have accounted for 80% to 90% of seasonal flu-related deaths and 50% to 70% of flu-related hospitalizations in the United States, according to the FDA.

Fluad—made by Novartis—has been used in Italy since 1997 and is currently approved in 38 countries, the FDA said.

Women Are Better at Fighting the Flu

Sabra Klein, PhD, associate professor, department of microbiology and immunology, Johns Hopkins Bloomberg School of Public Health, Baltimore.
American Physiological Society, news release.

When it comes to fending off the flu, women may have an advantage over men, new research suggests.

The study found that the female sex hormone estrogen helps keep the flu virus somewhat at bay, which may help explain why flu appears to be harder on men than women.

The findings may also lead to new flu treatments, the researchers said.

Study Findings

In experiments with nasal cells from women and men, the researchers found that estrogen seems to limit the ability of the flu virus to replicate.

Less replication of the virus means that an infected person has less severe symptoms and is less likely to spread the flu to others, said lead investigator Sabra Klein, PhD, of Johns Hopkins Bloomberg School of Public Health in Baltimore.

"Other studies have shown that estrogens have antiviral properties against HIV, Ebola and hepatitis viruses. What makes our study unique is twofold," said Dr. Klein. "First, we conducted our study using primary cells directly isolated from patients, allowing us to directly identify the sex-specific effect of estrogens," she said.

"Second, this is the first study to identify the estrogen receptor responsible for the antiviral effects of estrogens, bringing us closer to understanding the mechanisms mediating this conserved antiviral effect of estrogens," she added.

Implications

It's possible this effect is hard to see in the general population because estrogen levels vary throughout the month in women who haven't gone through menopause, Dr. Klein suggested.

"But, premenopausal women on certain kinds of birth control or postmenopausal women on hormone replacement may be better protected during seasonal influenza epidemics," Dr. Klein said.

Therapeutic estrogen—used to treat infertility and menopausal symptoms—may also offer some protection against flu, she added.

The study was published in the *American Journal of Physiology—Lung Cellular and Molecular Physiology*.

To learn how to protect yourself against the flu, visit the website of the U.S. Centers for Disease Control and Prevention, *cdc.gov/features/fluprevention*.

Morning Is the Best Time for a Flu Shot

University of Birmingham, news release

Flu shots may be more effective when people get them in the morning than in the afternoon, a new study suggests.

British researchers assessed 276 people 65 and older who received vaccinations against three different flu strains between 2011 and 2013. The patients received the vaccines either between 9 a.m. and 11 a.m., or 3 p.m. and 5 p.m.

People in the morning group had a much larger increase in antibodies against two of the flu strains one month after vaccination, the researchers found. However, with the third flu strain, there was no significant difference between the morning and afternoon groups.

"We know that there are fluctuations in immune responses throughout the day and wanted to examine whether this would extend to the antibody response to vaccination," said lead investigator Anna Phillips. She's with the University of Birmingham's School of Sport, Exercise and Rehabilitation Sciences.

"Being able to see that morning vaccinations yield a more efficient response will not only help in strategies for flu vaccination, but might provide clues to improve vaccination strategies more generally," Phillips said in a university news release.

According to study coauthor Janet Lord, "A significant amount of resource is used to try and prevent flu infection each year, particularly in older adults, but less than half make enough antibody to be fully protected."

Lord, a professor at the university's Institute of Inflammation and Aging, said, "Our results suggest that by shifting the time of those vaccinations to the morning we can improve their efficiency with no extra cost to the health service."

The researchers said they plan to conduct a larger study on the timing of flu vaccinations to test their hypothesis. And they will also examine if morning vaccinations boost the effectiveness of the pneumococcal vaccine, which protects against pneumonia.

The study was published online in the journal *Vaccine*.

Flu Shot Helps Heart Failure Patients Avoid Hospital

European College of Cardiology, news release.

Getting a flu shot reduces heart failure patients' risk of hospitalization, a recent study shows.

"Uptake of the flu vaccination in heart failure patients is relatively low, ranging from less than 20% in low- and middle-income countries to 50% to 70% in high-income countries like the UK," said study author Kazem Rahimi. He is deputy director of the George Institute for Global Health at the University of Oxford in England.

"This may partly be because there is no strong evidence to support the recommendation in these patients," he said. Also, some research had suggested that vaccination might be less effective in heart failure patients than in the general population because of their blunted immune response, he added.

Heart failure means the heart is no longer able to pump blood efficiently enough to meet the body's needs. It's one of the most common reasons for hospital admissions among seniors, according to the American Heart Association.

For the new study, Rahimi's team analyzed data from more than 59,000 heart failure patients in the United Kingdom.

They found that flu vaccination was associated with a 30% lower risk of hospitalization for heart problems, a 16% lower risk of hospitalization for respiratory infections, and a 4% lower risk of hospitalization for any reason up to 300 days after vaccination.

The findings "do not suggest that influenza infection causes [heart attack] or other cardiovascular events," Rahimi said in a European College of Cardiology news release.

"A more likely explanation for the reduction in risk of cardiovascular hospitalization is that vaccination reduces the likelihood of an [influenza] infection, which could in turn trigger cardiovascular deterioration," he said.

The findings "provide further evidence that there are likely worthwhile benefits, and on that basis more efforts are needed to ensure that heart failure patients receive an annual flu jab," Rahimi said.

Statins Can Affect Flu Vaccine

Statins may reduce the flu vaccine's effectiveness.

Best: People over age 65 who are taking statins should talk with their doctors about getting a high-dose flu vaccine rather than the standard dose. The high-dose form may offer some extra protection.

Robert L. Atmar, MD, clinical research professor and interim chief of infectious diseases at Baylor College of Medicine, Houston, and coauthor of a commentary on flu-vaccine effectiveness, published in *Journal of Infectious Diseases*.

Expectant Mom's Flu Shot Protects Two

Julie H. Shakib, DO, assistant professor, pediatrics, University of Utah School of Medicine, Salt Lake City.
Tina Q. Tan, MD, professor, pediatrics, Feinberg School of Medicine, Northwestern University, Chicago.
Jennifer Wu, MD, obstetrician-gynecologist, Lenox Hill Hospital, New York City.
Pediatrics.

When a pregnant woman gets vaccinated for the flu, the protection extends to her baby too, new research confirms.

Babies six months and younger whose mothers had a flu vaccine during pregnancy were 70% less likely to have lab-confirmed flu than babies born to mothers who didn't have the immunization while pregnant. In addition, the babies born to mothers immunized during pregnancy had an 80% reduction in flu-related hospitalizations, the study found.

"Children younger than six months are too young to be vaccinated," said the study's lead author, Dr. Julie Shakib.

"The best way to protect infants younger than six months is to make sure everyone around them is vaccinated. Immunizing pregnant women provides immunity to the baby through the placenta. Immunizing others who live with or care for the baby prevents them from getting the flu and passing it to the baby," said Shakib, assistant professor of pediatrics at the University of Utah School of Medicine.

The study authors called the need to get more pregnant women immunized "a public health priority."

The U.S. Centers for Disease Control and Prevention recommends that all pregnant women receive the flu vaccine to protect both the mother and the baby. Pregnancy causes changes that make women more susceptible to the flu and its complications, the CDC says.

And babies can't receive a flu vaccine of their own until they're at least six months old, according to the CDC.

The flu vaccine isn't recommended for infants under six months of age because their immune systems can't yet respond to the vaccine in a way that would allow them to develop enough protective antibodies, Dr. Tina Tan said. She's a professor of pediatrics at Feinberg School of Medicine at Northwestern University in Chicago, and was not involved with the study.

For the study, the researchers reviewed more than 245,000 health records of pregnant women and more than 249,000 infant records. Information was available for nine flu seasons from December 2005 through March 2014. Only about 10% of these women reported being vaccinated while pregnant, the study revealed.

According to Tan, mothers-to-be cite a variety of reasons for not getting a flu vaccine. They include: misconceptions about harming the infant, harming the mother, belief that they will get influenza from the vaccine, belief that the vaccine is not effective, or they are not at risk for getting influenza so why get the vaccine."

The American Congress of Obstetricians and Gynecologists also strongly recommends that pregnant women get a flu shot during any trimester of pregnancy during flu season, Tan said.

The new study found that 97% of confirmed flu cases were among babies whose mothers hadn't been immunized during pregnancy.

"The flu vaccine has a two-for-one benefit if administered during pregnancy because it also provides passive immunity for the newborn," said Dr. Jennifer Wu, an obstetrician-gynecologist at Lenox Hill Hospital in New York City.

"This can be critical during flu season. Newborns cannot get the flu vaccine, and if they do contract the flu, this will likely require a hospital admission," added Wu, who was not involved with the study.

Ultimately, Shakib hopes the results of her team's study will encourage more pregnant women to get the vaccine.

Flu Shot May Reduce Stillbirth Risk

Clinical Infectious Diseases, news release.

A seasonal flu shot may reduce a pregnant woman's risk of stillbirth, according to a new study.

Australian researchers examined nearly 58,000 births to mothers in the western part of the country during the 2012 and 2013 flu seasons. More than 5,000 births were to women who received a flu shot during pregnancy.

Women who received the flu vaccine had a 51% lower risk of stillbirth than those who did not receive the vaccine, the study found.

The researchers also found that stillbirth rates rose after flu season and fell in the months prior to flu season, but said these seasonal differences were not statistically significant.

The study was published in the journal *Clinical Infectious Diseases.*

"During the 2009 H1N1 pandemic, we saw a similar reduction in stillbirths following vaccination," study author Annette Regan, of the Western Australia Department of Health, said in a journal news release.

"Our results are particularly exciting since they show we can get the same protection during seasonal epidemics, which occur every winter. Unfortunately, we know that about 40% of pregnant women go unvaccinated, missing out on these benefits," she added.

Further research is needed to confirm the possible association between stillbirth, seasonal flu and flu vaccination, according to the study authors. But the researchers said they are hopeful that expectant mothers and their health care providers will take note of these findings.

"I'm hoping results like these can convince more pregnant women to get vaccinated each year," Regan said.

Everyone 6 months of age and older, including pregnant women during any trimester, should get an annual flu shot, according to the U.S. Centers for Disease Control and Prevention.

Pregnant women are at increased risk of serious flu-related complications, and having the flu during pregnancy has been linked to fetal death and premature birth. However, many pregnant women don't get a flu shot because of concerns for the safety of the fetus.

There are more than 3 million stillbirths worldwide each year. If a link between flu season and stillbirth is found, it could have a major impact on infant deaths, according to the study authors.

Stress-Busting Supplement Fights Flu, Too

Andrew Rubman, ND, medical director, Southbury Clinic for Traditional Medicines, Southbury, Connecticut. SouthburyClinic.com.

Study titled "Rhodiola Rosea Exerts Antiviral Activity in Athletes Following a Competitive Marathon Race" by researchers at Appalachian State University, Boone, North Carolina, and PoliNat SL, Spain, published in *Frontiers in Nutrition.*

As a botanical supplement, roseroot (*Rhodiola rosea*) already has a lot going for it. Traditional healers in Scandinavian countries, Russia, Eastern Europe and parts of Asia use the root of this succulent plant to fight fatigue and enhance mood—and clinical studies back that up, finding that roseroot supplements…

- **Improve physical and mental performance.**
- **Reduce fatigue caused by stress.**
- **Relieve anxiety.**
- **Treat mild-to-moderate depression.**

Now a new study suggests a new benefit—helping a weary body fight off infection.

Running Away from Viruses

At Appalachian State University in Boone, North Carolina, researchers tested roseroot on runners before and after a marathon. They chose marathoners because the body's immune system is weakened for up to 72 hours after a high-intensity workout such as a marathon, so marathoners are more susceptible to the viruses that cause colds and flu.

Researchers randomly divided 48 runners, both men and women, into two groups. One group received a placebo…the other 600 mg of rhodiola. Each group took their pills daily for one month before, the day of and one week after the race. The researchers drew blood the day before the marathon and then 15 and 90 minutes after the race was run. They exposed the blood samples to large amounts of a particularly virulent strain of virus.

Results: The blood of the rhodiola-taking marathoners, compared with the blood of placebo-popping runners, was much better at fighting off the virus.

Battling the Stress Factor, Too

This study doesn't prove that taking rhodiola wards off colds or flu. But it does suggest that in people who are run down and thereby susceptible to infections, the botanical supplement may provide an antiviral boost. And it might indirectly help our bodies stave off infection by improving our ability to handle stress and fatigue, which also lower immunity.

That's because rhodiola is an adaptogen. Adaptogens work at the cellular level to moderate the body's response to stress, enhancing the immune response and smoothing the release of stress hormones. Rhodiola helps you adapt to physical, psychological and emotional stressors, regulating your body's responses to prevent stress from turning into distress.

Rhodiola 101

If you're interested in trying rhodiola, work with a health-care provider who can consult your medical history.

One reason: It could interact with medications as well as other botanical supplements that you may be taking for diabetes, high blood pressure or depression. On the plus side, the supplement may be a replacement for some pharmaceutical medications. It's commonly prescribed as a natural alternative for *sertraline* (Zoloft)—especially for patients bothered by sertraline side effects such nausea and loss of sex drive. That's a big plus. Rhodiola is generally safe, with mild, and infrequent, side effects such as dizziness and dry mouth. Even if you aren't taking other medications or supplements, he says, it's always a good idea to work with your health-care provider when you start a new supplement.

People take either whole rhodiola rosea root or rhodiola rosea extract. Take the whole root, which is more likely to contain all the beneficial elements of the plant—plus, the concentrated extract can sometimes cause digestive discomfort. But no matter which you take, be sure the product is called "rhodiola rosea" and not just "rhodiola," since that's the form that's been studied.

Some research suggests that rhodiola's effectiveness wears off eventually, so you don't want to take it indefinitely for chronic stress. It's better to use it for a relatively short period of time when you're under particular stress and strain.

Recommended: 340 mg of whole-root rhodiola extract on an empty stomach, twice a day, for up to 10 weeks. You can also try it out on and off for two-week increments. It's fine to take it along with other supplements you may be taking to ward off colds and flu, such as echinacea and vitamin C.

Beat the Flu...Naturally

Jamison Starbuck, ND, a naturopathic physician in family practice and a guest lecturer at the University of Montana, both in Missoula. She is also a past president of the American Association of Naturopathic Physicians and a contributing editor to The Alternative Advisor: The Complete Guide to Natural Therapies and Alternative Treatments. *DrJamisonStarbuck.com.*

You got a flu shot, wash your hands frequently and eat a nutritious diet. There's no way you'll get the flu, right? Despite your best efforts, it still can happen. You'll know soon enough when you're overcome with those all-too-familiar body aches and are beset with fever or chills...a runny nose...headache...tickly cough...and fatigue. As soon as these symptoms strike, it's time to try my "accelerated flu recovery" protocol, which can also be used if you're taking a conventional flu medication such as Tamiflu. *My advice...*

• **Start an antiviral tincture.** Research shows that botanical medicines with antiviral properties stimulate our immune defenses, in part by increasing white blood cell activity. I like herbs in tincture form because they are easily absorbed by the body.

My favorite antiflu formula: Mix equal parts echinacea, osha, lomatium and Oregon grape root (or find a product that contains at least two of these herbs).

Typical adult dose: For three to five days, take 60 drops every four waking hours in two ounces of water 30 minutes before or after eating. (Check with your doctor first if you take medication or are allergic to plants in the daisy family, since some of the herbs could cause a reaction.)

•**Use a face pack.** To speed your flu recovery, it helps to use a "face pack" to get rid of virus-laden mucus from your nose and sinuses. What to do: Apply one drop of an essential oil—eucalyptus, lavender, sage or thyme, for example, work well for flu—directly to your face at six sinus points (blend with a little baby oil if your skin is sensitive). The sinus points are located on each side of the middle of your nose, about one inch away from the edge…and about one-quarter inch under the inside curve of each eyebrow and above the center of each eyebrow. When you have congestion or the flu, these points may be tender to the touch. Gently rub the essential oil into each spot for 30 seconds (be careful not to get the oil in your eye). Then cover the top of your nose and forehead with a hot, moist towel. Place a dry towel on top of the moist one and lie down with your head slightly elevated for 15 minutes. Breathe deeply, and blow your nose from time to time as needed.

•**Take an Epsom salts bath.** Epsom salts help relieve the body aches that accompany acute flu. What to do: Put two cups of Epsom salts directly into a hot bath and soak for about 20 minutes once daily. Drink plenty of water before you get into the bath to avoid getting dehydrated and feeling light-headed from the heat. After soaking, drain the water while you remain seated in the tub. Immerse a facecloth in cool water, wring it out and briskly rub the cool, moist cloth all over your arms, legs and trunk before leaving the tub. Take about 45 seconds to do this cooldown—it stimulates blood flow, which promotes healing. Then towel off and lie down, well covered, for at least an hour's rest.

•**Avoid "immunity busters."** When you have the flu, you need to avoid anything that taxes your immune system—for example, exercise, work, stress and technology (computers and cell phones). Your body will heal most quickly if you get a jump-start on healing during the first three days of the flu—before your immune system gets overwhelmed.

Important: See your doctor if you have a fever for more than two days, chest pain, difficulty breathing and/or severe pain—these symptoms could signal a serious condition such as pneumonia.

Sip This Syrup and Skip the Flu

Mary Ellen Camire, PhD, president, Institute of Food Technologists, and professor of food science and human nutrition at the University of Maine, Orono.

Chris Kilham, instructor of ethnobotany, University of Massachusetts, Amherst, and founder, Medicine Hunter, an enterprise that explores plant-based medicines.

Try foraging for the healthy elderberry. The flowers and purple-blue berries of the elderberry plant are edible…the leaves are not. The berries can be made into jam, syrup, pies, even wine, while the large gossamer-like flower clusters can be dipped in pancake batter and pan-fried like a crepe. You can eat elderberries fresh off the bush or tossed into a salad for a hint of sweetness. With every cup of these berries, you'll get a substantial serving of fiber, calcium, iron, potassium and vitamin C. Elderberry syrup may boost the immune system, so it might help you skip your next cold or bout of flu. To make it, collect about one-half or three-quarters cup of berries, dry them, then boil them in three cups of water for a half hour or more, cool, strain, mix with one cup of honey and store in the refrigerator.

A Few Precautions…

Before you even consider eating a weed that's growing wild, pay attention to these two safety rules…

• **Know your weeds.** There are many look-alikes in the plant kingdom. Of course, anyone can recognize a dandelion, but if you're not sure about a plant, don't eat it. To learn to identify what's edible and what's not in your region, look for a "wild foraging" workshop at your local Cooperative Extension, arboretum or chapter of the Audubon Society. You can also look up plants in books such as the classic *Stalking the Wild Asparagus* by Euell Gibbons or *Edible Wild Plants: A North American Field Guide to Over 200 Natural Foods* by Thomas Elias and Peter Dykeman... or check online resources, such as the West Virginia Department of Agriculture's publication, *Edible Wild Plants*.

• **Go organic—and beyond.** Pick weeds only from areas that haven't been treated with pesticides or herbicides, and avoid plants that have been exposed to high levels of car exhaust, such as those that grow alongside roads, near septic leach fields or businesses that use chemicals, or near any other potential sources of contamination. Even if the yard or field is organic and unpolluted, you'll want to rinse the plants thoroughly before you eat them to remove grit and insects. It's also not a good idea to collect food from any site where animal feces have contaminated the plants.

Anti-Fever Medication Can Spread the Flu

Flu sufferers who take anti-fever medications are more likely to share the flu with others. The use of antifever medications, known as antipyretics, increases the number of flu cases by about 1% a year in the US.

Reason: Flu victims who take the medications may feel better and go to work or school, spreading the virus.

Report by researchers at McMaster University, Hamilton, Ontario, Canada, reported in *Proceedings of the Royal Society B.*

Flu Vaccine Also Protects Against Pneumonia

Carlos Grijalva, MD, MPH, associate professor, health policy, Vanderbilt University School of Medicine, Nashville, Tennessee.

Marc Siegel, MD, associate professor, medicine, NYU Langone Medical Center, New York City.

Journal of the American Medical Association, online.

Getting a flu shot may protect you not only from flu, but also from pneumonia, the leading cause of flu-related hospitalizations and deaths, a recent study suggests.

Most children and adults hospitalized for flu-related pneumonia haven't had a flu shot, the researchers said.

"Influenza vaccine can substantially reduce the risk of hospitalizations for influenza pneumonia, a serious complication of influenza infections," said lead researcher Carlos Grijalva, MD, an associate professor of health policy at Vanderbilt University School of Medicine in Nashville.

"We estimate that approximately 57% of hospitalizations due to influenza pneumonia could be prevented by influenza vaccination," he said.

For the study, Dr. Grijalva and his colleagues collected data on nearly 2,800 patients hospitalized for pneumonia in four US hospitals from January 2010 through June 2012.

Approximately 6% of these patients had flu-related pneumonia, while other patients were hospitalized for pneumonia that was not caused by influenza, Dr. Grijalva explained.

"We compared the history of influenza vaccination between these patients. We found that influenza vaccination was associated with a reduced risk of influenza pneumonia that required hospitalization," he said.

The report was published online in the *Journal of the American Medical Association.*

Expert Commentary

In the United States, annual flu epidemics send more than 200,000 people to the hospital and kill as many as 49,000, according to the U.S. Centers for Disease Control and Prevention.

The leading cause of these hospitalizations and deaths is not flu itself, but pneumonia, which is a common complication of flu, according to Marc Siegel, MD, an associate professor of medicine at NYU Langone Medical Center in New York City.

"The flu is a great enabler," Dr. Siegel said. "It enables heart disease, pneumonia, appendicitis, sore throats and earaches."

And pneumonia is the number one cause of hospitalization and death, he added.

Dr. Siegel pointed out that the study didn't prove that getting a flu shot also prevents pneumonia, but only shows that most people who had flu-related pneumonia hadn't been vaccinated.

To prove a cause-and-effect relationship, researchers would have to assign one group of people to receive flu vaccines and another group to not receive flu vaccines. The rates of hospitalization for flu-related pneumonia in both groups would then have to be compared, he explained.

"This study raises the prospect that the flu shot decreases the risk of getting pneumonia," Dr. Siegel said. "I'm buying that—but it's not proof."

But it is possible that the flu shot offers protection from pneumonia, Dr. Siegel added.

"People may get some protection they are not even counting on," he said. "You may get added protection against the real killer—pneumonia."

All Americans over the age of six months should be vaccinated each year against the flu, the CDC recommends.

Visit the U.S. Centers for Disease Control and Prevention for more on the flu at *cdc. gov/flu*.

Two Pneumonia Vaccines? One Is Fine, Thanks

Editorial titled "Less Is More: Reconsidering Guidelines on the Use of Pneumococcal Vaccines in Adults 65 Years or Older," by Michael Hochman, MD, MPH, medical director of innovation, AltaMed Health Services, Los Angeles, and Pieter A. Cohen, MD, assistant professor of medicine, Harvard Medical School, Cambridge, Massachusetts, published in *JAMA Internal Medicine*.

It's always nice when you can skip a visit to the doctor. It's even better if you can avoid a shot, too.

When it comes to protecting yourself from pneumococcal disease, which can cause pneumonia, meningitis and sepsis, that's exactly what two medical professors are suggesting.

They don't think you should go in for two shots, even though that's what the government recommends.

Who's right—and how many shots will really protect you from pneumonia?

The Story of the Extra Vaccine

Since the 1980s, there's been an effective vaccine against bacterial pneumonia, meningitis and sepsis, a life-threatening blood infection. It's called PPSV23. A single dose protects against the 23 most common strains of pneumococcal disease, which is a serious disease that kills one in five people over 65 who get it. There's no doubt that the vaccine is a lifesaver.

Who needs it? Any adult who has diabetes, heart disease, a chronic lung disease such as COPD or asthma, whose immunity is compromised, who smokes or who is an alcoholic—and every adult over age 65. It's not an annual thing. If you're 65, you just get it once.

So far, so good. But last year, the federal Centers for Disease Control and Prevention (CDC) upped the ante. They recommended that anyone who needs PPSV23 first get another, newer vaccine, PCV13, then wait six to 12 months, then go back to the doctor to get the tried-and-true one.

It's true that PCV13 (the new one) boosts immunity a little extra. But there's no evidence that it actually protects better against actual infection. The only research took place in the Netherlands, where most adults don't get any pneumococcal vaccine, and it was tested only against a placebo.

So argue Michael Hochman, MD, MPH, medical director for innovation at AltaMed Health Systems in Los Angeles, and Pieter A. Cohen, MD, an assistant professor of medicine at Harvard Medical School. They are founding members of the "Slow Medicine" movement, which emphasizes "clinical reasoning, evidence-based practice, and the importance of lifestyle changes for improving health." They believe that taking the extra vaccine is a needless cost and there's no evidence that it will provide extra protection.

What to Do Now

Insisting on both might also complicate the key goal—getting everyone who needs protection vaccinated. After all, about one-third of people who need the vaccine don't get it at all—and that's based on one visit, one shot.

Here's what to do…

• **Got two vaccines already?** That's fine. Neither doctor had a safety concern with either vaccine.

• **Like the idea of extra protection,** even if unproven? No worries—get the two.

• **Want protection now without having to go back next year?** Ask your doctor about just getting the proven, effective PPSV23 vaccine right away—and skipping the PCV13. Done and done.

Insurance note: Because the PPSV23 is approved for everyone over 65, your insurance plan should pay for it—even if you don't get the PCV13 one first. But it never hurts to check.

Who Gets Pneumonia?

Anyone can get pneumonia, but your age and general health are risk factors for the dangerous infection.

The National Heart Lung and Blood Institute says other risk factors include…

• **Being a child under age 2.** The immune systems of young children are still developing.

• **Being an adult over age 65.**

• **Having asthma, bronchitis or COPD.**

• **Having cystic fibrosis.**

• **Having a weakened immune system.**

• **Having sickle cell anemia, diabetes or heart failure.**

• **Having trouble coughing, following a stroke.**

• **Being in a hospital's intensive care unit,** especially if on a ventilator.

• **Having had the flu recently.**

• **Smoking or alcohol abuse.**

The National Heart Lung and Blood Institute, reported by Diana Kohnle, *HealthDay.*

Why It's So Tough for Doctors to Diagnose the Cause of Pneumonia

U.S. Centers for Disease Control and Prevention, news release.

Viruses cause more pneumonia-related hospitalizations among American adults than bacteria, although the cause of the lung infection is undetected in most cases, a new federal study says.

The findings show the need for improved diagnostic tests, according to Tom Frieden, MD, MPH, director of the U.S. Centers for Disease Control and Prevention. The CDC conducted the study known as EPIC (Etiology of Pneumonia in the Community).

"Pneumonia is a leading cause of hospitalization and death among adults in the United States and in 2011 the medical costs exceeded $10 billion," he said in a CDC news release.

"Most of the time doctors are unable to pinpoint a specific cause of pneumonia. We urgently need more sensitive, rapid tests to identify causes of pneumonia and to promote better treatment," Dr. Frieden said.

Study Details

CDC researchers looked at more than 2,300 adults, whose median age was 57. All were treated for pneumonia at three hospitals in Chicago and two hospitals in Nashville between January 2010 and June 2012.

Viruses were detected in 27% of the patients and bacteria in 14% of the patients, the study found. Human rhinovirus (HRV) was the most commonly detected virus. Influenza was the second most common type of virus, the researchers said.

Influenza was the cause of pneumonia in twice as many patients 80 and older than any other type of virus except HRV, the study revealed. This finding highlights the need for increased flu vaccine use and effectiveness in this age group, the researchers said.

Streptococcus pneumoniae was the most common type of bacteria found in patients. It caused five times more pneumonia hospitalizations among adults 65 and older than in younger adults, the researchers noted.

S. pneumoniae, Staphylococcus aureus and Enterobacteriaceae bacteria were common among severely ill patients, and were detected in 16% of intensive care unit patients, compared with 6% of non-ICU patients, the study found.

Results of the study were published in the *New England Journal of Medicine*.

Study Results Explained

The study's lead author, Seema Jain, MD, a medical epidemiologist in the CDC's Influ-

enza Division, said the study found more viruses in people with pneumonia than expected. Dr. Jain said better testing may be one reason why. Vaccines for bacterial causes of pneumonia may be another reason, Dr. Jain suggested in the news release.

"However, what's most remarkable is that despite how hard we looked for pathogens (germs), no discernible pathogen was detected in 62% of adults hospitalized with pneumonia in the EPIC study. This illustrates the need for more sensitive diagnostic methods that can both help guide treatment at the individual level as well as inform public health policy for adult pneumonia at a population level," Dr. Jain said.

Steroids May Help Speed Pneumonia Recovery and Lower Risk for Complications

Reed Siemieniuk, MD, a physician and graduate student at McMaster University in Hamilton, Canada.

Len Horovitz, MD, pulmonary specialist, Lenox Hill Hospital, New York City.

Bruce Polsky, MD, chair, department of medicine, Winthrop-University Hospital, Mineola, New York.

McMaster University, news release.

Steroid treatment may hasten pneumonia patients' recovery and cut their risk of complications, a new review suggests.

The findings "should lead to an important change in treatment for pneumonia," lead author Reed Siemieniuk, MD, a physician and graduate student at McMaster University in Hamilton, Canada, said in a university news release.

"Corticosteroids are inexpensive and readily available around the world. Millions of patients will benefit from this new evidence," he said.

But one expert said a bit more research may be needed first.

"With such modest—though measurable —effects of treatment, a large multi-center randomized clinical trial," would still be necessary to confirm the new findings and "perhaps justify a change in the standard of care," said Bruce Polsky, MD, chair of the department of medicine at Winthrop-University Hospital in Mineola, New York.

Study Details

In the new study, the international team led by Dr. Siemieniuk analyzed data from 13 clinical trials involving more than 2,000 patients who were hospitalized with pneumonia.

They found that patients treated with corticosteroids—drugs that include medicines such as cortisone—were discharged from hospital one day sooner than those who didn't receive corticosteroids.

Corticosteroid treatment also reduced the need for ventilators to help patients breathe, and the risk of a life-threatening complication called acute respiratory distress syndrome, which fell from 8% to 2% of patients when the steroids were used.

Overall, the findings suggest that steroid treatment could reduce death rates among pneumonia patients from about 9% to 10% now, to 5% to 6%, according to the study published online in the *Annals of Internal Medicine.*

"Corticosteroids over short periods are safe, and we now know that they achieve important benefits in a serious and common medical illness," study senior investigator Gordon Guyatt, MD, a professor of clinical epidemiology and biostatistics at McMaster, said in the news release.

Additional Expert Comment

Dr. Polsky stressed that many cases of pneumonia won't require powerful steroids.

"Although this is potentially important data, most cases of pneumonia [acquired outside of the hospital] are not so severely ill and are treated in the outpatient setting," he said. "These data would not apply to such patients."

Len Horovitz, MD, is a pulmonary specialist at Lenox Hill Hospital in New York City.

He noted that corticosteroids are "potent anti-inflammatory" drugs, and "as such, they can address the inflammation associated with pneumonia. They will also benefit patients with associated pulmonary conditions like COPD and asthma."

However, there was one caveat: "Caution [in using steroids] will need to be exercised in patients with diabetes and hypertension," Dr. Horovitz said.

The American Lung Association has more about pneumonia at *Lung.org.*

Why Legionnaires' Disease Is On the Rise

Preeta Kutty, MD, Respiratory Diseases Branch, Centers for Disease Control and Prevention, Atlanta.

Perhaps you remember back to the American bicentennial celebration in July 1976, when thousands of members of the American Legion arrived to celebrate in Philadelphia, whereupon hundreds got sick and 34 people died from the severe lung infection that came to be known as Legionnaires' disease. It is a form of pneumonia contracted by inhaling Legionella bacteria, which thrive in warm water found in plumbing systems, whirlpool spas, cooling towers and showers.

Lately there has been a steep rise in the number of cases, according to figures released by the Centers for Disease Control and Prevention. The CDC estimates that about 5,000 cases of Legionnaires' disease are now reported every year. In 2000, the number was a little over 1,000 per year.

The reason for the increase remains unclear—Preeta Kutty, MD, a CDC medical epidemiologist, speculates it might relate to climate conditions that enable the bacteria that cause the disease to thrive, or it might be that diagnosis and reporting have improved. Even so, she said she believes that the disease remains both underdiagnosed and underreported.

Legionnaires' Disease: A Primer

Legionnaires' disease resembles other forms of pneumonia, with symptoms such as high fever, chills, coughing, muscle aches and headaches appearing two to 14 days after exposure to the bacteria. It's a serious illness, causing death in 5% to 30% of cases. Older people, smokers, people with chronic lung disease and those with weakened immune systems are particularly susceptible to infection and at greatest risk for complications. A milder form of the disease is known as Pontiac fever—collectively, Legionnaires' disease and Pontiac fever are often referred to as legionellosis.

Legionella bacteria enter the body via inhalation of contaminated water droplets in the air—for example, through air-conditioning systems in large buildings or whirlpool spas that have not been properly cleaned and disinfected. Another source of infection is by drinking contaminated water. Treatment is with antibiotics.

Guard Against Infection

Large-scale environments such as hotels or ships or hospitals are most likely to have Legionella lurking somewhere in their systems, but the bacteria can also be found in apartment building and hotel cooling towers…garden ponds and fountains…water heaters…and sometimes even in freshwater ponds and creeks. Dr. Kutty advises people at greatest risk to take precautions to limit exposure, especially when traveling or in a medical facility. *Her advice includes…*

• **Limit exposure to public hot tubs.** Studies have shown that these are one of the prime culprits in the spread of Legionnaires' disease.

• **Beware of long, hot, steamy showers—especially in big buildings, such as apartments or hotels, which are more likely to harbor Legionella bacteria.** The best defense is to make sure that water heaters bring temperatures above 140°F.

• **Follow a healthful lifestyle.** A robust immune system is your best protection against Legionnaires' as well as other diseases.

• **If you are immune-compromised and therefore especially vulnerable to such infections,** talk to your health-care provider about how to avoid infection. This is one more illness you don't need to get.

Chapter 9

REMEDIES FOR KIDNEY, BLADDER AND LIVER DISEASE

Millions Have This Deadly Disease and Don't Know It

I f you've never been tested for kidney disease, make an appointment now. An estimated 26 million American adults have chronic kidney disease (CKD), and millions more have a high risk of getting it. Kidney disease is on the rise in women over 65, with diabetes, high blood pressure and lupus being common risk factors. Yet many women with CKD don't realize that their kidneys are failing.

Important warning: CKD usually causes no symptoms until about 75% of kidney function is lost. At that point, you'll probably need dialysis—and possibly a kidney transplant—to survive. That's why everyone should have yearly kidney-function tests, starting at about age 60 or earlier if you are at risk for kidney disease.

Your two kidneys are the body's filters. Together they filter more than 40 gallons of blood daily, removing wastes that are then secreted in the urine. CKD is caused by ongoing damage to the nephrons, the kidneys' filtering units. When CKD reaches an advanced stage, you will have a dangerous buildup of fluid, electrolytes and wastes in your body.

But you may be able to halt the progression of CKD with timely intervention. The blood tests for CKD—serum creatinine and glomerular filtration rate—are simple and inexpensive. If you have CKD, your doctor likely will treat the underlying causes (see risk factors on next page) and put you on a diet that stabilizes kidney function and slows or stops further damage. There are no studies to prove that this diet will prevent CKD, but many of the recommendations, such as consuming less salt and fewer soft drinks, offer health benefits for us all...

•**Less protein overall.** The average American adult gets about 0.55 grams (g) of protein for every pound of body weight. A 176-pound man, for example, probably consumes at least 96 g of protein a day. That's about 33% too much for someone with early-stage chronic kidney disease—and about double the amount recommended for someone with advanced disease.

Mandip S. Kang, MD, a nephrologist at Southwest Kidney Institute in Phoenix and a former clinical assistant professor at the University of Utah School of Medicine. He is author of *The Doctor's Kidney Diets: A Nutritional Guide to Managing and Slowing the Progression of Chronic Kidney Disease.*

A high-protein diet delivers too much nitrogen, which stresses the kidneys and can accelerate progression of CKD. Most patients are advised to limit their daily protein to 0.34 g per pound of body weight—for a 176-pound man, that is about 60 g of protein.

How much protein are we talking about? *Examples:* A five-ounce serving of salmon has 36 g of protein...a three-ounce serving of lean chicken has 28 g...one cup of pinto beans has 11 g...and a large egg has 6 g.

My advice: Limit your total protein from animal foods to about 50%. Get the other half from high-protein plant foods, such as tofu, grains and beans. Plant-based proteins are easier on the kidneys, and these foods also provide important fiber, nutrients and antioxidants.

•**Watch for phosphorus.** This is an important mineral for bone health, but it can rise to dangerous levels in people with CKD. Too much phosphorus can cause bone pain, bone thinning and an increased risk for fractures. It also increases the risk for heart disease.

The body absorbs relatively little of the organic phosphorus in meats, vegetables and other natural foods. However, you'll absorb up to 100% of the inorganic phosphorus that's used in preservatives in packaged foods, fast foods and processed meats.

Helpful: To avoid products that contain phosphorus, look for any form of "phos" on the label—sodium phosphate, phosphoric acid, calcium phosphate, etc.

•**Leach out potassium.** Like phosphorus, the mineral potassium can rise to unsafe levels. Patients with CKD should limit their daily consumption to 2,000 mg to 2,700 mg.

Chronic Kidney Disease Risk Factors

The following may increase your risk for chronic kidney disease...

•**Diabetes.** More than 40% of diabetics will eventually develop CKD.

•**High blood pressure.** This is the second-leading cause, accounting for nearly 30% of all cases.

•**Family history of kidney disease.**

•**Heart disease or cancer.**

•**Obesity.**

•**High cholesterol.**

•**Smoking.**

•**Regular use of certain over-the-counter medications,** including aspirin, ibuprofen and acetaminophen.

Many fruits and vegetables, such as bananas, oranges, potatoes, beets, Brussels sprouts and dark, leafy greens are high in potassium. One potato, for example, has nearly 900 mg.

You can use a leaching process to reduce the potassium in some high-potassium vegetables before using. Peel and place the vegetables in cold water so that they don't darken... slice the vegetables about one-eighth-inch thick... rinse them in warm water...then soak them in warm water for at least two hours, using 10 cups of water for every one cup of vegetables.

A two-hour soak is enough for most vegetables, but root vegetables such as potatoes or beets need to soak longer, preferably overnight. If soaking longer, change the water every four hours.

Or choose lower-potassium foods, such as apples, asparagus, celery, green beans, grapes and blueberries.

•**Limit dairy.** People with CKD may need to limit their dairy intake. Milk, cheese and other dairy foods are high in potassium and phosphorus. You can get healthy amounts of calcium from other foods, such as soy milk or almond milk.

•**Get much less salt.** Too much sodium can increase blood pressure along with kidney damage and cause swelling of the extremities.

The average American consumes more than 3,000 mg of sodium daily. Lower that to 1,500 mg to 2,000 mg, especially if you have CKD. Because packaged/prepared foods often are high in sodium, get in the habit of reading labels. It's also helpful to rinse certain prepared foods (such as canned vegetables) in water. And use herbs and spices to bump up the flavors of foods instead of using table salt.

Don't depend on salt substitutes. Most contain potassium or other ingredients that can be hard on the kidneys.

• **Give up soft drinks.** Studies have shown that people who drink more than a few sodas a week may be more likely to get kidney disease. If you have been diagnosed with CKD, soft drinks—particularly "dark" sodas—are a problem. They're high in phosphorus as well as sodium.

My advice: I advise everyone to give up sodas (including diet beverages and "clear" soft drinks) and switch to drinking water instead. It dilutes the blood and puts less strain on the kidneys. Most people should drink about 64 ounces of water daily.

Are Green Smoothies Bad for Your Kidneys?

Andrew Rubman, ND, medical director, Southbury Clinic for Traditional Medicines, Southbury, Connecticut. SouthburyClinic.com.

While eating cooked greens, or even eating plenty of raw greens in salads, is fine, it is possible to get into trouble if you drink large amounts of raw greens in daily juices or smoothies. But rest assured— if you like green smoothies, there are ways to enjoy them safely, even daily.

Some greens—spinach and beet greens in particular—are very high in oxalates, which can produce kidney stones. In rare cases, a very high oxalate diet can even produce kidney failure. In one medical case, an 81-year-old man who replaced all his meals with oxalate-rich green juices developed kidney failure.

It's easy to avoid that fate if you follow a few commonsense tips. Unless you have been told to avoid oxalate-rich foods by your doctor, it's fine to eat plenty of greens, even raw. Cooked greens are even better, since steaming or boiling greens removes some of the oxalates. Vitamin C, also in spinach, binds some oxalates in the gut so that they're less absorbed. Foods rich in calcium also bind oxalates.

Even having a daily green drink can be done safely: Just limit yourself to no more than one 10- to 12-ounce serving a day. You may also want to use lower-oxalate greens such as kale…add in an additional 1,000 mg of powdered vitamin C…follow the green drink with a healthy meal…and consume plenty of water throughout the day. Your kidneys will thank you for it.

Surprising Risk Factors That Can Clobber Your Kidneys

Orlando Gutiérrez, MD, an associate professor of medicine in the division of nephrology and assistant professor of epidemiology at The University of Alabama at Birmingham School of Medicine. He is also the chair of the Medical Affairs Committee for the American Kidney Fund. KidneyFund.org

Your kidneys are two of your body's best friends. Besides filtering and cleaning your blood, they also regulate fluids, acidity and key minerals…produce hormones

Can't Sleep? You May Be at Risk for Kidney Disease

Women who consistently slept five hours or less a night had a 65% greater risk for rapid decline in kidney function compared with women who regularly slept seven to eight hours a night. Men were not evaluated, although it is reasonable to expect a similar effect in both genders. If you have trouble sleeping: Ask your doctor about being tested for renal impairment.

Ciaran J. McMullan, MD, a nephrologist at Brigham and Women's Hospital, Boston, and leader of a data analysis presented at an American Society of Nephrology meeting in San Diego.

that control blood pressure...and manufacture a form of vitamin D that strengthens bones.

But modern life can really clobber your kidneys—high blood pressure, elevated blood sugar and obesity all can damage these vital organs and are major risk factors for chronic kidney disease (CKD).

The Best Defense

Controlling the big risk factors mentioned above are the best ways to prevent or control CKD. But recent studies have revealed several new risk factors that might threaten your kidneys. *These include...*

• **Proton Pump Inhibitors.** Americans spend about $11 billion yearly on acid-reducing, heartburn-easing proton pump inhibitors (PPIs), such as *esomeprazole* (Nexium) and *omeprazole* (Prilosec).

New finding: Researchers at Johns Hopkins University studied more than 10,000 people with normal kidney function. After 15 years, those using PPIs were 20% to 50% more likely to develop CKD.

Possible explanation: PPIs may cause interstitial nephritis—inflammation and scarring in the kidneys.

What to do: The researchers found that people who took an H2 blocker—such as *ranitidine* (Zantac) or *famotidine* (Pepcid)—instead of a PPI for heartburn did not have a higher risk for CKD.

Note: Many of my patients find that TUMS and lifestyle changes, such as avoiding spicy

Should You Be Tested for Kidney Disease?

More than 25 million Americans have chronic kidney disease (CKD)—but only 6% know it!

Beware: The symptoms of kidney disease (such as swollen legs, feet and/or ankles...frequent urination...fatigue...and/or dry, itchy skin) are not likely to be noticed until you reach end-stage renal disease because the body is very good at adapting to loss of kidney function until most of the function is gone.

Blood test for measuring kidney function: Estimated glomerular filtration rate (eGFR). A filtration rate of less than 60 mL/min for more than three months means that you have CKD. Most insurance companies pay for the cost of the test if the patient has a risk factor for kidney disease—such as high blood pressure...type 2 diabetes...obesity...age (65 or older)...or a family history of the disease (a parent or sibling who has CKD). If you have a risk factor for CKD, get the test every year. Otherwise, there's usually no need for testing, but be sure to consult your doctor for advice.

and fatty foods and eating more slowly, can greatly reduce heartburn.

• **High Acid Diet**

Just as our oceans are becoming more acidic and threatening marine life, scientists are finding that an acidic diet threatens our kidneys.

New finding: When researchers analyzed 14 years of health data for nearly 1,500 people with CKD, they found that those who ate a high-acid, junk food–laden diet that included red meat, processed foods, sweets and few fruits and vegetables were three times more likely to develop kidney failure.

What to do: Adopt a more alkaline diet. In a recent study, researchers from Columbia University Medical Center followed 900 people for nearly seven years and found that those who routinely ate a Mediterranean-type diet—rich in alkaline foods such as vegetables, fruits, beans and heart-healthy fats like olive oil—were 50% less likely to develop CKD than those who didn't eat these foods.

• **Sitting Too Much**

It's not just lack of regular exercise that contributes to chronic health problems such as heart disease— it's also excessive sitting. And sitting takes a toll on your kidneys, too.

New finding: In a study of nearly 6,000 people, every 80-minute period of sitting during the day increased the likelihood of CKD by 20%, according to research from the University of Utah School of Medicine. That was true whether or not the person exercised regularly or had diabetes, high blood pressure or obesity.

What to do: When the same team of researchers looked at people with CKD, they found that standing up and/or walking around for just two minutes an hour lowered the risk for death by 41%. Research also shows that regular exercise is good for your kidneys.

My advice: Walk at least 30 minutes, three times a week (in addition to getting up every hour you sit)…or check with your doctor for advice on the best type of exercise for you.

Poor Leg Circulation Hits Women With Kidney Disease Earlier Than Men

Grace Wang, MD, assistant professor of surgery, division of vascular and endovascular surgery, Hospital of the University of Pennsylvania, Philadelphia.
Reese Wain, MD, chief, division of vascular surgery, Winthrop-University Hospital, Mineola, New York.
Suzanne Steinbaum, MD, director, Women's Heart Health, Lenox Hill Hospital, New York City.
Circulation: Cardiovascular Quality and Outcomes.

Compared to men, women under the age of 70 who have kidney disease are at higher odds for peripheral arterial disease (PAD), an often disabling impairment of blood flow in the legs.

That's the finding from a new study of almost 3,200 people with chronic kidney disease. Researchers led by Grace Wang, MD, of the Hospital of the University of Pennsylvania in Philadelphia, found that women under 70 with kidney disease had a 53% higher risk of PAD compared to their male peers.

However, after age 70 the difference between the sexes evened out, the researchers noted.

About Peripheral Arterial Disease (PAD)

PAD involves a narrowing of vessels that carry blood to the arms or legs. Left unchecked, PAD can cause serious disability and even limb loss or death, according to the American Heart Association. About 8 million people in the United States aged 40 and older, and up to 20% of Americans over 65, are affected by PAD, the heart association says.

According to Dr. Wang's team, prior research has shown that women with PAD have even greater functional impairment and worse quality of life compared to men with the disease.

Study Findings

In their study, the Philadelphia team looked at rates of PAD in nearly 3,200 patients with chronic kidney disease. Average age was about 57.

They found that women had 53% higher odds for PAD than men, but this gap was most pronounced for patients under the age of 70.

The study was published in the journal *Circulation: Cardiovascular Quality and Outcomes.*

Possible Explanation

Why would PAD affect women earlier? According to the study authors, "females are known to have smaller diameter vessels compared to men." That could mean that, given similar amounts of plaque buildup in vessels, women's might close off earlier than men's.

Recommendations

The findings show that women with kidney disease may need closer monitoring at younger ages, two experts said.

"Based on these results, it is imperative that we maintain a higher index of suspicion for diagnosing such vascular problems in women sooner," said Reese Wain, MD, chief of vascular surgery at Winthrop-University Hospital in Mineola, New York.

Suzanne Steinbaum, MD, directs women's heart health at Lenox Hill Hospital in New York City. She said there is now "a greater and greater understanding of the profound differences between men and women's arteries."

According to Dr. Steinbaum, "women's arteries are significantly affected by kidney disease, and this correlation emphasizes the critical importance of early screening and detection for those women at the greatest risk."

Dr. Wang's team believes that, based on the new findings, current recommendations to begin screening people at age 50 (if they have smoked or have diabetes) or 65 (without such risk factors) "is likely 'too late' for women."

Find out more about PAD at the website of the Society for Interventional Radiology, *irweb.org*. Search "PAD."

Hormone Replacement May Protect Your Kidneys

American Society of Nephrology, news release.

Hormone-replacement therapy may be good for a woman's kidneys, a preliminary study suggests.

"The risks and benefits of hormone-replacement therapy in postmenopausal women are still an area of active debate, and the effect of hormone-replacement therapy on the kidney has shown variable results," said study author Dr. Andrea Kattah of the Mayo Clinic in Minnesota.

Her study compared nearly 700 older women taking hormone replacements with more than 1,500 who were not.

Rates of two indicators of kidney disease—microalbuminuria and decreased estimated glomerular filtration rate—were much lower in the women taking hormone replacements, the study found.

Microalbuminuria occurs with higher-than-normal levels of a protein called albu-

min in urine that could be a sign of kidney damage.

After they adjusted for known kidney and heart disease risk factors, the researchers found that hormone replacement was still strongly associated with lower rates of microalbuminuria.

But only an association and not a cause-and-effect link was seen in the study.

The study was presented at an American Society of Nephrology meeting in San Diego. Data and conclusions should be considered preliminary until the results are published in a peer-reviewed medical journal.

"Clarifying the role of hormones on kidney function may have implications for explaining gender differences in chronic kidney disease, counseling women on the use of hormone-replacement therapy, and future therapeutic targets for patients with chronic kidney disease," Dr. Kattah said in a society news release.

Because of potentially dangerous side effects, hormone-replacement therapy should only be taken for as long as necessary at the lowest effective dose, doctors say. It is typically prescribed for managing symptoms of menopause.

The American Academy of Family Physicians has more about hormone-replacement therapy at *familydoctor.org*.

Making CT Scans Safer If You Have Kidney Disease

I have chronic kidney disease (CKD), but my doctor says I need a CT scan with contrast dye. Is there anything I can do to protect my kidneys?

Many imaging tests—such as CT or MRI scans—use contrast dyes to help create more detailed images. But the dye used in a CT scan can further damage the kidneys, and gadolinium used in MRIs can cause scar tissue to form in skin or other organs. If you have stage 3, 4 or 5 CKD, always ask if a CT scan can be done without dye.

If it is absolutely necessary to use dye, intravenous fluids containing sodium bicarbonate should be given before and after the procedure to minimize risk to the kidneys. MRIs with gadolinium should not be done at all.

Mildred Lam, MD, a nephrologist at MetroHealth Medical Center in Cleveland.

New Kidney Transplant Drug Cuts Risk of Earlier Death

Flavio Vincenti, MD, kidney and pancreas transplant specialist, University of California, San Francisco.
Eliot Heher, MD, medical director, kidney transplant program, Massachusetts General Hospital, Boston.
New England Journal of Medicine.

A newer drug used for preventing organ rejection might improve the long-term outlook for kidney transplant recipients, a recent study finds.

Over seven years, patients given the drug *belatacept* (brand name: Nulojix) were 43% less likely to die or see their donor kidney fail compared to patients given an older drug called *cyclosporine*.

Experts said the findings should encourage more doctors and patients to choose belatacept over standard anti-rejection medications.

"This is a potentially transformational drug," said study lead researcher Flavio Vincenti, ND, a transplant specialist at the University of California, San Francisco.

The study—funded by the drug's maker, Bristol-Myers Squibb—was published in the *New England Journal of Medicine*.

Belatacept was first approved by the U.S. Food and Drug Administration in 2011 for preventing organ rejection after a kidney transplant. That was based on a three-year trial showing that the drug can prevent rejec-

tion in the shorter term, according to background information in the study.

Now the new findings prove what experts had hoped—that belatacept would be better than cyclosporine in the long run, doctors said.

Eliot Heher, MD, cowrote an editorial published with the study. "When belatacept was approved, there was promise that it would bring longer-term benefits," he said. "But until now, we didn't have the data."

Cyclosporine and similar anti-rejection drugs such as *tacrolimus* are effective at suppressing the immune system's response against donor kidneys, explained Dr. Heher, medical director of the kidney transplant program at Massachusetts General Hospital, in Boston.

Unfortunately, he said, they have substantial downsides over the long term, potentially causing damage to the kidney they are supposed to protect. The drugs can also raise the risk of high blood pressure, heart disease and diabetes, according to Dr. Heher.

Belatacept works differently from those older drugs, and doesn't appear to harm the kidneys or carry the same cardiovascular risks, Dr. Heher said.

On top of that, the recent study found it may do a better job of preventing the immune system from eventually creating antibodies against the donor kidney.

"That was more of an unexpected finding," Dr. Heher said.

Kidney Rejection Is Rare... In the Short Term

As of early 2016, nearly 133,000 Americans were on waiting lists for an organ transplant —with the large majority in need of a kidney, according to the U.S. Department of Health.

The past few decades have seen major advances in the short-term outlook after a kidney transplant, Dr. Heher said: In the 1980s, anywhere from 50% to 80% of patients had an episode of rejection within one year of receiving a new kidney.

These days, over 90% of donor kidneys are still well-functioning after a year, according to the U.S. National Kidney Foundation.

And yet, Dr. Heher said, there's been relatively little change in the long-term outlook —kidneys from a deceased donor last 10 to 15 years, on average, while those from living donors typically function for 15 to 18 years. "The question has been, why don't they last?" Dr. Heher said.

One reason, he said, has become clear: Damage from cyclosporine, tacrolimus and other anti-rejection drugs eventually causes some kidneys to fail.

Another reason is that there are different types of organ rejection. In the long run, Dr. Heher explained, there can be a "slow, insidious" form of rejection—where the immune system produces antibodies against the donor kidney, which gradually reduces its function.

That happens to about 20% of patients within five years, Dr. Vincenti said. In this study, less than 5% of belatacept patients developed antibodies against their kidneys over seven years.

The new trial included 660 transplant patients who were randomly assigned to receive either one of two belatacept doses, or cyclosporine.

Downsides to the New Drug

There are downsides to belatacept: Like all immune suppressors, it puts people at risk of infections. It also carries an FDA-mandated warning about the risk of a blood-cell cancer called lymphoproliferative disorder. The cancer developed in five belatacept patients in this trial, and in two on cyclosporine.

Another issue is "inconvenience," Dr. Heher said. Older anti-rejection drugs come in pill form, but belatacept has to be given by IV once a month.

There's also cost. All anti-rejection drugs are expensive; a 3-milligram daily dose of tacrolimus costs around $7,000 per year, according to Dr. Heher. Belatacept is even pricier, with hospitals paying $21,000 yearly to get the drug. Then there's the added costs

of nursing time and supplies to do the infusions, Dr. Heher pointed out.

"This drug is not for everyone," Dr. Vincenti said. "But it does offer a good alternative."

A limitation to this study, Dr. Heher said, is that it compared belatacept only to cyclosporine. After the trial started in 2006, tacrolimus became the anti-rejection drug of choice. So it would be helpful to compare those two drugs head-to-head, Dr. Heher said.

New Research Shows This Expensive Treatment May Not Work!

Navdeep Tangri, MD, PhD, Seven Oaks General Hospital Renal Program, Winnipeg, Manitoba, Canada.
Jeffrey Berns, MD, president, National Kidney Foundation, and professor of medicine and pediatrics, Hospital of the University of Pennsylvania, Philadelphia.
Annals of Internal Medicine, online.

The pricey anemia drugs often given to people with chronic kidney disease appear to make no difference in how they feel day to day, a new research review confirms.

Researchers said the study results back up current guidelines on how to use the drugs, called erythropoietin-stimulating agents (ESAs).

These include the injection drugs marketed under the names Procrit, Epogen (*epoetin alfa*) and Aranesp (*darbepoetin alfa*).

Patients may still benefit from the medications because they reduce the need for blood transfusions to treat severe anemia, said Navdeep Tangri, MD, senior researcher on the study.

"But this should close the book on the idea that these drugs help with exhaustion and improve patients' quality of life," said Dr. Tangri, an attending doctor at Seven Oaks General Hospital Renal Program in Manitoba, Canada.

Background on CKD and Anemia

People with chronic kidney disease often develop anemia, which hinders the blood's ability to transport oxygen. So doctors have long prescribed ESAs to boost blood levels of hemoglobin, the oxygen-carrying protein in red blood cells.

But in recent years, the drugs have come under closer scrutiny: Research has shown that using them to boost kidney patients' hemoglobin beyond a certain level—around 11 grams per deciliter of blood—can raise the risks of heart attack, stroke and blood clots.

So guidelines now recommend lower hemoglobin "targets," of no higher than 10 or 11. And the U.S. Food and Drug Administration says the only reason to prescribe the drugs to kidney disease patients is to curb the need for blood transfusions.

Study Details

For their study, Dr. Tangri and his colleagues pooled results of 17 clinical trials that tested ESAs and aimed for either relatively higher or lower hemoglobin targets. On average, patients in the higher-target groups got their hemoglobin to between 10 and 14, while those with lower targets had levels between 7 and 12.

Overall, the researchers found, patients with higher hemoglobin reported no bigger gains in quality of life.

There was some evidence that among patients not on dialysis, higher hemoglobin led to bigger improvements in their physical functioning and energy levels. But, Dr. Tangri said, the average differences did not appear "clinically meaningful."

He said the evidence does not support the idea that for certain patients, treatment should be "individualized" to reach a relatively higher hemoglobin level.

Expert Comment

One expert argued that while on average, overall exhaustion and quality of life are not improved, some patients do feel better on the medications—particularly younger, more active people.

"They're not recommended for treating quality-of-life issues," said Jeffrey Berns, MD, president of the National Kidney Foundation and a professor of medicine at the University of Pennsylvania.

In Dr. Berns's view, it makes sense that these medications would not change day-to-day life for many people with chronic kidney disease, especially those on dialysis. Patients are often older, have heart disease or other medical conditions, and are mostly sedentary.

"It's not realistic to expect that you'll improve their quality of life by raising their hemoglobin a little," Dr. Berns said.

But, he added, younger patients who are still physically active and have full-time jobs or families to take care of may feel the difference when their hemoglobin is at 9 instead of 11.

"One of the challenges we have is that a study, or a meta-analysis of studies, tells us about the average for a group of patients," Dr. Berns said. "That doesn't necessarily tell me what to do with the patient in front of me."

He said kidney disease patients on ESAs who don't feel better than they did before should ask their doctor whether it makes sense to stay on the drug.

It may, Dr. Berns said, since the drugs can help limit blood transfusions. That's a particular concern for patients awaiting a kidney transplant. Multiple transfusions can cause the immune system to generate antibodies with the potential to attack a donor kidney, he explained.

That still leaves the question of how to improve exhaustion and other quality-of-life issues for patients with chronic kidney disease.

"The search for effective options needs to continue," Dr. Tangri said. He added that those options could include diet changes and physical therapy, not just medication.

Is Poor Diet Causing a Rise in Kidney Stones for Women and Teens?

The Children's Hospital of Philadelphia, news release.

A growing number of teens, women and blacks are being diagnosed with kidney stones, and the trend is cause for alarm, researchers report.

Historically, middle-aged white men have been most likely to develop the painful condition, which involves small, hard mineral deposits that form in the kidneys, often when urine becomes concentrated.

Research Details

The researchers analyzed data from South Carolina from 1997 to 2012, and found that the annual incidence of kidney stones among children and adults rose 16% during that time. The largest increases were among teens (4.7% a year), females (3% a year), and blacks (nearly 3% a year).

During the study period, the risk of kidney stones doubled among children, and there was a 45% increase in the lifetime risk for women.

Teen girls had the highest rate of increase in kidney stones, and they were more common among females aged 10 to 24 than among males in the same age group. After age 25, kidney stones were more common in men, the study authors said.

Kidney stone incidence rose 15% more in blacks than in whites during each five-year period of the study, according to the findings, published online in the *Clinical Journal of the American Society of Nephrology*.

Treatments for Children Limited

"The emergence of kidney stones in children is particularly worrisome, because there is limited evidence on how to best treat children for this condition," said study leader Gregory Tasian, MD, a pediatric urologist and epidemiologist at The Children's Hospital of Philadelphia.

"The fact that stones were once rare and are now increasingly common could contribute to the inappropriate use of diagnostic tests such as CT scans for children with kidney stones, since health-care providers historically have not been accustomed to evaluating and treating children with kidney stones," he explained in a hospital news release.

"These trends of increased frequency of kidney stones among adolescents, particularly females, are also concerning when you consider that kidney stones are associated with a higher risk of chronic kidney disease, cardiovascular and bone disease, particularly among young women," Dr. Tasian added.

There may be a number of reasons for the rise in kidney stone rates, including not drinking enough water and poor eating habits, such as increased salt and decreased calcium intake, the researcher said.

Even Small Declines in Kidney Function May Affect Your Heart

Hypertension, news release.

Even a slight decline in kidney function can lead to heart damage, a recent study suggests.

"Mild chronic kidney disease is common, affecting over 10% of the US population, so if kidney disease really is a cause of heart disease it may be a major public health problem," said study senior author Jonathan Townend, MD, a professor of cardiology at Queen Elizabeth Hospital Birmingham in England.

Study Details

The study, published in the journal *Hypertension*, included 68 living kidney donors, average age 47, who were followed for a year after donating their kidney. They were compared with a control group of 56 people, average age 44, who did not donate a kidney.

Compared to those in the control group, the kidney donors had an expected decrease in kidney function, an increase in the mass of the heart's left ventricle (a strong predictor of heart disease risk), and a rise in heart damage markers in blood tests, the study found.

There was no difference in blood pressure between the two groups, according to the study.

"Even in very healthy people, a small reduction in kidney function from normal to just a bit below normal was associated with an increase in the mass of the left ventricle, a change that makes the heart stiffer and impairs its ability to contract," Townend said in a journal news release.

It has long been known that kidney disease patients are at increased risk for heart disease. But many of them have other health problems such as high blood pressure and diabetes, making it difficult to assess the effect that declining kidney function has on the heart.

The kidney donors in this study had no chronic health conditions, making it possible to assess how a small reduction in kidney function affects the heart, the researchers explained.

"This is evidence that reduction in kidney function itself leads directly to measurable adverse effects on the heart and blood vessels, even without other risk factors. More research is needed to know just what aspects of reduced kidney function are responsible for the effects," Townend said.

Kidney Donors Need Not Worry

However, kidney donors should not be alarmed by these findings, he and his colleagues said.

"Kidney donors are already highly selected as healthy individuals. Our paper has shown that kidney donation causes very small adverse effects on the heart and blood vessels that took careful and accurate measurements

to detect. We do not yet know if these effects are maintained over the long term," Townend said.

Even if there is a small increase in your long-term risk of heart disease after donation, it is still likely that you will be at lower-than-average risk, he added.

No More Running to the Bathroom!

Tomas L. Griebling, MD, MPH, the John P. Wolf 33° Masonic Distinguished Professor of Urology at The University of Kansas (KU) School of Medicine, Kansas City. Dr. Griebling is a professor and vice-chair in the department of urology and faculty associate in The Landon Center on Aging.

For millions of American women (and men) who suffer from overactive bladder (OAB), going to the bathroom is a stressful part of daily life. They urinate much more frequently than they should and suffer from a "got to go now" feeling multiple times a day.

Latest development: There are recently approved FDA drugs and high-tech treatment options that help sufferers overcome their troubling symptoms.

Important: Behavioral approaches (see next page) can effectively treat OAB in some people and should typically be tried first for six to eight weeks. If these approaches don't adequately improve symptoms, then one or more of the following treatments can be added to the regimen.

Even if you're already taking an OAB drug, there are newer options that may be more effective or convenient than your current treatment. *What you need to know…*

How the Bladder Should Work

Normally, when the bladder is relaxed, it fills up like a balloon, stretching but not leaking. Then when you urinate, it gets squeezed empty. But in people who have OAB, the bladder starts squeezing even when it's not full. If it squeezes hard enough, you leak urine.

OAB causes one or more of the following symptoms…

• **Urgency**—Sudden episodes of having to get to the toilet very fast. This may involve leakage.

• **Frequency**—On average, adults without OAB urinate roughly every three or four waking hours—about six times a day. But individuals with OAB need to urinate more than that and consider their frequent urination bothersome.

• **Nocturia**—Having to get up from sleep to urinate. More than once a night is not normal.

Is There a Problem?

If you suspect that you have OAB, see your primary care doctor. He/she will take your medical history…perform a physical exam—to check for a prolapsed (dropped) uterus in women, for example—and test for a urinary tract infection.

Make sure your doctor also: Rules out other medical conditions that can lead to frequent and/or urgent urination—including diabetes, a history of stroke or a neurological condition such as Parkinson's disease, multiple sclerosis or Alzheimer's disease. Once you're sure you have OAB, treatment can begin.

Treatment Developments

A number of prescription medications, including *darifenacin* (Enablex), *fesoterodine* (Toviaz), *oxybutynin* (Ditropan, Oxytrol) and *tolterodine* (Detrol), are commonly used in pill form to help improve bladder control in OAB patients. Now, there are new options that may cause fewer side effects and/or be more convenient to use.

Recent development I: In 2013 the FDA approved for women with OAB an over-the-counter version of Oxytrol in a patch that is placed on the skin every four days. A patch is more convenient than pills for some people. (The drug is available only by prescription for men.)

The patch's possible side effects, including dry mouth and constipation, are believed to be milder than those that can occur with the pills, since the dose is lower. The patch may cause minor skin irritation where it is placed.

Recent development II: Also in 2013 the FDA approved Botox injections for patients with OAB who do not respond to medication. Small amounts of botulinum toxin are injected at various sites in the bladder. The treatment may need to be repeated in nine to 12 months if symptoms persist. Side effects could include urinary tract infection and incomplete emptying of the bladder.

Other OAB treatments now covered by some insurance companies (check with your insurer)…

• **Peripheral tibial nerve stimulation** involves inserting a small needle electrode near the ankle to stimulate the tibial nerve, which helps control urination. The electrode is then charged with electrical current (it is not painful). Thirty-minute sessions are typically scheduled once weekly for 12 weeks. Thereafter, maintenance sessions are usually required every two to three weeks.

• **Sacral neuromodulation (SNM).** This treatment, also known as sacral nerve stimulation (SNS), and sometimes referred to as a "pacemaker for the bladder," involves implanting a device near the tailbone where it can send electrical signals to the sacral nerve, which helps control the bladder and muscles that are related to urination. A handheld remote control device is used to change the settings, allowing patients to adjust it to their symptoms.

Clinical trial: Researchers often recruit women for clinical trials for OAB. To find a trial applicable to your specific condition, ask your doctor or go to *clinicaltrials.gov* and search "Overactive Bladder."

Overactive Bladder: Natural Care

The following natural approaches, used alone or in conjunction with the treatments described in the main article, can help relieve overactive bladder (OAB)…

• **Keep tabs on yourself.** Write down how often you go to the toilet to urinate…how often you experience urgency (this may not precede each urination)…what you eat and drink (dietary factors can play a role in OAB) and when. Doing this for at least three days can help pinpoint some lifestyle factors that might be making your OAB worse—for example, drinking fluids right before bedtime.

For a printable bladder diary or information on bladder diary applications for smartphones, go to the American Urological Association website (*urologyhealth.org/OAB/patients.cfm*) and click on "Assess Your OAB Symptoms."

• **Do pelvic-floor exercises the right way.** With these exercises, also known as Kegels, you train the muscles that stop and start the flow of urine. This can reduce the urgent sensations and give you more time to get to the toilet.

What to do: Squeeze your muscles as if you are trying to stop yourself from urinating. Hold the muscle for five seconds, then relax for five seconds. Repeat this 10 times, three to five times a day. Work up to holding each contraction for 10 seconds, then relaxing for 10 seconds between contractions.

Common mistakes to avoid: Contracting the wrong muscles, such as abdominal, thigh or buttock muscles…bearing down as if you're going to have a bowel movement and straining the abdominal muscles (this may actually worsen symptoms)…and doing too many repetitions, which can fatigue the muscles and cause discomfort.

Important: Some women learn to do the exercises, feel improvement and then quit. Unfortunately, the symptoms often come back when patients stop the exercises.

• **Watch your diet.** Avoid foods and beverages that trigger symptoms. For example, caffeine, carbonated beverages, alcohol and, in some people, acidic foods, such as citrus and tomatoes, bother the bladder. *Also*…

• **Drink more water, not less.** Many patients think that if they cut way back on the amount they drink, their bladder symptoms will improve because they'll need to urinate less. But it can make things worse—urine becomes concentrated, which has an irritating effect and increases urgency.

• **Prevent constipation—it can make bladder problems worse.** Eat a high-fiber diet. If you take a fiber supplement, drink plenty of water with it. A stool softener also may help.

Important: People who smoke tend to have more OAB problems and urinary urgency. There's also a strong link between cigarette smoking and bladder cancer.

• **Bladder training.** The goal is to increase the time between urinations to minimize urgency incontinence.

What to do: When you get a sensation of needing to urinate, the natural reaction is to rush to the toilet, but the bladder is often contracting while you do that so you may leak on the way.

Better: Stop everything—don't head for the bathroom—and do a series of rapid Kegels until the sense of urgency passes. It may take several weeks for urgency to improve.

Best Surgery for Incontinence or Dropped Bladder

Women with incontinence or pelvic organ prolapse (dropped bladder) should consider corrective surgery using their own tissue instead of synthetic mesh. Synthetic mesh allows for quicker surgery but is riskier long-term.

Possible complications of synthetic mesh: Severe, prolonged abdominal pain…painful sex…need for additional surgeries. Complications of using your own tissue are minor. A small incision in the lower abdomen can leave a scar that can result in a hernia.

Jerry Blaivas, MD, a urologist in private practice and clinical professor of urology at Weill Cornell Medical College, New York City, and author of *Conquering Bladder and Prostate Problems*.

Test Could Eliminate Need for Catheter

Measuring the bladder with a portable, pocket-size ultrasound device effectively diagnosed postoperative urinary retention in a group of 100 patients who had recently undergone surgery.

Benefit: Patients who did not have urinary retention were able to avoid unnecessary catheterization (a common cause of infection).

If you need surgery: Ask your doctor about this simple test.

Aurelien Daurat, MD, anesthesiologist and critical care physician, Lapeyronie University Hospital, Montpellier, France.

5 Secrets for a Super Liver

Michelle Lai, MD, MPH, hepatologist at Beth Israel Deaconess Medical Center, Boston. Dr. Lai is coauthor of *The Liver Healing Diet.*

Most people assume that liver disease happens only to people who abuse alcohol. But that is not true.

Surprising facts: More than 30 million US adults suffer from chronic liver disease—and many of these people don't even know that they have it. Liver problems can be caused by a number of conditions such as fatty liver disease (see below) and hepatitis C and hepatitis B. The result can range from mild dysfunction to cirrhosis, liver failure and liver cancer.

An under-recognized problem: A condition called nonalcoholic fatty liver disease (NAFLD). Affecting as many as one in four adults in this country, it is marked by a build-up of extra fat in the liver cells. This can allow a more serious condition to develop that can result in liver scarring and cirrhosis—prob-lems that may lead to liver failure or cancer, requiring a liver transplant.

Keeping Your Liver Healthy

Your liver is one of the hardest-working—and underappreciated—organs in your body. It's responsible for more than 500 critical functions, ranging from digesting and storing nutrients to processing and excreting toxic substances that sneak into your body via food, drink and air. If your liver gets sick, you get sick—it's that simple.

Fortunately, there are simple steps you can take to help protect your liver health. *My advice…*

•**Fight unwanted weight gain.** This is key to liver health. For most people, a crucial part of maintaining a healthy body weight is to cut back on their sugar intake.

Besides promoting system-wide inflammation and weight gain, excessive sugar (typically from sweets, soda, fruit drinks and other flavored beverages) can cause your liver to become fatty and inflamed—thus contributing to NAFLD.

Important: The just-released 2015–2020 edition of the federal Dietary Guidelines calls

New Cirrhosis Danger Uncovered

Women who drank up to one alcoholic drink daily and men who had up to two drinks every day were 11% more likely to develop cirrhosis (scarred liver tissue that can lead to liver failure) than those who drank alcohol more heavily but not daily, according to a recent study. A standard drink is 12 ounces of beer…5 ounces of wine…or 1.5 ounces of liquor.

Ramon Bataller, MD, PhD, associate professor of medicine and nutrition, University of North Carolina at Chapel Hill School of Medicine.

for us to limit our added sugar intake to less than 10% of daily calories—the equivalent of roughly 10 to 15 teaspoons of sugar per day.

Some easy ways to cut back on sugar in your diet: Switch from flavored yogurt to plain Greek yogurt topped with fruit...and substitute unsweetened applesauce for refined white sugar when baking.

• **Drink coffee.** Scientific evidence continues to shore up coffee's protective effect on the liver—perhaps due to its inflammation-fighting properties.

Important recent findings: A March 2015 World Cancer Research Fund study found that each cup of coffee you drink per day reduces your risk for liver cancer by 14%. An analysis of other studies showed that drinking two cups of coffee per day may reduce risk for cirrhosis by 44%.

Helpful: Opt for caffeinated coffee and, if possible, have it black. Sugar, of course, causes inflammation, and decaf java has not been shown in research to have the same liver-friendly benefits.

• **Try wheat germ.** With its mild, nutty taste, wheat germ is an excellent source of vitamin E. Two tablespoons of ready-to-eat wheat germ provide 5.4 mg of vitamin E—about one-third of your daily needs. Why is this vitamin so important? Animal studies suggest that wheat germ can help protect the liver against toxins. While human data is limited, a study of 132,000 Chinese adults found

Household Toxins

A healthy liver functions like a fortress, defending your body from toxins. A frequently overlooked source of toxins: Household cleaning agents.

Every time you spray your counter or wipe down a table, you release irritating chemicals (such as chlorine, ammonia, alcohol and others), which are inhaled. *Fortunately, safer alternatives are readily available...*

• **For an all-purpose cleaner,** (good for appliances, counters and inside the refrigerator), dissolve four tablespoons of baking soda in one quart of warm water.

• **To polish stainless steel, olive oil works great.**

Still want the convenience of a store-bought cleaner? Choose brands labeled "phosphate-free" ..."VOC-free"...and/or "solvent-free." Also, look for products with the green-and-white USDA Organic Seal or ones with nontoxic, plant-derived ingredients.

that as vitamin E intake rose, the likelihood of liver cancer dropped.

Wheat germ is also rich in essential fatty acids, potassium and magnesium—all of which help ease oxidative stress on the liver by protecting the body's cells from free radical damage.

Helpful: Sprinkle wheat germ over oatmeal, yogurt or popcorn...or mix it into meatloaf or smoothies. For other good sources of vitamin E, try almonds, spinach, avocado and sunflower seeds.

• **Choose seafood wisely.** Fish is an excellent source of protein, vitamins and minerals and heart-healthy omega-3 fatty acids. However, many types of fish can accumulate heavy metals, such as mercury, lead and cadmium, from the water and the aquatic life they consume. When we eat such fish, we ingest these toxins, which, over time, can cause liver damage.

Self-defense: Select seafood that is less likely to contain heavy metals. For example, you can safely enjoy 12 ounces a week of smaller fish such as anchovies...catfish... flounder...herring...perch...wild salmon...sardines...and trout.

Caution: Limit your intake of fish that may contain higher levels of heavy metals such as Chilean sea bass...grouper...mackerel...and yellowfin and white albacore tuna to less than 18 ounces per month.

Avoid large fish such as marlin...orange roughy...ahi tuna...and swordfish—these fish usually contain the highest levels of heavy metals.

Helpful: Visit the Natural Resources Defense Council at *NRDC.org* for a complete list of the safest seafood options.

•Don't forget water! Water makes the liver's job easier by helping flush toxins out of the body. It's also a sugar-free substitute for juice, soda, sweetened tea and other sugar-enhanced beverages.

Helpful: Keep a glass of water on your nightstand, and start your morning with it, then continue sipping all day long. To jazz up your water, try adding freshly cut slices of citrus.

Green Tea Danger? Your Liver Might Be at Risk

Shannon M. Clark, MD, MMS, associate professor, University of Texas Medical Branch-Galveston, fellow, The American College of Obstetricians and Gynecologists.

Andrew Rubman, ND, medical director, Southbury Clinic for Traditional Medicines, Southbury, Connecticut. SouthburyClinic.com

C ould green tea, linked to so many health benefits ranging from cardiovascular health to preventing dementia to weight loss, actually be bad for pregnant women and green tea extracts bad for everyone?

For more information, we checked with obstetrician Shannon Clark, MD, MMS, an associate professor in the division of maternal-fetal medicine at University of Texas Medical Branch at Galveston, and naturopathic doctor Andrew Rubman, ND. *Here's what they said…*

Pregnancy and Green Tea

Adequate folate in the months before pregnancy and during the first trimester is indeed critical in reducing the likelihood of neural tube defects such as spina bifida. And it's true that tea, particularly green tea, contains catechins, antioxidants that have an inhibitory effect on an enzyme that converts folic acid to folate, the active form that the body uses.

However, according to Dr. Clark, the most current research does not find that drinking green tea decreases levels of folate concentration in pregnant women. Additionally, any woman who is pregnant or may become pregnant should be taking a supplement that contains 400 mcg of folic acid/folate, which will further protect her.

One caveat: Pregnant women should limit their caffeine intake to no more than 200 mg per day, says Dr. Clark. (There is conflicting evidence that higher levels may increase miscarriage risk.) That's what's in about two or three cups of green tea.

Bottom line: Green tea in moderation is safe for pregnant women.

Extract Concerns

There have been reports of liver injury and even liver failure linked to green tea extracts, says Dr. Rubman. Green tea is not a concern, he emphasizes.

The ingredient in questions is, again, catechins. In small amounts they act as antioxidants and are responsible for many of green tea's health benefits, but in large concentrated doses, they can harm the liver. To put it in perspective, the American College of Gastroenterology recommends a daily limit of 500 milligrams (mg) of catechins. One cup of green tea may have between 50 mg and 150 mg, and in the study we reported, the subjects took either standardized green tea extract totaling only 375 mg or a placebo. In contrast, some supplements, such as those sold for weight loss, contain as much as 700 mg in a single pill—and the labels recommend taking several pills a day.

Dr. Rubman is particularly concerned about "enhanced" products—those that combine green tea extracts with other, often undisclosed, ingredients, which may be harmful on their own as well. While extracts made from whole tea leaves, consumed in doses that are consistent with normal daily use, are likely to be safer, he still favors the beverage. "The best advice is to drink brewed green tea rather than use extracts," he says. "This practice has been followed safely by the Japanese, including pregnant and nursing women, for centuries."

Bottom line: Skip the extracts—drink green tea instead.

Natural Ways to Protect Your Liver

Gerard E. Mullin, MD, an internist, gastroenterologist and nutritionist. He is an associate professor of medicine at Johns Hopkins University School of Medicine and director of Integrative Gastroenterology Nutrition Services at The Johns Hopkins Hospital, both in Baltimore. Dr. Mullin is also author of *Integrative Gastroenterology* and *The Inside Tract.*

When it comes to vital organs in the body, it often seems like the heart and brain get all the attention.

But the liver also plays a crucial role in maintaining good health. Liver disease, which affects one person in 10, is among the top 12 causes of death in the US (primarily from cirrhosis).

Fortunately, there are plenty of steps you can take to help safeguard the health of your liver. *What you need to know...*

Antioxidant-Rich Foods

All tissues of the body are subject to damage by highly reactive molecules known as oxygen free radicals, which are produced by natural metabolic processes. In the liver, free radicals can trigger an inflammatory response that may result in scarring and culminate in the tissue destruction that characterizes cirrhosis.

The body has built-in defenses against free radicals—enzyme systems that neutralize these dangerous chemicals. But they can be overwhelmed without the help of additional antioxidant compounds provided by the diet. To help protect your liver, make sure that your daily diet includes at least some of the foods with the highest antioxidant levels—

especially if you have liver disease or are at risk for it (due to such factors as obesity or alcohol abuse)...*

- **Cinnamon.**
- **Berries** (especially wild blueberries, which are particularly high in antioxidants), cranberries, blackberries, raspberries and strawberries (frozen berries also are a good choice).
- **Red, kidney or pinto beans.**
- **Pecans.**
- **Artichoke hearts.**
- **Russet potatoes** (with the skin).
- **Apples.**
- **Plums.**

Also: For a concentrated source of liver-shielding antioxidants, drink fresh raw juices made from beetroot, dandelion leaf, wheatgrass and/or barley grass. Antioxidant-rich green tea also promotes liver health.

Detoxifying Foods

The liver plays a central role in ridding the body of toxins produced by bacteria and derived from external sources such as air pollution, heavy metals, pesticides, hormones in foods and natural wastes such as metabolic by-products.

The liver's detoxification process is complex. Enzymes first alter the toxic chemicals into more reactive compounds that can ultimately dissolve in bile for excretion through the digestive tract.

Certain foods stimulate the enzymes that catalyze detoxification. These include cruciferous vegetables, such as broccoli, cauliflower, cabbage and kale.

A key ingredient of cruciferous vegetables, sulforaphane, also protects the liver as an anti-inflammatory and antioxidant. Sulfur-containing foods that have a similar effect include eggs, garlic, onions, leeks and shallots.

The amino acid L-arginine also stimulates the liver's detoxification mechanism.

*There are no current guidelines on the amounts of these foods to consume for liver protection—add them to your diet in liberal amounts whenever possible.

Kidney beans and pea-nuts are good sources of L-arginine.

Bile flushes toxins out of the liver into the intestine en route to excretion. Choloretic foods—artichokes and ginger, for example—help stimulate the production and flow of bile.

Healthful Bacteria

Regularly taking medications including nonsteroidal anti-inflammatory drugs, such as *ibuprofen* (Motrin), can create inflammation that may allow bacterial toxins to leak through the intestinal wall, triggering oxidative stress that can progress to scarring and even tissue destruction of the liver. Excessive alcohol consumption aggravates this disruption of the intestinal lining.

Beneficial bacteria found in the large intestine help keep harmful germs and their toxins from seeping through the intestinal wall. Probiotics (foods and supplements containing "good" bacteria) and prebiotics (foods that feed these bacteria) protect the liver indirectly by promoting the overall growth of healthful bacteria. Prebiotics include bananas, artichokes and fermented foods such as miso.

You can also use probiotic supplements, such as lactobacillus gg, or eat yogurt containing live cultures.

Healthy Liver Lifestyle

Excessive alcohol disrupts the liver's metabolism and causes inflammation that leads to fatty deposits, scarring and the irreversible tissue destruction of cirrhosis.

While moderate alcohol intake (up to two drinks daily for men and no more than one drink daily for women) offers general health benefits for most people without endangering

---

Key Facts About the Liver

The liver, which weighs about three pounds, is the second-largest organ in the body (only the skin is larger). *A metabolic and biochemical powerhouse, the liver...*

- Converts food into energy and building-block nutrients.
- Stores excess carbohydrates for endurance.
- Filters out toxins.
- Breaks down medications for absorption.

---

the liver, excessive amounts must be avoided.

Also: Exercise and watch your weight. Obesity and diabetes increase the risk for nonalcoholic fatty liver disease, which affects up to 23% of the population. Although it usually causes no symptoms, this buildup of fat deposits in the liver can, over time, lead to inflammation, a condition called nonalcoholic steatohepatitis (NASH) that may ultimately cause the same kind of lasting liver damage as alcohol.

Exercise goal: Two and a half hours of moderately strenuous exercise per week—spread over four or more days—will protect your liver while also improving your overall health.

Key Supplements

There is no definitive research to support vitamin or herbal supplements to preserve liver health, but some studies suggest that they may help in treating liver disease. *If you are being treated for liver disease, ask your doctor about...*

- **Vitamin E.** Previous research is mixed, but a major two-year clinical trial recently published in *The New England Journal of Medicine* found significant improvement in NASH symptoms among patients who took 800 international units of vitamin E daily, compared with those who were given placebos or received a diabetes drug used to treat NASH.
- **Betaine.** A pilot study involving seven patients with NASH suggested that a year of treatment with this nutritional supplement could reduce fatty deposits, inflammation and fibrosis in the liver.

Chapter 10

INFECTIOUS DISEASES

A Hidden Cause of Chronic Disease

Everyone gets infections from time to time—a swollen cut...a tooth abscess...or simply a common cold. Most infections come on quickly, cause a brief period of discomfort and then disappear, either on their own or with medication.

What research is now finding: The acute illnesses that we get from infections might be just the tip of the iceberg. Experts now believe that some of the most serious chronic diseases are actually old infections in disguise.

Simmering Damage

If you're struck with a nasty infection, you probably assume that once you start feeling better, everything is fine. But that may not be true. Even after your symptoms are gone, some bacteria and viruses have the ability to linger almost indefinitely—you can have a subclinical infection that persists months or even years after the initial illness is gone.

When Infection Lingers

Some infections, such as those caused by the human papillomavirus (discussed on the next page), have a proven link to chronic diseases. Others may be part of a constellation of risk factors that may also include genetics or immune system vulnerabilities. *Examples…*

• **Atherosclerosis.** Up to half of those with atherosclerosis (the accumulation of cholesterol and other fats on artery walls) have none of the usual risk factors, such as smoking or high blood pressure. Yet something causes the fats to accumulate.

Arterial inflammation is a known trigger for atherosclerosis—and inflammation is often due to infection. When researchers examined the blood vessels of patients with atherosclerosis, they repeatedly discovered Chlamydophila pneumoniae (a bacterium that causes pneumonia and bronchitis), Helicobacter pylori (a bacterium that causes ulcers) and other infection-causing organisms. This doesn't prove that the organisms were responsible for the atherosclerosis. Some bacteria or viruses may have been innocent bystanders that just happened to be there.

What's more, if the microbes caused atherosclerosis, eliminating them should have

Bennett Lorber, MD, a professor of microbiology and immunology and the Thomas M. Durant Professor of Medicine at Temple University School of Medicine in Philadelphia, where he specializes in anaerobic infections, the interaction of society and infectious diseases and the infectious causes of "noninfectious" diseases.

been helpful—but heart attack patients who were treated with antibiotics were just as likely to have a second heart attack as those who weren't given the drugs. It's possible, however, that the bacteria were eliminated after the arterial damage was done.

What is known: It's been proven that patients with periodontal disease (a gum infection) are more likely to get heart disease. So are people with high levels of C-reactive protein (CRP), an inflammatory "marker" that may be elevated by any type of infection.

My advice: Since CRP is a heart disease risk factor—one that may be caused by infection—it's worth getting it checked. Ask your doctor for advice on the frequency of CRP testing. People who test high might be motivated to take better care of themselves— stopping smoking, eating a healthier diet, lowering blood pressure, etc. Be sure to get regular dental checkups, too.

Also helpful: If you have been diagnosed at any time with C. pneumoniae, H. pylori or another serious infection, tell your doctor so that he/she can consider this as a potential risk factor for atherosclerosis.

• **Rheumatoid arthritis.** It occurs when the immune system attacks the membrane that lines the joints, usually in the hands and feet. Periodontal disease appears to increase risk for rheumatoid arthritis.

What may happen: One of the bacteria (Porphyromonas gingivalis) that causes virtually all periodontal disease produces enzymes that allow the infection to survive in crevices between the teeth and gums. These enzymes then trigger a chemical reaction that produces immunogens, molecules that activate an immune response in the body's joints.

Scientific evidence: A study of more than 6,600 men and women found that those with moderate-to-severe periodontitis were more than twice as likely to have rheumatoid arthritis as those with no or only mild periodontitis.

Even though not everyone with periodontal disease will develop rheumatoid arthritis (or have worse symptoms if they've already been diagnosed), there's strong evidence that the two are related.

My advice: In addition to daily brushing and flossing, get your teeth checked at least once a year. Periodontal disease can be treated with professional care. It will help you save your teeth—and possibly your joints as well.

• **Cervical and anal cancers.** Virtually all of these malignancies—along with many cancers of the oral cavity—are caused by the human papillomavirus (HPV), the most common sexually transmitted infection in the US.

HPV is so common that most sexually active men and women will get at least one form of the virus. Most people will never know they're infected (your immune system usually eliminates the virus with time), and there's no blood test to detect it. Most HPV viruses have oncogenic (cancer-causing) potential. Two of the highest-risk strains, types 16 and 18, account for the majority of cervical cancers. (The viruses that cause genital warts do not cause cancer.)

My advice: The HPV vaccine is recommended for young men and women before they start having sex, but it's effective for anyone who hasn't yet been exposed. Even if you've already been infected with HPV, the vaccine may protect you against a strain that you haven't yet been exposed to. Talk to your doctor for advice.

Also important: Women between the ages of 21 and 29 should have a Pap test every three years, and starting at age 30, they should have a Pap and HPV test at least every five years until age 65. (The HPV test may detect the virus before cell changes can be seen with the Pap test.) A form of the Pap test can also be done for men and women who engage in anal sex.

Get the Shingles Vaccine

Shingles vaccine reduces long-term pain in women. Shingles patients often develop postherpetic neuralgia (PHN), long-term pain that is a complication of the condition. More than 10% of unvaccinated women developed PHN. But only 4% of vaccinated women developed PHN. (Vaccinated and unvaccinated men had a roughly 6% chance of developing PHN.) The US Advisory Council on Immunization Practices recommends that all people age 60 and older be vaccinated against shingles.

Study of 2,400 people over age 60 who developed shingles by researchers at Kaiser Permanente Southern California, Pasadena, published in *Journal of Infectious Diseases.*

Mosquitoes Aren't the Only Zika Transmitters

The Zika virus, suspected of causing devastating birth defects, is not spread just by mosquitoes. The CDC now recommends abstinence/condom use for women with male partners from Zika-affected areas. Zika has also been detected in saliva, but it's not known if kissing can spread infection.

Centers for Disease Control and Prevention.

Zika: Should I Change My Travel Plans?

Phyllis Ellen Kozarsky, MD, professor of medicine at Emory University School of Medicine, board-certified in tropical and travel medicine.

Zika is terrifying. The mosquito-borne illness is expanding rapidly throughout Central and South America and the Caribbean—where many Americans vacation—and will almost certainly spread in the US. (At press, local infections are being investigated. Several infections have been caused by travel to South America or the Caribbean.) It is strongly linked to serious birth defects, including babies born with tiny heads (microcephaly). There's a possible link to the paralyzing autoimmune disease Guillain-Barré. There's no vaccine, no readily available test to determine if you've been infected and, worst of all, no treatment. It's a public health emergency, perhaps a global one.

So what if you're planning a vacation to an infected area such as Puerto Rico, the Virgin Islands, Barbados, Mexico, Panama or Brazil?

Time to reconsider?

Surprisingly, for most adults, unless you're pregnant or planning to get pregnant, it's fine to go ahead with your travel plans.

"It's generally a very mild disease," says board-certified travel medicine expert Phyllis Kozarsky, MD, a professor of medicine at Emory University School of Medicine. "Zika represents a horrifying illness for women who are pregnant—but for most people, it's either asymptomatic or mild."

Here's the nitty-gritty…

•**Women who are pregnant or planning to get pregnant should not travel to affected areas.** If you have a male partner who lives in or has traveled to an area where Zika transmission is ongoing, either use condoms or do not have sex during your pregnancy. The Centers for Disease Control and Prevention (CDC) has expanded its travel alert to dozens of countries. Find out more at *http://wwwnc.cdc.gov/travel/page/zika-information.*

•**For all other adults, the travel risk should be minimal.** "It's a nuisance," said Dr. Kozarsky. Indeed, 80% of the people who get infected don't ever have symptoms. Even if you do get sick—symptoms may include a fever, rash, joint pain and red eyes—"you'll likely just stay home for a few days and then feel better. Most people don't even go to a doctor." However, we don't know everything about this virus, and as time goes on, we may find that there are other concerns.

A possible exception: If you're immunocompromised—you're taking high-dose steroids, for example, or undergoing chemotherapy—you may want to avoid any travel to a locale where there are serious infectious disease risks. In that case, said Dr. Kozarsky, it's best to travel more locally.

• **What about infants and children?** Dr. Kozarsky commented that because we don't know enough about how the virus might affect them, you may want to keep children and infants away from infected countries.

• **If you do go to an affected area, though, by all means protect yourself.** Wear insect repellent all the time. "We used to say between dusk and dawn, but the Aedes mosquito, which carries Zika, can bite indoors or outdoors, as well as during the day," she said. Zika isn't even the only reason why you want to avoid mosquito bites in the first place, she said—this mosquito also can carry other diseases including dengue fever and chikungunya, which may be more serious than Zika, and potentially deadly. You can use a repellent that contains DEET or, if you want to avoid it, there are CDC-recommended repellents such as those that contain oil of lemon eucalyptus. "Make sure you follow directions on the container telling you how often to reapply it," said Dr. Kozarsky.

• **What about Guillain-Barré disease?** The link has not been confirmed, but even if Zika can trigger the autoimmune disease, it's one of many viruses that under certain circumstances might do so. In sum, it's a low risk.

If you do go on vacation or on business to a country that has Zika, you'll want to take precautions when you return. (That's also true if you're welcoming a friend or relative just back from, say, Brazil.) If you get symptoms that might be related to Zika, tell your doctor—and try to avoid getting bit by a mosquito back home for at least a week. This isn't to protect you, but to protect others, especially pregnant women—by helping to prevent the disease from spreading via mosquitoes in the US.

Bottom line? It's true that Zika might become a public health crisis in the US just as it now is in other areas. However, it is thought that like dengue and chikungunya, it may not become a serious public health problem here. But for now, unless you're pregnant or might soon become pregnant, Zika is just a nuisance—unless we learn otherwise, said Dr. Kozarsky. So stay tuned. "The major preventable cause of death in travelers isn't an exotic disease at all—it's auto accidents."

Planning a trip to the Virgin Islands? By all means, go.

Just drive safely.

Vaccines You Need Before Going Overseas

Many US travelers fail to get vaccinations before going overseas. Outbreaks of infections such as measles and hepatitis A could be prevented if more people were vaccinated against the diseases. Many people do not realize how prevalent these diseases are outside the US. Measles outbreaks occur in developed countries, including Europe, and while hepatitis A is rare in the US, it is common in places with poor sanitation and limited access to clean water.

Self-defense: Visit a travel clinic four to six weeks before an international trip, or see your doctor to get recommended shots.

Study of more than 40,000 US travelers by researchers at Harvard Medical School and Massachusetts General Hospital, both in Boston, reported at a recent meeting of specialists in infectious illness during Infectious Diseases Week in San Diego.

Is the Zika Virus Harming Our Blood Supply?

The Red Cross has implemented the FDA's updated blood donation guidelines to help reduce risk of transmission of the Zika virus through blood transfusions. The Zika virus (which has been linked to birth defects) has recently spread through Central and South America. As a precaution, people who have traveled to Mexico, the Caribbean, or Central or South America within the past 28 days should not donate blood.

Donors who have traveled to these countries and developed Zika symptoms (such as fever, rash, joint pain and conjunctivitis) within 14 days after donation, or have been diagnosed with a Zika infection, should immediately notify the Red Cross so that their donation can be quarantined.

The Red Cross screens all blood donors and accepts donations only from those who are healthy and feeling well. Anyone with Zika symptoms, even though they have not traveled to an area with the outbreak, should not donate blood.

Susan Stramer, PhD, vice president of scientific affairs, American Red Cross, Washington, DC.

Are You a Mosquito Magnet?

In warm weather, do mosquitoes keep biting you but no one else?

Some people are highly attractive to mosquitoes—those who emit a lot of carbon dioxide (tall and/or overweight people, pregnant women and those who exercise heavily) and people whose metabolism results in excess lactic or uric acid or high amounts of cholesterol on the skin. But people with high cholesterol in their blood are not more likely to be bitten. Cholesterol on the skin results not from how much is in the blood but from how quickly it is metabolized.

To protect yourself, the Centers for Disease Control and Prevention recommends repellents that contain one of these ingredients—DEET, picaridin, IR3535 or oil of lemon eucalyptus. You can also spray a product containing permethrin on clothing, which helps keep these pests away.

Joseph Conlon, MA, technical advisor, American Mosquito Control Association, Mount Laurel, New Jersey.

The 7 Germiest Spots in Your Home

Charles Peter Gerba, PhD, professor of microbiology and environmental sciences who specializes in virology, parasitology and risk assessment at University of Arizona College of Agriculture and Life Sciences, Tucson. He is coauthor, with Allison Janse, of *The Germ Freak's Guide to Outwitting Colds and Flu.*

Even if you are a germaphobe when you are out in public, you probably relax on your own turf. Don't be fooled—germs are lurking in the average home, and they spread amazingly fast.

In one study, we coated the hands of just one person in a family with bacteriophage (a benign surrogate for common gastrointestinal and respiratory viruses). Within eight hours, the hands of every family member had been contaminated, along with things like the refrigerator handle, stove knobs and countertops.

Disease-causing germs, called pathogens, include cold and flu viruses and food-borne bacteria such as E. coli and Salmonella that can cause dangerous intestinal tract infections. According to the Centers for Disease Control and Prevention (CDC), about 20% of food-poisoning outbreaks are related to food handling in the home.

Here's where germs are most likely to hide in your home...

• **Kitchen sponge.** It's the dirtiest thing in the house. When we tested sponges, we found that 15% tested positive for Salmonella. Sponges often are contaminated with E.coli as well. The more you use the sponge—such as for wiping counters and cleaning the microwave—the farther germs will spread.

My advice: Disinfect your wet sponge by zapping it for 30 seconds in the microwave, running it through a dishwasher cycle or soaking it in a bleach-water solution at least once a week.

• **Cutting boards.** We found that the average cutting board had 200 times more fecal bacteria than toilets. You're safer making a sandwich on a typical toilet seat than on a typical cutting board!

My advice: After cutting meats or uncooked produce, wipe a wooden board generously with a sponge that has been soaked in a solution of two tablespoons of bleach to one gallon of water. Let it sit for a few minutes, then wipe off the excess. You can clean plastic cutting boards by running them through the dishwasher. Some cutting boards are impregnated with triclosan, an antimicrobial product. But there's no good evidence that it makes a difference.

• **Kitchen towels.** In a recent study, researchers observed 132 people preparing meals from raw chicken or ground beef. The participants were frequently seen touching their kitchen towels after handling the raw meats and before washing their hands. When they did wash their hands, they used the contaminated towels to dry them.

My advice: Don't wipe your hands on towels after handling raw meat. Wash your hands first or use paper towels.

• **Bars of soap.** Germs can live quite comfortably in the "slime" on any bar of soap, even antibacterial soap. This can be risky for people with compromised immune systems—the elderly…transplant patients…and those with serious underlying diseases, such as diabetes.

My advice: Use an alcohol-based hand sanitizer, even when you are at home, whenever you would wash your hands (unless your hands are very dirty—then wash them first). People who use a hand sanitizer daily can reduce their risk for infection by 70% to 80%. If you prefer not to use a hand sanitizer, at least switch from bar soaps to liquids.

• **Bathroom towels are loaded with germs.** That's partly because people don't

---

Germy Desk Danger for Women

In a study, we found that the desks of female workers harbor three to four times more bacteria than men's desks. Women tend to be neater than men, but about 70% kept food at their desks—and it tended to be fresh food that can be contaminated. (Men are more likely to stock their drawers with things such as candy bars.)

It's a good idea to clean desk surfaces with a disinfecting wipe at least a few times a week.

---

wash their hands thoroughly enough. A scant 16% follow the CDC's advice to lather the fronts and backs of the hands, between the fingers and under the nails, taking a full 20 seconds to do a thorough job.

And people who wash their hands well after "Number 2" often give them just a ritual rinse after urinating because they believe that urine doesn't contain germs. Not true. Urine can be loaded with viruses, including adenoviruses (which cause colds, sore throats and other symptoms) and even the virus that causes encephalitis. I'd estimate that up to 70% of the population is excreting viruses in urine at any given time.

Also, every time you flush the toilet with an open lid, bacteria spray as far as six feet into the air around the toilet and can migrate to your towels. And because towels tend to stay moist, they harbor large populations of pathogens. Studies have shown that hand towels can have more E. coli than a toilet bowl after the toilet is flushed.

My advice: Wash bathroom towels every two to three days. Close the toilet lid before you flush. Thoroughly wash your hands or use hand sanitizer after every trip to the bathroom.

• **Phones, remotes, computer keyboards.** When was the last time you wiped down your cell phone, computer keyboard or mouse or TV remote control? When someone in your family has the flu or a cold, about 60% to 80% of household gadgets are probably contaminated with the virus.

Don't assume that germs can't survive on inanimate objects. In fact, they may live longer on your cell phone than on your skin (which has antimicrobial properties). And because we use phones frequently, they're a common source of reinfection.

Example: Suppose that while working in the kitchen, you touch raw chicken that has Salmonella. Your phone rings. When you take the call, the germs will be transferred to your cell phone.

Later, after you have washed your hands, you'll pick up the same germs when you use the phone again.

My advice: If you use your phone after touching raw meat, use a disinfecting wipe to clean your phone immediately after washing your hands. At least once a week, wipe down your devices (including computer keyboards) with an alcohol sanitizer. Do it daily during cold and flu season.

•**Laundry.** Sure, it's dirty, but it's even dirtier than you think. The average pair of used underwear contains one-tenth gram of fecal material. When you load clothes into the washer, you could be picking up huge amounts of pathogens if someone who wore them was ill—and there's no guarantee that clothing will be germ-free when the washing cycle is complete. About 95% of households save energy with cold-water settings, which do not kill all germs.

My advice: Wash your clothes in hot water. And wash underwear separately from the other clothes, and after the cycle, run the machine empty, using two cups of bleach, to kill any remaining germs.

Cleaner Cooking Tips

When 132 home chefs were observed in a recent study, they were frequently seen touching cloth kitchen towels after handling raw chicken or ground beef and then spreading germs by using the towels to dry their hands after washing them. Tests revealed that 89% of the towels were contaminated with coliform bacteria and 26% with Escherichia coli.

Takeaway: Always wash towels in hot water with bleach after preparing raw meat, and use paper towels after washing your hands.

Charles Gerba, PhD, professor of microbiology and environmental sciences, The University of Arizona, Tucson.

Disgusting Stuff Found in Reusable Grocery Bags

Reusable grocery bags can make you sick. A recent study found that 97% of people never clean their bags—and most were crawling with bacteria, such as Escherichia coli, that can cause gastrointestinal ailments. Bags may collect pathogens from, say, a package of meat or raw produce, and then spread them to other foods.

Self-defense: Don't carry meat in reusable bags…and keep meat, as well as produce, separate from other foods. Wipe bags with bleach or machine-wash them after every use.

Charles Gerba, PhD, professor of microbiology and environmental sciences, The University of Arizona, Tucson.

Shocking Danger for Contact Lens Wearers

Jennifer Cope, MD, MPH, a medical epidemiologist with the Centers for Disease Control and Prevention's Division of Foodborne, Waterborne and Environmental Diseases in Atlanta. CDC.gov

There has been an increase in recent years in the number of eye infections caused by the rare but dangerous Acanthamoeba parasite. These infections can be very difficult to treat and sometimes lead to blindness.

Contact lens wearers usually are the victims, because Acanthamoeba can attach itself to the surface of a contact lens and then enter the eye through tiny cuts in the cornea.

Contact lenses can cause some of these tiny cuts (microtrauma).

Three things contact lens wearers can do to stay safe…

• **Remove your lenses before showering, bathing and swimming.** Acanthamoeba can live in tap water…swimming pool water… hot tub water…and even in natural bodies of water, both fresh and salt. This danger exists even if the water has been treated by a local water district and is perfectly safe to drink…and even if swimming pool water has been chlorinated. Acanthamoeba can survive these treatments, and infections have been increasing since 2004. Previously there were one to two cases per million American contact lens wearers. Now there are about 15 cases per million. It is not clear what is causing the increase.

• **Remove and thoroughly disinfect your lenses as soon as possible if they are exposed to water.** Peroxide cleaning systems are the only type that have been shown to kill Acanthamoeba.

• **Never use tap water to rinse off lenses or lens cases.**

Dead Disease Alive Again?

Plague has been on the rise. Cases in humans have been reported in Arizona, California, Colorado, Georgia, Michigan, New Mexico, Oregon and Utah. Plague is a bacterial infection carried by a rodent flea.

Self-defense: Wear insect repellent. Use flea-control products on pets. If you develop fever, chills, weakness and swollen lymph nodes—and have been in areas where plague is a concern—see your doctor immediately. Plague is treatable with antibiotics.

Natalie Kwit, DVM, MPH, an epidemic intelligence service officer at National Center for Emerging and Zoonotic Infectious Diseases, Centers for Disease Control and Prevention, Atlanta.

Urgent Lyme Disease Updates

One Tick Can Cause Two Infections

Deer ticks that carry Lyme disease bacteria can also be infected with *babesiosis*, a less common disease that infects red blood cells. A single bite from a doubly infected tick can cause a person to develop both diseases. In an area of New York State where tick-borne disease is common, nearly one-third of ticks were found to be infected with the bacteria that cause Lyme disease…and one-third of the infected ticks—or about 7% of all the ticks studied—also carried a second disease. Most people bitten by ticks do not develop Lyme or other tick-borne diseases.

Study of 7,643 ticks by researchers at Bard College, Annandale-on-Hudson, New York, published in *PLOS One*.

Lyme Transmitted Via Sex?

The risk of transmitting lyme disease sexually appears to be low but possible. Preliminary studies have found that among sexually active couples in which one person had Lyme (from a tick bite), the Borrelia bacterium that causes the disease was present in the genital secretions of both partners. But researchers don't know if certain Borrelia strains are more likely to grow in the uninfected partner or the role that immunity may play. Much more research is needed before Lyme can be considered a sexually transmitted disease.

Richard Horowitz, MD, Lyme disease specialist in Hyde Park, New York. CanGetBetter.com

New Species of Lyme Disease Discovered

A new species of Lyme disease bacteria discovered in the Midwest causes a spotted rash, not the well-known bull's-eye rash. New species of bacteria that cause Lyme and Lyme-like illnesses are being identified nearly every year. Look for a constellation of symptoms including fatigue…headaches…muscle and joint pain…nerve pain (tingling, numbness and burning)…sleep problems…and memory and concentration problems.

Richard Horowitz, MD, medical director of Hudson Valley Healing Arts Center, Hyde Park, New York, and author of *Why Can't I Get Better? Solving the Mystery of Lyme & Chronic Disease.*

You Can Cure Hepatitis C…The Trick Is Paying For It

Paul J. Thuluvath, MD, gastroenterologist, chief of the division of gastroenterology at Mercy Medical Center in Baltimore. He is the author of *Hepatitis C: A Complete Guide for Patients and Families.*

For those with hepatitis C, the good news is that the FDA recently approved new medications that eliminate the virus in nearly 100% of those who take them. That's roughly double the cure rate of older hepatitis C medications—and without the dreaded side effects, such as debilitating fatigue, nausea, skin rashes, anemia and depression, commonly caused by ribavirin and interferon, long used as the standard treatments.

Here's the catch: Many people can't afford to take these powerful new drugs, which can cost more than $100,000 for a recommended course of treatment. What you need to know about hepatitis C and the new—but costly—medications…

Getting Tested

Up to 75% of the people infected with hepatitis C are baby boomers (those born between 1945 and 1965). For this reason, the Centers for Disease Control and Prevention recommends that all people in this age group get tested for the virus.

Remember: Many people with hepatitis C have no symptoms—jaundice (yellowing of the skin and eyes), dark-colored urine, fatigue and loss of appetite are among the red flags that can (but don't always) occur during the acute (initial) or chronic (more than six months after infection) phase of hepatitis C infection. The only way to know if you carry the hepatitis C virus is to receive a blood test.

Typical cost: Up to $150, which is usually covered by insurance.

Because it is a blood-borne virus, some Americans were infected with hepatitis C during blood transfusions or organ transplants that were done before the blood supply was screened for the virus. Others were infected by contaminated needles (from drug use—the most common cause—or tattoos) or, less commonly, from unprotected sex with an infected partner.

Best Treatment Options

If you test positive for hepatitis C, you should talk to your doctor about getting treated. When choosing a drug, doctors look at viral genotypes (the specific type of virus that's causing infection), along with the severity of liver disease and other factors, such as viral counts. *New treatments…*

• **Harvoni.** This drug, a once-daily combination pill that includes the antiviral drugs sofosbuvir and ledipasvir, is for people with hepatitis C genotype 1, which affects up to 75% of those who carry the virus. Depending on the severity of the patient's liver damage, the medication costs about $63,000 (for an eight-week course) to $94,000 (for a three-month course). Side effects include fatigue, headache and insomnia, but they're usually tolerable.

• **Viekira Pak.** This "pak" contains two different pills—one combines the antiviral drugs *ombitasvir, paritaprevir* and *ritonavir*…the second pill is *dasabuvir*, another antiviral. Viekira Pak is prescribed for patients with or without cirrhosis who are infected with genotype 1. The cure rate for this

*Caution: All of the direct-acting antiviral drugs can interact with other medications and supplements—tell your doctor about all the drugs/supplements that you're using.

medication is close to 100% for genotype 1b and about 95% for genotype 1a.

Typical cost: About $83,000 to $168,000. Viekira Pak causes some of the same side effects as Harvoni.

Note: Viekira Pak has been linked to liver failure, so the FDA has recently warned that it may not be appropriate for patients with advanced liver damage.

•*Sofosbuvir* (Sovaldi) plus ribavirin. This drug combination is mainly used for patients with genotype 2 or genotype 3 infections, which account for about 20% of all hepatitis C patients. The cure rate is about 80% to 90%. Side effects are similar to those linked to Harvoni, plus possible anemia caused by ribavirin.

Typical cost: $84,000.

Coping With Costs

Most people who are exposed to hepatitis C develop a chronic infection that slowly (over decades) causes liver damage, so early treatment is preferable to avoid permanent liver damage. But for now, most insurers will approve treatment only for patients who already have advanced scarring or cirrhosis. Since cirrhosis increases the risk for liver cancer, it is better to get treated before cirrhosis develops.

Note: Even though up to 80% of people who are prescribed one of the costly hepatitis C drugs are initially denied coverage, some of them may get the medication after repeated appeals. If you have hepatitis C…

•**Get tested for liver damage.** Your insurer won't pay for the new treatments until you get a needle liver biopsy (a small piece of liver is removed with a needle) to determine the extent and severity of liver damage. If a biopsy shows that you have some liver damage but not enough to get insurance coverage, you'll have to make some hard choices—get another biopsy and subject yourself to a repeated invasive procedure or wait until symptoms develop, which indicates irreversible and advanced liver disease.

What helps: Even though health insurers require a biopsy, you can get some information about liver damage with a blood test or FibroScan, which is similar to an ultrasound. These tests aren't as accurate as biopsies but can help your doctor decide if you need the more invasive procedure.

•**Ask about clinical trials.** If you are denied insurance coverage and can't afford to pay out of pocket, you might qualify to participate in a study that will provide the new drugs at no cost to you. Most hepatitis C clinical trials are done without a placebo group, so everyone participating gets medication. For drugs that have already been approved, sometimes the FDA will request Phase 4 trials to gather information on any side effects with long-term use. Consult your doctor or check *ClinicalTrials.gov.*

•**Look into PAPs.** Pharmaceutical companies and other organizations sponsor patient-assistance programs (PAPs) that offer discounted drug prices for people without health insurance or for those with insurance who can't afford prohibitively expensive co-payments. Your doctor will have information.

Other resources: GoodRx.com…HelpRx. info…and NeedyMeds.org.

Another STD Spurs Concern

Betsy Foxman, PhD, professor, epidemiology, and director, Center for Molecular and Clinical Epidemiology of Infectious Diseases, University of Michigan, Ann Arbor.

Philip Tierno, PhD, professor, microbiology and pathology, NYU School of Medicine, NYU Langone Medical Center, New York City.

International Journal of Epidemiology.

There's yet another sexually transmitted infection that doctors and patients need to watch out for—Mycoplasma genitalium.

Recent research from England adds to evidence that the bacteria Mycoplasma genitalium, or MG, is transmitted through sexual contact. Until now, researchers weren't sure how the often-symptomless infection, identified in the early 1980s, was spread.

But the current study of more than 4,500 British residents found MG prevalent in 1% of participants and linked to risky sexual behaviors, such as multiple sex partners.

This finding suggests MG warrants more attention than it has received to date, said epidemiology professor Betsy Foxman, PhD, who specializes in infectious diseases at the University of Michigan.

The bacteria infects the mucus membranes of the urethra, cervix, throat or anus. Untreated, MG infection among women appears to raise the risk for infertility, preterm delivery or ectopic pregnancy (a potentially fatal pregnancy that occurs outside of the uterus). With men, the infection can lead to inflammation of the urethra (urethritis), the tube that carries urine and semen through the penis, according to the U.S. Centers for Disease Control and Prevention.

Few Symptoms Reported

Few study participants had symptoms, however.

Nearly 95% of infected men reported none of the symptoms generally associated with a sexually transmitted disease, such as penile irritation, inflammation, discharge, pain or odor. The same was true for 56% of women with MG who lacked any vaginal irritation, inflammation, bleeding or discharge.

Some women, however, reported bleeding after sex.

The researchers also analyzed results of an accompanying survey and concluded that, despite few classic STD symptoms, the risk for MG infection was "strongly associated" with sexual activity.

The study "strengthens evidence" that MG should be classified as a sexually transmitted disease, the authors wrote in a recent issue of the *International Journal of Epidemiology*.

Many American clinics already test for MG, said Philip Tierno, PhD, a professor of microbiology and pathology with the NYU School of Medicine in New York City.

"It used to be an organism that we couldn't easily diagnose," he said. "It would take days or weeks to grow, if at all, in a laboratory. But now it's much easier."

Currently, it's included in the standard STD molecular analysis done when a doctor suspects a possible sexually transmitted disease, Dr. Tierno said. That means it's tested alongside chlamydia, gonorrhea, syphilis, herpes simplex 1 and 2, and several other infections.

But the new study results suggest that only testing people with symptoms would miss the majority of infections, the authors said.

MG Prevention

So what about prevention? Drs. Foxman and Tierno agreed that, as with any STD, the more sexually active you are, the greater the risk.

Dr. Tierno cautioned that condom effectiveness "is limited"—given that even handling condoms after sex can expose users to MG. But, Dr. Foxman said "using condoms and other safe sex practices are good ways to minimize risk."

For those diagnosed with MG, the antibiotic *azithromycin* is the treatment of choice, according to the U.S. Centers for Disease Control and Prevention. In some cases, however, antibiotic resistance has forced clinicians to try alternatives, including the experimental antibiotic *moxifloxacin*.

New Health Threat: Antibiotic-Resistant Gonorrhea

Kirsten Bibbins-Domingo, MD, PhD, co-vice chair, U.S. Preventive Services Task Force, Rockville, Maryland., and professor, school of medicine, University of California, San Francisco.

Robert D. Kirkcaldy, MD, MPH, epidemiologist, division of STD prevention, U.S. Centers for Disease Control and Prevention.

Public health experts are expressing growing anxiety over the prospect of antibiotic-resistant gonorrhea.

Health officials in Great Britain recently cautioned their physicians and pharmacies about the dangers posed by drug-resistant strains of the sexually transmitted infection.

That concern is now being echoed by Robert Kirkcaldy, MD, a U.S. Centers for Disease Control and Prevention epidemiologist in the division of STD prevention.

"Resistant gonorrhea and the prospect of untreatable gonorrhea are real threats," he said, with resistant strains now detected in many parts of the world.

"The threat of untreatable gonorrhea underscores the importance of identifying new treatment options, ensuring adherence to screening and treatment guidelines—including treatment of (infected) partners—and increasing awareness among individuals on how they can best protect themselves from infection," Dr. Kirkcaldy added.

Gonorrhea spreads through unprotected vaginal, anal and oral sex. More than 350,000 new cases were reported in the United States in 2014, according to the CDC. But, the agency believes that the exact number is much higher. Young people, especially those under 24, appear to be most at risk of gonorrhea, the CDC says.

Women Should Be Routinely Screened

Symptoms of the infection are often absent. Undiagnosed and untreated gonorrhea may lead to pelvic inflammatory disease, infertility, ectopic pregnancy (a pregnancy that occurs outside of the uterus) and/or chronic pelvic pain, the CDC reports.

To prevent such complications, the U.S. Preventive Services Task Force vice chair Kirsten Bibbins-Domingo, MD, PhD, said that at-risk older women and all sexually active women aged 24 and younger should be routinely screened for the infection.

The task force didn't issue specific guidance for men. But the CDC said that anyone who's sexually active is at risk of gonorrhea.

Currently, gonorrhea is curable.

Since 2012, the CDC has advised doctors and other health professionals to use a combination therapy to treat the infection. The combination includes the injectable antibiotic *ceftriaxone* along with the antibiotic pill *azithromycin*. By 2014, more than 97% of U.S. cases were treated this way, up from 9% in 2006, the CDC said.

Is Antibiotic-Resistant Gonorrhea a Threat in the US?

The bad news? The CDC estimates that at least 2 million Americans contract infections—including gonorrhea—that are resistant to at least one antibiotic.

Still, "no patients have had confirmed failures of (gonorrhea) treatment with the currently recommended combination of ceftriaxone and azithromycin in the United States," Dr. Kirkcaldy stressed.

"However, a small but growing number of gonorrhea infections that were unsuccessfully treated with cefixime, ceftriaxone, or azithromycin by themselves have been observed in other countries," he said.

"And at least one azithromycin treatment failure has occurred in the US," Dr. Kirkcaldy added. This means that "it is only a matter of time before gonorrhea becomes resistant to the only remaining treatments currently available," he said.

The alarm in the United Kingdom followed antibiotic-resistant cases that popped up earlier in 2015 in the British city of Leeds. That government's letter urged medical professionals to adhere to the recommended two-drug combination treatment, given that antibiotic misuse could open the door to resistance.

In the US, antibiotic overuse or misuse "is probably not the largest contributor to the problem," Dr. Kirkcaldy said. Instead, he suggested, the threat more likely stems from resistant strains being imported from abroad.

Regardless, the fear of a "post-antibiotic era" remains.

"Losing effective treatment will cripple our ability to fight and prevent gonorrhea, and will also leave patients at greater risk of serious health complications from untreated gonorrhea," Dr. Kirkcaldy warned.

Chapter 11

PAIN AND AUTOIMMUNE DISEASE

Why a Woman Should Sit Like a Man to Prevent Pain

Ladies, the way you were taught to sit may be polite but could be contributing to a long list of orthopedic problems that cause hip and knee pain.

The solution: SLAM! It stands for "Sit Like a Man," a phrase coined by Texas orthopedic surgeon Barbara Bergin, MD, who believes that the approach is key to treating—even better, preventing—painful conditions of the knees and hips that are particularly common in women, especially as they age.

What problems can sitting like a man help prevent? *They include…*

•**Hip bursitis,** caused by inflammation of the tiny fluid-filled bursa near the hips, which serve as cushioning for the hip bones.

•**Patella malalignment,** a kneecap "tracking" condition in which the knee has a tendency to slip out of the "knee groove."

•**Chondromalacia,** sometimes called "runner's knee," in which the cartilage under the kneecap (the patella) deteriorates.

•**Gluteal tendonitis,** an inflammation of the tendons that attach the gluteal muscles on the butt to the thighs.

•**Piriformis syndrome,** in which the piriformis muscle in the butt compresses the sciatic nerve.

The Downside to a Ladylike Demeanor

What's wrong with sitting like a lady? It exacerbates a natural female anatomical tendency to rotate the femur (thighbone) inward, which pushes the knees inward. "When we sit 'lady like,' we further exaggerate that movement," explains Dr. Bergin. *Here's how…*

Keeping your knees and thighs together when you sit pulls the tendons that attach the buttocks to the hip across the hip bone. That puts tension on both the piriformis and the gluteal tendon, which can become inflamed—and can also irritate the bursa sac.

Crossing your legs is bad in its own way—contorting the tendons along the knee and overstretching the hip tendons, which puts pressure on the sciatic nerve.

Barbara Bergin, MD, orthopedic surgeon, Texas Orthopedics, Sports & Rehabilitation Associates, Austin. She is currently writing a book based on the SLAM concept. DrBarbaraBergin.com

In treating her patients for these conditions, Dr. Bergin became frustrated because the known treatments didn't always work. Standard options included certain strengthening and stretching exercises, cortisone treatments, anti-inflammatory medications, braces and other orthotic aids.

So she added specific exercises to encourage the femur to rotate outward—and found that this helped reduce her patients' pain. The problem, she surmised, was that women too often rotate their legs inward.

Herself included. "As I started aging, I got hip bursitis, and I started being mindful of my pain and realized that it had to do with the way I was sitting. It was worse when I was shoving my legs inward," she says.

If you want to try it, the good news is that you don't need to slouch like a teenage boy with your legs splayed out—aka manspreading—to get the benefits of SLAM. It's a subtle change, although it may be easier to get in the habit when you're wearing pants rather than a skirt or dress.

How to SLAM

When sitting, let your knees drop slightly apart, with your knees at about the 11:00 and 1:00 positions. Your knees should align with your feet.

It's a slight relaxation of your legs. You may notice that when you sit the way you've been trained, there's a little tension in your legs—when you SLAM, it's a more natural position for your legs. Be especially attentive to using this positioning when you get in and out of your chair, because sitting and standing puts a lot of stress on your kneecaps. When you get up, keep your feet flat on the ground and don't allow your legs to collapse into a knock-kneed position.

While Dr. Bergin's approach hasn't been proven scientifically, she has seen many of her female patients improve from simply sitting differently. "When I have patients start the SLAM program, they start to feel relief in their hips and their knees," says Dr. Bergin. "Most are getting better."

She typically combines the SLAM technique with other recommendations. For kneecap-tracking issues and knee pain, Dr. Bergin recommends also doing physical therapy and avoiding stairs, squats, deep-knee bends and lunges. For hip pain, she recommends physical therapy and avoiding activities that are painful, such as squatting, sleeping on the painful side, power walking and getting in and out of chairs quickly.

Her mission is to help women prevent these painful conditions—so they don't have to see orthopedic experts like her. She understands that it's not always possible to SLAM, but she encourages women to wear pants when they can and to take every opportunity, when seated, to sit like a man. She'd like moms to pass on the new approach to their daughters, too.

Eat Your Way to Pain Relief

Mel Pohl, MD, a physician who specializes in treating addiction and chronic pain. He is the medical director of the Las Vegas Recovery Center and author, with Katherine Ketcham, of *The Pain Antidote: The Proven Program to Help You Stop Suffering from Chronic Pain, Avoid Addiction to Painkillers—and Reclaim Your Life.*

Most people don't realize that dietary changes—eating certain foods and avoiding others—can have a big effect on chronic pain, such as joint pain, back and neck pain, headaches and abdominal pain. I've seen for myself with patients who have a variety of chronic pain conditions (as well as my own back pain) just how effective dietary changes can be.

Where to start...

• **More cherries and berries.** All fruits contain healthy amounts of antioxidants, which are important for reducing inflammation and pain. Inflammation is associated with tissue swelling, pressure on nerves and decreased circulation, which contribute to pain. Cherries (along with blueberries, cranberries and blackberries) are particularly helpful because they're rich in anthocyanins, chemicals that relieve pain even more effectively than aspirin. Cherries do have a fairly short season, but frozen cherries and 100% cherry juice offer some of the same benefits, though nothing takes the place of fresh organic produce.

In a study, researchers at University of California-Davis found that men and women who ate a little more than a half pound of cherries a day had a 25% reduction in C-reactive protein (CRP), a clinical marker for inflammation.

Bonus: The vitamin C in cherries and other berries has additional benefits. It's used by the body to build and repair joint cartilage, important for people with joint pain caused by osteoarthritis. Like anthocyanins, vitamin C also is a potent antioxidant that can reduce CRP.

•**Give up sugar.** By now, many of the hazards of sugar, including weight gain and cardiovascular damage, are well known—but most people don't know that consuming sugar increases pain.

What's the link with chronic pain? A high-sugar diet causes the body to produce advanced glycation end products (AGEs), which trigger massive amounts of inflammation.

And it isn't only sugar per se that does the damage. The American College of Clinical Nutrition has reported that foods with a high glycemic index—these include white bread, white rice and other "simple" carbohydrates that are quickly converted to glucose during digestion—increase inflammation even in healthy young adults. For those with arthritis or other ongoing painful conditions, even a slight increase in inflammation can greatly increase discomfort.

My advice: Try to eliminate added sugar and processed carbohydrates from your diet. Give up candy, soda, baked goods and highly refined grains. If you really enjoy a bit of sugar in your morning coffee, go for it. Treat yourself to the occasional sweet dessert. But in my experience, people with chronic pain usually do better when they give up sugar altogether.

•**Cooler cooking.** You might struggle with pain control if grilling is one of your favorite rituals. Meats and other foods exposed to prolonged, high-heat cooking—on the grill, in the broiler, pan-frying and deep-fat frying—generate high levels of AGEs. Increased pain is just one of the risks—some research has linked AGEs to heart disease, diabetes and possibly even Alzheimer's disease.

You'll do better with cooler cooking methods, such as simmering and sautéing and moderate-heat (around 350°F) roasting. Slow-cookers are another good choice. I don't advise patients with chronic pain to give up grilling, broiling or pan-frying altogether. Just remind yourself to use these methods less often—say, once a week. Let your pain be your guide. If it's getting worse, make bigger changes.

•**Less alcohol.** Actually, no alcohol is the best choice for people with chronic pain. Alcohol irritates intestinal tissue and allows bacteria to pass into the blood more readily. The presence of bacteria will increase inflammation even if you don't develop obvious symptoms of infection.

Listen to your body. Some people can have an occasional beer or a glass of wine without noticing any change in their pain levels. If you're one of them, go ahead and imbibe on occasion.

•**Switch to olive oil.** The heart-healthy benefits aren't the only reasons to use extra-virgin olive oil in place of polyunsaturated vegetable oils (such as canola). Olive oil contains a substance called oleocanthol, which interferes with the inflammatory COX-1 and COX-2 enzymes. People who consume olive oil have lower levels of prostaglandins, the same pain-causing neurotransmitters that are blocked by aspirin.

Use olive oil just as you would other cooking oils—by drizzling some on pasta or salads, for example, or using it when you sauté vegetables or fish.

•**Eat seafood twice a week.** The omega-3 fatty acids in cold-water fish (such as salmon, sardines and trout) are among the most potent anti-inflammatory agents. Studies have shown that people who suffer from morning stiffness and joint tenderness do better when they consume more omega-3s. You can get by with fish-oil supplements, but they're unnecessary if you eat fatty fish at least twice a week.

•**Drink plenty of water—between eight and 10 glasses a day.** It helps the kidneys and liver filter toxins (such as pesticide residues) from the body. Even though the liver breaks down about 95% of the toxins you ingest, the by-products can linger in the blood and other tissues. Water dilutes the concentration and reduces the inflammatory effects.

Also helpful: Green tea. It provides extra water along with catechins, antioxidants that reduce inflammation and pain.

Stop Pain with a Soothing Ginger Compress

When placed on the lower backs of people with osteoarthritis for 30 minutes daily, a warm ginger compress reduced overall pain and fatigue by half after just one week. The ginger compress was a cotton cloth soaked in a hot ginger infusion (two teaspoons of ground ginger to one-half cup of very hot water), squeezed well so that it was just moist.

Theory: Topical ginger seems to warm and relax the musculoskeletal system, increasing mobility. The compress likely will work on pulled muscles and achy joints, too.

Study by researchers at Edith Cowan University, Perth, Western Australia, published in *Journal of Holistic Nursing.*

Shingles Vaccine Eases Long-Term Pain

Shingles vaccine reduces long-term pain in women. Shingles patients often devel-

Common Pain Relievers May Undermine Fertility

Pain killers known as nonsteroidal anti-inflammatory drugs (NSAIDs), such as *naproxen* (Aleve), may hinder ovulation and reduce levels of the female hormone progesterone. Women who are trying to get pregnant should ask their doctors about alternative pain relievers.

Study by researchers at University of Baghdad, presented at the European League Against Rheumatism Congress in Rome.

op postherpetic neuralgia (PHN), long-term pain that is a complication of the condition. More than 10% of unvaccinated women developed PHN. But only 4% of vaccinated women developed PHN. (Vaccinated and unvaccinated men had a roughly 6% chance of developing PHN.) The US Advisory Council on Immunization Practices recommends that all people age 60 and older be vaccinated against shingles.

Study of 2,400 people over age 60 who developed shingles by researchers at Kaiser Permanente Southern California, Pasadena, published in *Journal of Infectious Diseases.*

Powerful PMS Prevention

Green veggies prevent PMS. Three daily servings of cooked green cruciferous vegetables such as kale, broccoli and brussels sprouts cut risk of developing premenstrual syndrome (PMS) by up to 40%, according to a 10-year study of nearly 3,000 women.

Why: Green cruciferous vegetables are high in iron, which is necessary to produce mood-elevating neurotransmitters in the brain.

Patricia Chocano-Bedoya, PhD, visiting scientist, Harvard School of Public Health, Boston.

Jump Up on Knee Pain

Jumping—yes, jumping!—may help knee arthritis.

Recent study: Postmenopausal women with minor knee osteoarthritis who did high-impact exercise (step aerobics with quick turns and jumps) three times a week had improved stability and stronger knee cartilage than those who didn't do this exercise.

Why: Jumping and other high-impact movements build collagen and bone.

Implication: Men and women with knee osteoarthritis may benefit from high-impact exercise but should get an OK from a doctor first.

Jarmo Koli, MSc, physiotherapist, University of Jyväskylä, Finland.

Aching Knees? It Could Be Low Vitamin D

Low vitamin D levels are linked to progression of knee osteoarthritis. Patients found to be clinically deficient in vitamin D were twice as likely to experience worsening knee osteoarthritis as people with sufficient vitamin D.

Fang Fang Zhang, PhD, MD, an assistant professor in the Friedman School of Nutrition Science and Policy, Tufts University, Boston, and leader of a data analysis, published in *Journal of Nutrition.*

Helpful Headband Halts Headaches

BioTrak Health Halo senses subtle head and neck muscle tension that can presage the onset of migraines and tension headaches. The headband sends a gentle vibration to alert its wearer to the potential problem. Then an app guides the wearer through relaxation techniques designed to ward off the headache. BioTrak says Halo users eventually learn to

Migraines Can Worsen as Menopause Approaches

The frequency of migraine headaches increases as women go through perimenopause, during which hormone levels change and menstrual cycles become irregular. The chance of high-frequency migraines—10 or more per month—increases by 60% during this transition and is highest in the later stage of perimenopause. Hormone therapy may help reduce migraine frequency.

Study of more than 3,600 women led by researchers at University of Cincinnati and Albert Einstein College of Medicine, New York City, published in *Headache: The Journal of Head and Face Pain.*

sense an oncoming headache themselves, reducing the need to wear the headband. Halo has not yet been subjected to independent studies, but research suggests that biofeedback and relaxation techniques can control certain headaches. Halo should be available by early 2017. Visit *HaloCalm.com* for more information and to sign up for alerts.

Gary Kaye, founder and chief content officer of Tech50+, an Internet site that covers consumer electronics–related topics. Based in Oxford, Connecticut, he has reported on technology for more than 30 years at *NBC News, ABC News, CNN, Fox Business Network* and other organizations. Tech50Plus.com

Release the Kinks of a Stressed-Out Neck

Jill Miller, fitness therapy expert based in Los Angeles, author of *The Roll Model* and creator of the exercise program YogaTuneUp.com.

If the pain in your neck is…a real pain in the neck, then your head is probably not in the right place—literally. *Los Angeles–based fitness therapy expert Jill Miller has an easy, stress-releasing move to fix that…*

How to tell if that's the problem: You constantly want to rub the back of your neck...or crack your neck...or you frequently get neck aches.

What you should do: Place your hands, fingers interlaced, on the back of your head where it would touch the headrest on a car seat. Push your head back against your hands while resisting the push. Hold for 10 seconds...rest for 30 seconds...then repeat twice more.

This isometric exercise will strengthen your neck muscles and align your head over your rib cage—where it should be. "Do this every time you recognize that your head is leaning in front of your rib cage," Miller advises.

Soon you'll train your neck to stay in a relaxed, neutral position...where it belongs.

Stop Shoulder Pain Without Surgery

Beth E. Shubin Stein, MD, an associate attending orthopedic surgeon and a member of the Sports Medicine and Shoulder Service at the Hospital for Special Surgery in New York City.

Most people are quick to chalk up shoulder pain to tendinitis, a nagging form of inflammation. But that's usually a mistake.

New thinking: The shoulder pain thought of as tendinitis is typically a result of tendinosis, a related condition that occurs when the tendons (ropelike cords connecting muscle to bone) begin to deteriorate. Tendinosis can usually be diagnosed with a physical exam and an X-ray and/or MRI.

Red flag for the patient: The pain may be barely perceptible while the arm is at rest—but if you extend the arm outward, in front of the body or overhead, the pain can range from dull to excruciating.

Rotator cuff tendinosis develops when tendons in the rotator cuff (a group of tendons and muscles that attach the upper arm to the shoulder joint) break down over time. This can occur due to age...repetitive use...or weakness of the rotator cuff muscles.

What works best: During the first week or two, to "quiet" the inflammation around the tendon, apply ice (for 15 to 20 minutes several times daily)...and take a nonsteroidal anti-inflammatory drug (NSAID), such as *ibuprofen* (Motrin).

If pain continues, your doctor should also refer you to a physical or occupational therapist, who can recommend exercises (such as those on the next page) to strengthen the rotator cuff and shoulder blade (scapula) muscles. If pain worsens or lasts longer than a week or two, a cortisone injection into the bursa surrounding the rotator cuff tendons can help.

Good news: Within six weeks, this nonsurgical regimen alleviates the pain 90% of the time.

Beware: Chronic use of cortisone can damage tendons, so surgery (see below) should be considered if two or three injections (given no more than every three months) have not relieved the pain.

If you don't get relief after six weeks or the pain returns after cortisone therapy wears off, you may want to consider surgery. Arthroscopy (inserting a tiny camera via small incisions) allows the surgeon to assess the shoulder joint and correct the damage that has led to rotator cuff tendinosis. When performed by an experienced surgeon, the procedure has a high success rate. Complications are rare but may involve infection or stiffness.

To find an experienced surgeon, consult The American Orthopaedic Society for Sports Medicine, *SportsMed.org*.

Two approaches that are less invasive than surgery...

•**Platelet-rich plasma (PRP) injection involves the use of platelets from a patient's blood.** The platelets are separated from the blood with a centrifuge and reinfused into the affected tendons. The platelets are rich in growth factors that aid healing, and the technique is considered safe, since the patient's own cells are used.

A small study published in 2013 in *Global Advances in Health and Medicine* found that a single PRP injection significantly improved pain and function at a 12-week follow-up. More research is needed, however, for definitive evidence of its effectiveness. Some patients opt to have a series of PRP injections. Insurance rarely covers the cost—typically about $1,500 per injection.

• **Stem cell treatment.** With this therapy, which is currently experimental, certain bone marrow cells are reinjected into the shoulder area, where they can help replace degenerated tendon tissue. Though promising, this therapy is not yet widely available. Several clinical trials are now ongoing. To find one, go to *ClinicalTrials.gov.*

Frozen Shoulder

Frozen shoulder (or adhesive capsulitis), which usually occurs for unknown reasons, develops when the capsule surrounding the shoulder joint gets inflamed and then stiffens. A dull ache in the shoulder can come and go, slowly worsening to a ferocious pain that may awaken you during sleep or hurt even when your arm is at your side.

In the past, doctors recommended physical therapy to "thaw out" the joint and restore range of motion. But the physical therapy typically aggravated the condition—and it often did not improve for more than a year.

New thinking: With a two-part approach—a cortisone injection given early on into the joint and gentle exercises—sufferers can get pain relief and restore their range of motion within a matter of weeks to months.

Surgery is rarely needed if frozen shoulder is promptly diagnosed and treated at this stage. Cortisone injections are usually not helpful when frozen shoulder has progressed to severe stiffness, but physical therapy may help restore mobility.

After receiving a cortisone injection, the following exercises should be performed on the recovering shoulder three times a day. *Gently hold each for five seconds and do 10 reps of each exercise…*

• **Overhead stretch.**

What to do: Lie on your back with your arms at your sides. Lift your arm straight up in the air and over your head. Grab your elbow with your other arm and gently press toward your head.

• **Cross-body reach.**

What to do: Stand and lift your arm to the side until it's a bit below shoulder height, then bring it to the front and across your body. As it passes the front of your body, grab the elbow with your other arm and exert gentle pressure to stretch the shoulder.

• **Towel stretch.**

What to do: Drape a towel over the unaffected shoulder, and grab it with your hand behind your back. Gently pull the towel upward with your other hand to stretch the affected shoulder and upper arm.

This Little-Known Joint Could Be Causing Your Back Pain

Jo Ann Staugaard-Jones, MA, an advanced Pilates and Hatha yoga instructor and trainer based in Andover, New Jersey. She is author of *The Vital Psoas Muscle* and *The Concise Book of Yoga Anatomy.* Move-Live.com

It's easy to blame nagging low-back pain on a muscle strain or even a disk problem. But that's not always the real cause.

A surprising culprit: Up to one-third of chronic low-back pain can actually be traced to pelvic instability. The sacroiliac (pronounced sak-ro-il-ee-ak) joints, commonly called the SI joints, are located on both sides of the pelvis, connecting it to the lower part of the spine (sacrum).

If this little area of the body gets out of whack, that is when the trouble begins. Unlike other joints throughout the body, a healthy SI joint doesn't flex and extend. Instead, it's considered a "gliding" joint, meaning that the ligaments holding it together can shift, but that

211

shifting is ideally kept to a minimum. The SI joint's main job is to hold the lower spine and pelvis together to increase stability.

Certain life events can cause excess movement in the SI joint, however. Pregnancy is a big one—the SI joints can be affected when ligaments and joints in the pelvic area loosen before giving birth.

For women who are years beyond childbearing age—and men, too—SI joint pain is slightly different. Usually affecting only one side of the pelvis, this type of SI joint trouble leads to a chronic, nagging pain in the lower back, which typically worsens when bending over from a standing position. Sitting, which the average American does for up to 13 hours per day, is another risk factor for SI joint pain—it weakens these joints and promotes inflammation.

Easy Steps That Help

If you have SI joint pain (marked by a consistent ache on either side of the base of your spine) or suspect that your SI joints may be contributing to low-back pain, see an orthopedic specialist to confirm your diagnosis. Movement tests and an X-ray or a CT scan will be performed.

A clue to watch for: If your pain improves when lying down, this is a sign that the SI joints may be involved. (This can also be a sign of spine degeneration, which can affect the SI area.)

In addition to the exercises on the next page, most doctors recommend the following to help relieve pain due to one or both SI joints...

● **Ice.** It reduces inflammation and produces a brief numbing effect that temporarily relieves pain. Ideally, ice the affected area for 15 minutes three times a day.

What to do: Lie on your belly with an ice bag on the painful area. You can alternate ice packs with a heating pad after the first 24 hours of treatment, when inflammation has subsided, to increase blood flow to the area.

● **Massage.** For some people, this helps... for others, it can aggravate the problem. If you would like to try massage, ask the therapist to use gentle pressure to promote circulation but avoid deep tissue work.

● **SI belt.** It is designed to relieve overtaxed ligaments by decreasing motion in and around the pelvis. The research on these belts is mixed. One study reported significant pain reduction in those wearing the belt, while other research found no such benefit or a worsening of pain for a small number of people.

If you want to try an SI belt, a good product is the New Serola Sacroiliac Hip Belt (about $45, depending on size). But if pain seems to worsen with a belt, stop using it.

● **Pain-relief medication.** If the therapies described above and exercise routine below don't give you adequate relief, you may need to add pain medication such as *ibuprofen* (Advil) or topical arnica gel.

Exercise for Your SI Joints

The main goal of a workout to relieve SI pain is to balance the strength of the muscles and tendons surrounding the joints so they can provide stability. Exercises that work the transverse abdominis (the deep ab muscles that support internal organs)...the deep external hip rotators that connect the sacrum to the thighbone...and the gluteus muscles will also help the SI joints remain strong yet supple. If you're in pain, relax the muscles and do these exercises when pain has lessened. Try the following 10-minute routine three

Simple Exercise Prevents Back Pain

Do this simple exercise to strengthen your back: Stand, sit or lie on your back, and exhale all your breath while pulling your navel in and up toward your head. Hold for 10 seconds, and release. Repeat 12 times.

Todd Sinett, DC, a chiropractor and founder/owner of Midtown Integrative Health & Wellness in New York City. He is author of *3 Weeks to a Better Back.*

times a week—you should get relief within three to six weeks…*

● **Squats.**

What to do: While holding a light weight (five pounds to start, working up to 10) or a 10-pound bar overhead (keep your shoulders down), stand in front of a mirror with a chair behind you to assist with the exercise.

(Holding a bar or weights overhead helps keep the body in correct alignment.) Engage your abdominal and back muscles as you bend your knees, lowering yourself toward a sitting position. (If your lower back begins to sway, you have gone far enough and need to pull your naval in toward your spine.) Allow your hips to fall back toward the chair until your buttocks lightly touch the chair, but do not sit down. Aim for your upper thighs to be parallel to the floor. Hold the squat for 10 to 20 seconds, while breathing deeply, then slowly return to a standing position. Repeat three to five times.

● **Hand/knee balance.**

What to do: Get down on all fours in a tabletop position with your back as level and flat as possible. Your hands should be directly under your shoulders and your knees under your hips. Begin by stretching your right leg back and lifting it to hip height, then slowly lift your left arm forward in line with your ear. Keep your pelvis stable and centered and your core muscles tight. Hold for 10 seconds. Then return to the tabletop position and repeat on the other side. Alternate sides for one minute.

● **SI stretch.**

What to do: Lie on your back on an exercise mat or carpeted floor with your legs straight and your arms outstretched to your sides. Bend your right knee toward your chest, then let it fall across your body to the left, letting your hips roll with it. (Keep both your shoulders on the floor.) Relax and breathe in and out for a minute before repeating on the other side.

*As with any exercise program, check with your doctor first.

Stress-Busting Move for Tense Hips and Buttocks

Jill Miller, fitness therapy expert based in Los Angeles, author of *The Roll Model* and creator of the exercise program, YogaTuneUp.com

I f getting up after hours of sitting is a slow, painful unfolding process, it's likely that you're holding stress in your hips and buttocks.

How to tell if that's the problem: Your hips are stiff and ache or your lower back hurts when you stand up after sitting for a long time…or you have pain along the sciatic nerve, which extends from the lower back down the back of each leg.

What you should do: Lie on your back on the floor with your legs extended and the soles of your feet against a wall. Slide a yoga block or a three- or four-inch-thick book under your hips. Keeping your left leg straight and your left foot against the wall, draw your right knee toward your chest, getting as close as you can. Hold this position for one minute while "breathing deeply from your abdomen so that your belly and ribs swell," Miller advises. Then switch legs. This move targets the psoas muscle, which runs from your hips into the tops of your thighs and helps support your lumbar spine (lower back). Do it during an afternoon break from your desk and at the end of the day.

Surprising Causes of Back Pain

Todd Sinett, DC, chiropractor and founder/owner of Midtown Integrative Health & Wellness in New York City. He is author of *3 Weeks to a Better Back: Solutions for Healing the Structural, Nutritional and Emotional Causes of Back Pain.*

P eople blame all sorts of things for back pain. Maybe it started when you were lugging suitcases from the car or hauling boxes from the garage. These may seem like obvious culprits, but most cases of back pain are caused by things that you would never suspect, including…

• Oversized Bags

When you carry a heavy bag—a gym duffel, a purse, a computer bag—the working shoulder elevates and puts the spine out of alignment.

Another danger: "Bag jerk" occurs when a heavy bag abruptly falls off the shoulder, causing a jerk to the body. The resulting neck, shoulder and back strain can be comparable to a sports injury.

The best evidence that women's handbags have gotten too big comes from the American Chiropractic Association. It now advises women to limit the weight of their handbags to 10% of their body weight. But should a 150-pound woman be carrying even 15 pounds over her shoulder? That's a lot of weight!

My advice: Put your bag on a diet—take out whatever you really don't need. When you're walking, shift the bag from shoulder to shoulder now and then. You also might consider a backpack.

• Flip-flops

These casual slip-ons give almost no support. The thin soles are a common cause of heel and arch problems. The lack of heel support forces people to take shorter steps and to scrunch up their toes to keep the shoes on, both of which can lead to pain in the knees, hips and lower back. Walking in flip-flops is worse for you than walking barefoot.

My advice: Wear flip-flops only in the venues for which they were designed—at swimming pools, in locker rooms, at the beach, etc.

• Too Much Sitting

Sitting has been called the "new smoking" because it has been linked to type 2 diabetes, cancer and heart disease. It's also hard on the back because it exerts more pressure on the spine than standing. People who slouch when they sit—or hunch forward when watching TV or working on the computer—experience even more pressure.

My advice: Don't just sit when you're sitting. Shift your weight every few minutes. Arch your back. Lean back when you notice that you have been hunching forward. At least twice an hour, get up and walk around for a few minutes.

Also helpful: A reclining chair. Recliners lengthen the spine and cause less pressure than upright chairs.

• Chewing Gum

Too much jaw action stresses the temporomandibular (jaw) joint, which stresses the muscles throughout your back, leading to tension and pain.

Jaw-related problems may be accompanied by tightness all along the back and spine.

Possible signs of jaw problems: You can't open your mouth very wide…your jaw occasionally clicks or "sticks"…and you grind your teeth or clench your jaw a lot.

My advice: Give up chewing gum altogether. It's also helpful to stretch the jaw muscles. Place your hand under your jaw. Push with just a little resistance while you open/close your mouth. Repeat the stretch 10 times, three times a day.

Also helpful: Wearing a mouth guard when sleeping reduces pressure on the jaw from clenching. If an over-the-counter mouth guard doesn't fit properly, ask your dentist for a customized one.

• Constipation

Believe it or not, constipation is a common cause of back pain. A lack of regular bowel movements causes buildups of inflammatory wastes that irritate the large intestine, which in turn irritates muscles in the back.

My advice: When you notice that "things aren't moving," drink a big glass of cold water. It will stimulate the urge to have a bowel movement.

Also important: Regular exercise and plenty of beans, fruits, vegetables and other high-fiber foods.

Caution: Don't depend on high-powered "digestive cleanses"—colonics, supplements, extreme fasts, etc.—for regular bowel movements. They can trigger irritation that is just as hard on the back as constipation.

• Stress Breathing

People with stressful lives take rapid, shallow breaths often or even all the time, and they aren't really aware of it. Rapid breathing can't deliver all the oxygen your body needs. Muscles that are deprived of oxygen get tight and sore...and the stress that causes rapid breathing makes muscle tension even worse. Back pain can result.

Self-test: Turn your head all the way to the right or left—and see how far it goes. Then, take slow, deep breaths for about 30 seconds. Turn your head again. Did it go farther this time? If it did, you need to relax and get more oxygen.

My advice: Every day—particularly when you're stressed—take a few moments to breathe deeply.

Back Pain? Relief Is in the Palm of Your Hands

Deborah Flanagan, certified reflexologist and founder, Center for True Health, New York City.

If you have back pain, relief may lie in the palms of your hands. Reflexology involves applying mild pressure to specific spots on the hands and feet that are believed to correspond with different body organs. While it hasn't been extensively studied, there is scientific evidence that reflexology can help with chronic back pain.

This move is one that you can perform for yourself—any time, anywhere—to get speedy relief.

How it works: Relieve a tense, aching back by stimulating the spine reflex. This is the area on each thumb that extends down the outside, along the base to the wrist.

What to do: Press with the pad of your left thumb along the outside edge of your right thumb, inching from the top of the thumb, down across the base and across to the mid-

dle of your wrist. Then use your right thumb to do the same thing to the outer edge of your left thumb. Repeat this exercise three or four times on each hand, several times a day. Spend a little more time on any spot that feels tender.

Surprising Cure for Back Pain: It's Not Drugs, Exercise or Surgery

Todd Sinett, DC, chiropractor and founder/owner of Midtown Integrative Health & Wellness in New York City. He is author of *3 Weeks to a Better Back: Solutions for Healing the Structural, Nutritional and Emotional Causes of Back Pain.*

If you have persistent back pain, most doctors look for structural problems—a herniated disc, for example, or a misaligned spine. These can be real issues, but they point to a solution for only a small percentage of patients.

Surprisingly, back pain can be the result of poor nutrition and poor digestion, which causes chronic inflammation that irritates muscles, ligaments, tendons and/or nerves. A recent study in *Asian Spine Journal* found that nearly one-third of women and one-quarter of men with back pain also had food intolerances or other gastrointestinal complaints.

Dietary changes won't always eliminate back pain (although they might), but they often reduce pain significantly. If you rate your pain as an eight, for example, changing your diet could reduce it to a manageable two or three. *What to do...*

• Get enough fiber. If you're often constipated or have infrequent bowel movements, you'll have buildups of toxins that increase inflammation and back pain. A high-fiber diet can fix this and reduce your back pain.

My advice: Look at your stool. It should be more or less smooth (and should pass easily). If it is lumpy and hard, you probably need more fiber. Increase your water, fruit and vegetable intake.

●**Cut back on caffeine.** Caffeine is a stimulant that increases levels of cortisol, a hormone that triggers inflammation. People who drink a lot of coffee or other caffeinated beverages are more likely to have painful muscle cramps and spasms.

My advice: Eliminate caffeine for two to three weeks. If this makes a big improvement, give it up altogether. If it doesn't help, you can go back to it because caffeine isn't the culprit.

●**Stay well hydrated.** Many of my patients don't drink water very often. This is a problem because you need water to improve digestion and reduce inflammation—and because people who don't drink much water often consume less healthful beverages, such as sodas. Water also helps lubricate the spinal discs and can help prevent fissures, cracks in the discs that can allow the soft middle portion to bulge out and press against a nerve.

Everyone with back pain should drink between four and 10 glasses of water a day. The first thing I do every morning is drink a big glass of water. If you're not a fan of plain water, you can spruce it up with a squeeze of lemon or lime or substitute watered-down juice (half juice, half water).

●**Eliminate all added sugar.** The average American consumes about 175 pounds of sugar a year—from soft drinks, desserts and even packaged foods that you wouldn't imagine are loaded with sugar, such as white bread, salad dressing, ketchup and pasta sauce.

The rapid rise in glucose (blood sugar) that occurs when you eat sweetened foods triggers the production of cytokines, proteins secreted by immune cells that increase inflammation. A high-sugar diet also irritates the digestive tract, which can lead to back pain.

My advice: Give up all added sugar for at least three weeks. It takes about two weeks for existing inflammation to "calm." Staying off added sugar for an additional week will help reinforce the change in your usual habits. After that, you can reintroduce a small amount of sugar—by having an occasional dessert, for example, or adding a small amount of sugar to your morning coffee.

If you add back a bit of sugar and your pain doesn't increase, you'll know that you can enjoy some sugar. On the other hand, you might notice that you're having more back pain again, in which case you'll want to cut out sugar.

●**Eat more organic produce.** Most people know that antioxidants in fruits and vegetables—substances such as vitamin C, lycopene and indole-3-carbinol—can reduce levels of cell-damaging molecules (free radicals) that cause inflammation. In my experience, getting more antioxidants isn't as effective for pain as improving digestion (with fiber, cutting back on sugar, etc.), but it can help. I tell patients to buy organic produce because it won't be tainted with pesticides or other inflammatory chemicals. Also, a recent study found that organic corn contained 58% more antioxidants and that organic marionberries (a type of blackberry) had up to 50% more antioxidants than their nonorganic counterparts.

Look for sensitivities. The healthiest diet in the world won't improve back pain if you're eating foods that trigger a reaction in you. Many foods (including foods considered healthy, such as broccoli) can trigger symptoms in some people. In addition to pain, these symptoms could include digestive irritation, sleepiness after a meal, fogginess, achiness and/or congestion.

To find out whether you're sensitive to one or more foods, track what you eat with

Non-Addictive Painkiller

A new harder-to-abuse narcotic painkiller has been approved. Targiniq ER is a combination of the narcotic oxycodone and naloxone, which blocks the euphoric effects of oxycodone. Naloxone is activated if the pill is crushed, snorted, dissolved or injected, but Targiniq still can be abused by swallowing too many pills. Targiniq is approved for use by patients with chronic pain that has not responded to other medications.

US Food and Drug Administration, Silver Spring, Maryland.

a journal. When you notice an increase in pain, you can review the journal and find the food(s) that might be responsible. In addition to the foods mentioned in this article, dairy and gluten are common offenders.

My advice: When you identify a likely food suspect—maybe you drank a beer on the day your back got worse—give it up for a few weeks. If your symptoms improve, test your conclusion by having a small amount of that food or beverage. If the pain increases again, you'll know that you have to avoid that food in the future. Or you can go to a gastroenterologist, allergist, nutritionist or integrative medical doctor for food-sensitivity testing.

Got Knee Pain?

Jordan Metzl, MD, a sports medicine physician at the Hospital for Special Surgery in New York City. He is coauthor of *The Exercise Cure: A Doctor's All-Natural, No-Pill Prescription for Better Health & Longer Life*. DrJordanMetzl.com

Why live with a bum knee when you can have less pain and more mobility with a new one? With such great promises and the relative ease of knee-replacement surgery, it's no surprise that this is now one of the most popular procedures in the US.

It's true that the procedure can be a blessing for those with severe arthritis (the main reason for surgery) that impairs their ability to live an active, pain-free life. But the decision to have surgery should not be made casually—and if you do end up getting a knee replacement, there are facts you should know before choosing between the tried-and-true approach and the newer, less invasive surgical procedure.

To Avoid Surgery

If you have mild-to-moderate knee pain, but you're still able to work and do normal activities, chances are you can greatly improve without surgery by following these steps...

•**Stretch and strengthen the muscles.** Studies have shown that simply strengthening the muscles that support the knees (the quadriceps in the front of the thighs and the hamstrings in the backs) can reduce damage, pain and disability.

My advice: Work those muscles three or four times a week for at least six to eight weeks before making a decision about surgery.

Examples: Leg extensions, hamstring curls and clamshells. Even if your knee is hurting, it's worth taking an over-the-counter painkiller, such as *ibuprofen* (Advil) or *acetaminophen* (Tylenol), about 30 minutes before your workout so that you can do the exercises. Curcumin supplements have also been shown to decrease inflammation and arthritis pain. A physical therapist or personal trainer can help design a workout that includes targeted stretches and strengthening exercises that are right for you.

•**Drop some excess weight.** Every pound of body weight equals several pounds of "loading force." This means if you are 10 pounds overweight, for example, your knees get an extra 40 pounds of pressure. That's enough to increase pain and limit mobility—and accelerate arthritis-related damage.

My advice: If you're overweight—even by a few pounds—it's affecting your knees. Get serious about losing those extra pounds!

•**Try hyaluronic acid.** This naturally occurring substance acts as a lubricant to the joints and may work as well as painkillers and steroids (without the side effects) for some people. It's usually injected into the affected joints once a week for three to five weeks.

My advice: There's no way to predict who will benefit from these injections. Consider them if exercise and weight loss haven't given you adequate relief. Insurance typically covers the cost.

What Next?

If you've given the strategies described earlier your best shot and still have serious knee pain, surgery is usually the next step. *What to consider…*

• **Partial knee replacement.** This approach, also known as uni-compartmental knee replacement, is newer than total knee replacement and gets a lot of attention because it is less invasive. The advantages include an incision that is roughly half the size (about three to 3.5 inches) of that used for total knee replacement. Patients also are hospitalized for just a day or two rather than three to five days for a total knee replacement. With the partial approach, the knee may feel more "natural"—for example, it may have less "creakiness" and better range of motion—than it would after a more extensive procedure.

But a partial knee replacement isn't for everyone. To be a candidate for this procedure, the damage is generally isolated to only one part of the knee. Also, the research is not yet clear, but patients who have partial procedures may be more likely to require subsequent "revision" surgery—because of continuing arthritis, for example, or because the first procedure didn't improve pain and/or mobility. For many patients, the risks from repeat surgery could outweigh the benefits of a less traumatic initial procedure.

• **Total knee replacement.** This procedure is called a "total" replacement because the damaged surfaces of the knee bones are replaced—the tibia (shinbone)…femur (thighbone)…and sometimes the patella (kneecap). The surgery requires a large incision (usually seven to eight inches) and typically takes about two hours.

The majority of patients who opt for knee surgery require a total replacement. Surgeons have a lot of experience with the procedure—and there's strong evidence that it works. More than 90% of total knee-replacement patients report that they have a lot less pain…and about 85% of these artificial knees are still going strong after 20 years. While patients who receive total replacements have somewhat less flexibility than those who go the partial route, most are able to do light hiking, ballroom dancing and biking.

The Bottom Line

No matter which approach your surgeon suggests, make sure you're comfortable with the plan. Some patients will feel best about the decision if they get a second opinion.

Until more is known about the long-term benefits and risks of partial knee replacement, most surgeons advise their patients with severe arthritis to get it over with and have a total replacement.

Patients with osteoarthritis in all areas of the knee and those with inflammatory arthritis (such as rheumatoid arthritis), which tends to affect the entire knee, are not candidates for a partial approach and require a total knee replacement.

Consider a partial procedure only if you mainly have damage in just one part of the knee, you haven't improved after physical therapy, weight loss and the other suggestions described above, and your pain prevents you from sleeping through the night and/or performing your normal daily activities.

Sore, Achy Feet? Take the Ball Cure

Jill Miller, fitness-therapy expert based in Los Angeles, author of *The Roll Model* and creator of the exercise program YogaTuneUp.com.

If your feet get tender and achy, you might be holding stress in your feet, says fitness-therapy expert Jill Miller. Her easy-to-do move releases foot tension and makes for happy feet. All you need is a small, hard ball such as a racquetball—and a wall.

Here's how to tell if that is your problem: You have heel pain, achy arches or soreness in the balls of your feet.

What to do: Stand next to a wall for balance, and place a racquetball under your right foot. Load your weight onto the ball, then move the ball from side to side, and up and down, under the sole of your foot. If you'd like to, you can place your left foot on

Don't Take Tylenol for This

Tylenol doesn't relieve two common types of pain. Acetaminophen, found in Tylenol, is ineffective for low-back pain—it worked no better than a placebo—and provides only minimal, short-term benefit for knee/hip osteoarthritis. What may help more: Oral or topical nonsteroidal anti-inflammatory drugs (NSAIDs), such as ibuprofen and naproxen… weight loss…and exercise.

Gustavo Machado, PhD candidate, The George Institute for Global Health, University of Sydney, Australia, and lead author of an analysis published in *BMJ*.

top of your right foot to sandwich it and massage your right foot from above, helping it to destress, Miller says. Do this for one minute, then switch feet. Do this at the beginning and end of each day as well as anytime you sense tension building up in your feet.

Important note: If you have persistent foot pain, see a health-care professional.

Shoes for Hammertoe

Johanna Youner, DPM, podiatric surgeon in private practice in New York City. HealthyFeetNY.net

There are actually many fashionable choices for hammertoes and leg pain. You need a shoe with maximum support, so look for a more rigid shoe with a sturdy heel and cushioned footbed to help support your feet. A high toe box (vertical room at the front of the shoe) protects hammertoes from additional friction.

The best shoe for hammertoes is a tie-up oxford, since the foot does not have to work to keep it on. Other trendy styles that give good support are low-height "flatforms" (flats on a platform)…and booties (a cross between boots and shoes).

Expect to pay at least $75 for a good pair of shoes. Look for shoes that have the seal of acceptance from the American Podiatric Medical Association, which means they have been found to promote good foot health. Good brands (for women and men) include Clarks, Ecco, Rockport, Asics and Vionic.

Drug-Free Cure for Underactive Thyroid

Pamela Wartian Smith, MD, MPH, MS, codirector of the Master's Program in Medical Sciences with a concentration in metabolic and nutritional medicine at Morsani College of Medicine, University of South Florida. She is author of *What You Must Know About Thyroid Disorders & What to Do About Them*. Center ForPersonalizedMedicine.com

Do you feel tired or cold much of the time? Are you anxious, irritable, depressed? Maybe you have trouble losing weight. If so, you may have an underactive thyroid (hypothyroidism)—and you're not alone. The American Association of Clinical Endocrinologists estimates that about 27 million adults, close to 10% of the population, suffer from thyroid disease. Hypothyroidism (underactive thyroid) is the most common form, accounting for about 90% of all cases.

What to do? Hormone replacement always is an option—but you might not need it.

My advice: Start with these lifestyle changes and other natural treatments. If you're currently taking thyroid medication, you may need less medication—so be sure to let your doctor know that you're taking these steps…

•**Add iodine.** You've probably heard that iodine deficiency is rare in the US because iodine is added to salt—and because many foods contain it. Not true. There's been an increase in iodine deficiency because many people avoid iodized salt (or are eating less salt in general). In addition, many people eat diets that are high in pasta and bread. These foods often contain bromide, a compound that decreases iodine absorption.

My advice: Get tested for iodine. Low levels are easily corrected by using iodized salt…eating sea vegetables (such as nori) a few times a week…or by taking an iodine supplement.

Important: Don't take an iodine supplement unless you need it. Too much iodine can cause thyroid inflammation and increase your risk of developing Hashimoto's thyroiditis (a kind of hypothyroidism) or thyroid cancer.

• **Eat Brazil nuts.** They're high in selenium, a mineral that helps the body convert thyroxine (T4, a less active form of thyroid hormone) to triiodothyronine (T3, the active form). One study found that low-thyroid patients given selenium supplements later tested normal on a thyroid test. A few Brazil nuts a day will provide enough selenium. Other high-selenium foods include fish, chicken, turkey and beef.

Note: If you live in North Dakota or South Dakota, then you already have a lot of selenium in your diet because the ground in these states is rich in selenium. Therefore, you probably will not need additional selenium as a food or supplement.

• **Take probiotics.** I recommend them for everyone with low-thyroid function. Studies have shown that probiotic supplements—Lactobacillus, Bifidobacterium, etc.—improve the body's ability to absorb the nutrients that are needed for thyroid health. I've had patients who were able to avoid using medication simply by optimizing their digestive health with probiotics.

My advice: Buy probiotic supplements that contain at least 20 billion colony-forming units per dose (available at health-food stores and pharmacies). Research has shown that people tend to do better when they rotate bacterial strains about every six months.

• **Take a daily multi.** Many different nutrients are required for the body to convert T4 to the more active form of thyroid hormone, T3. Even if you eat a nutritious diet, you might not be getting enough. For insurance, take a multinutrient supplement that includes all the basics, such as potassium, selenium, B vitamins and zinc. Ask your health-care provider if you need iron in your multivitamin.

• **Don't skip breakfast.** The pancreas ramps up insulin production in the morning and again in the evening. You need to synchronize meals with high-insulin times to improve insulin sensitivity—the ability of cells to respond to insulin and absorb blood sugar. One study found that people with improved insulin sensitivity had lower TSH (see box below) and higher T4. An example of a good breakfast would be turkey sausage and berries. The sausage is a protein that slows the absorption of the carbohydrate (the berries), which is better for blood sugar levels.

Don't Trust the Thyroid Test

The standard test for low thyroid might not provide a clear answer. You could test normal but still have thyroid function that's at the lower end of the range—which, for some people, is enough to cause problems.

Low thyroid is diagnosed with a simple blood test for thyroid-stimulating hormone (TSH). If you have low thyroxine, a thyroid hormone, your body will produce high levels of TSH to compensate. People with significantly elevated TSH—say, a reading of 5.0 mIU/L (milli-international units per liter) or higher—have obvious hypothyroidism.

What if you test within a normal range but still are having symptoms? It doesn't mean you're imagining things. Laboratories have different reference ranges, the measurements that are considered normal. In 2004, endocrinologists suggested a change in the normal range so that a TSH reading of 2.5 was the upper limit. But for some people, normal isn't optimal. I've found that patients can suffer from thyroid-related symptoms even when they "pass" the TSH test.

This is why it is very important to have a complete thyroid panel done when you see your doctor and not just a TSH and free T4. An entire thyroid panel includes TSH, free T3, free T4, reverse T3 and thyroid antibodies.

•**Avoid harmful foods and ingredients.** Sugar, refined carbohydrates (such as white bread and white rice) and soft drinks can contribute to hypothyroidism by decreasing the levels of important minerals in your body. Opt for healthier choices—a Mediterranean-style diet is ideal, along with plenty of purified water.

If Your Symptoms Don't Improve...

If your symptoms don't improve from lifestyle changes and natural treatments, you'll probably need a thyroid medication. The good thing about these prescription drugs is that they precisely mimic the effects of your body's natural hormones. You're unlikely to experience any side effects after your doctor has determined the correct dose. Until then, you might have the same symptoms that you had before (if you're taking too little). Or, you might have shakiness, insomnia, rapid heartbeat or an increased appetite (if you're taking too much).

The standard prescription hormones, such as Synthroid or Levothroid, contain only T4.

My advice: Ask your doctor to prescribe one of the powdered thyroid hormones—such as Armour Thyroid, Euthroid or Liotrix—that contains T3 along with T4. They usually come in a standard ratio of four parts T4 to one part T3. Studies have shown that most patients who are given both tend to do better than those who take only T4.

Real Help for Fibromyalgia

Daniel Clauw, MD, professor of anesthesiology, medicine (rheumatology) and psychiatry, and director of Chronic Pain and Fatigue Research Center, both at the University of Michigan, Ann Arbor.

Effective treatment for fibromyalgia is finally possible now that there is a better scientific understanding of this painful condition, which affects about five million Americans.

The new insights explain a lot, in fact—including how prescription painkillers often make fibromyalgia pain worse...which medications can provide relief...and why the real route to fibromyalgia recovery lies in non-drug approaches that retrain the brain. For the answers that fibromyalgia patients need, we spoke with one of the top specialists in the country, Daniel Clauw, MD, director of the Chronic Pain and Fatigue Research Center at the University of Michigan.

Key insight: The primary source of fibromyalgia pain is not in the back or neck or head or stomach or legs, where the pain is typically felt—but rather is inside the brain. And that points to solutions.

Where the Pain Is Really Coming From

While people with fibromyalgia may suffer pain all over their bodies, the primary cause of the pain stems from the way the central nervous system interprets sensory input. Painful stimuli...or even just touch...gets intensified in the brain and spinal cord. It's like a stereo system that keeps turning up its own volume.

The evidence: Two neurotransmitter chemicals—glutamate and substance P, which increase the transmission of pain signals—are too high in people with fibromyalgia. Other neurotransmitters, including serotonin, norepinephrine, and GABA (gamma-aminobutyric acid), which decrease pain transmission, are—you guessed it—too low in people with the condition. Brain imaging studies show that when patients with fibromyalgia are given a mild pressure or heat stimulus, the pain-processing areas of their brains light up. In people without fibromyalgia, they don't.

There is still debate, of course. There are new findings that people with fibromyalgia have abnormalities in the peripheral nervous system, which sends signals from the arms, legs and organs to the brain. However, even proponents of peripheral involvement now agree that the central nervous system plays an important role.

Why Opioids Backfire

Patients with fibromyalgia often don't get relief from traditional pain relievers, such as nonsteroidal anti-inflammatory drugs (NSAIDs), which can be effective for peripheral pain syndromes such as typical headaches or muscle aches but help only about one-third of patients with chronic pain such as fibromyalgia.

Opioid drugs are even worse.

The reason: The body is already overproducing its own natural opioids released in response to chronic pain. These natural painkillers are flooding the system, filling up the body's opioid receptors, so there are few places for synthetic opioids to land. This chronic overstimulation of the body's opioid system, originating in the brain, may contribute to the progress of fibromyalgia.

There has never been a study showing that opioids are effective for fibromyalgia. In fact, by contributing to this overstimulation, synthetic opioids may even increase pain in people with fibromyalgia. Indeed, in some studies, a low dose of the opioid-blocking medication naltrexone has provided fibromyalgia relief. Heaping on synthetic opioids, as many doctors have tried (and patients have asked for), just makes the overstimulation worse. Giving more opioids might be akin to throwing kerosene on a fire.

The more effective treatments have included drugs that target neurotransmitters. These include the three drugs currently approved by the FDA for fibromyalgia—*pregabalin* (Lyrica), which reduces brain glutamate levels, and the antidepressants *duloexitine* (Cymbalta) and *milnacipran* (Savella), which increase both serotonin and norephinephrine.

But even these drugs shouldn't play the primary role in a fibromyalgia treatment plan. Rather, the focus should be on lifestyle modification and mind-body therapies that help manage stress, incorporate exercise and help improve sleep.

It's not just general "healthy living" advice, but based on rigorous research on what works for this specific medical condition. In a clinical review of all relevant studies on fibromyalgia from 1955 through 2014, the treatments that have the best scientific evidence were evaluated. Treatment approaches were then rated based on the quality of the studies. Pharmacological therapies can be helpful in alleviating some symptoms, but patients rarely achieve meaningful improvements without adopting these core self-management strategies.

Retraining Your Brain Without Drugs

Lifestyle and mind-body approaches that help with fibromyalgia have something in common—they all help restore a balance of neurotransmitters in the brain and central nervous system. They literally change the brain. Brain imaging studies are showing more and more that these approaches can affect brain function. They are not only just as effective as medication, he says, but almost always are safer and less expensive.

The following approaches are particularly effective in treating fibromyalgia…

• **Exercise.** It's not easy to become more active when you're in pain—not to mention often sleep-deprived because of your discomfort—but it really helps. The best approach is to "start low, go slow," focusing first on increasing daily activity such as walking a little more than you usually do, then building up slowly so that you develop more aerobic endurance. While aerobic exercise has been best studied for fibromyalgia, strength-training and stretching have also been shown to be of value. Exercise boosts brain levels of norepinephrine and helps reduce stress.

• **Cognitive Behavioral Therapy (CBT).** Fear of pain can make pain worse. This form of "talk therapy" helps patients learn new ways to think about how they feel, and that affects brain function and can reduce pain. CBT is effective in fibromyalgia whether it's one-on-one, in groups or even through online programs. It is important to understand that CBT is not primarily a "psychological" intervention in this context, but an approach that can help change how the brain interprets pain signals.

• **Complementary and alternative therapies.** These include tai chi, yoga, water-based massage such as Watsu and acupuncture. While these have not been rigorously studied for fibromyalgia, Dr. Clauw believes that they are effective for many patients.

Getting a good night's sleep is also key to balancing neurotransmitters and feeling better...which is easier said than done. When pain keeps you up at night, it's awfully tough to get the sleep you need. To help fibromyalgia patients understand how to work through the challenges of this disease and reduce stress, get more exercise, sleep better and use other nondrug strategies, as well as help you personalize your plan, check out the free online Fibroguide (*https://fibroguide.med.umich.edu/fibromodules.html*).

Relieve the Pain, Sleep and Anxiety Problems of Fibromyalgia with Qigong

Mary Lynch, MD, a professor of anesthesiology, pain medicine and perioperative care at Dalhousie University in Halifax, Nova Scotia. Her pain research focuses on the use of complementary therapies such as qigong and acupuncture as well as art therapy.

If you have fibromyalgia, or know someone with this chronic condition that can make even the lightest touch excruciatingly painful, it's easy to get frustrated. But there is hope for lasting relief. As modern science uncovers the key role the central nervous system plays in this disease, we are discovering that the best approaches aren't drugs at all but ancient mind-body disciplines that literally "retrain the brain." There are many ways to retrain your brain, including yoga and tai chi.

The key is to find a practice that you like and can do regularly.

That's why it's great to find that yet another gentle movement system has now been shown to relieve fibromyalgia symptoms.

It's called qigong.

Qigong Against Chronic Pain

Qigong, a form of "meditative movement," involves fluid, dynamic movements along with quieting breath work. It's already been shown to relieve chronic neck pain, help in recovery from mild traumatic brain injury and reduce symptoms of chronic fatigue syndrome.

In the new study, researchers from Dalhousie University in Halifax, Nova Scotia, assigned 100 people with fibromyalgia to learn and practice qigong—or to be put on a waiting list for treatment (the control group). Most were women (average age 52) who had been suffering for about 10 years. Those in the qigong group spent three half-days learning the practice from a qualified instructor and then were asked to practice for 45 to 60 minutes every day for eight weeks.

Results: After eight weeks, those in the qigong group improved significantly in their pain levels, sleep quality, anxiety levels and ability to function, physically and mentally. But the study didn't end there. They were encouraged to keep practicing on their own and, four to six months later, the women reported that the benefits continued.

Those who practiced the full 45 minutes a day got the most benefit. Exactly how it works isn't known, but lead author Mary Lynch, MD, a pain medicine expert, notes that the mindful, meditative state that you reach through qigong releases neurochemical and immunological messengers that improve healing and reduce pain.

"We do know that it works," she says. "Some people in the study reduced the amount of medications they were using or got off meds completely. But you have to continue to practice it. This is not an as-needed treatment."

Exploring the Qigong Way

The best way to find a qigong training program near you is to look at community centers with recreational offerings, mindfulness centers, alternative healing centers and women's centers, Dr. Lynch says.

Why Lupus Patients Need Gene Testing Before Taking Certain Drugs

Claudia Mauri, PhD, professor, immunology, University College London, UK.

Rosalind Ramsey-Goldman, MD, DrPh, professor, medicine, Northwestern University Feinberg School of Medicine, Chicago.

Immunity, online.

Scientists have found new clues that help explain what's going wrong in the immune systems of people with lupus—insight they hope will lead to new therapies, or help guide current treatment choices.

Lupus has several forms, but the most common is *systemic lupus erythematosus* (SLE). In SLE, the immune system mistakenly produces antibodies against the body's own tissue. The onslaught can have widespread effects, damaging the skin, joints, heart, lungs, kidneys and brain, according to the Lupus Foundation of America.

The disease mostly strikes women, usually starting in their 20s or 30s, the foundation says.

Study Details

In the recent study, the researchers found evidence that in people with lupus, some of the immune system's "B cells" mature the wrong way—so that they promote inflammation instead of fighting it.

The findings, published online in the journal *Immunity,* could help in developing new lupus therapies, said senior researcher Claudia Mauri, PhD.

In people without lupus, anti-inflammatory B cells appear to prevent excessive production of a protein called interferon-alpha, explained Dr. Mauri.

That's a critical job because too much interferon-alpha leads to too many B cells that produce antibodies, the study authors said. Antibodies are necessary soldiers in the body's defense against infection, but in lupus, some of those antibodies target the body itself.

The findings are based on blood samples from nearly 100 healthy volunteers and 200 people with lupus. Dr. Mauri's team found that lupus patients seemed to have an imbalance among three types of immune cells: B cells that produce antibodies; B cells that regulate inflammation; and cells that produce interferon-alpha. The root cause of it all remains a mystery, however, Dr. Mauri said.

"We will continue to work to develop new [treatment] strategies that harness the anti-inflammatory B cells in patients with SLE," Dr. Mauri said.

Gene Testing for Lupus Patients

Right now, a number of drugs are used to treat lupus, including immune-system suppressors such as *cyclophosphamide* and *tacrolimus*, and anti-malaria drugs like *hydroxychloroquine*—which can ease the fatigue, joint pain and skin rash that lupus commonly causes, according to the Lupus Foundation of America.

In some cases, doctors try a drug called *rituximab*, an IV medication designed to kill off certain B cells. Rituximab is approved to treat certain cancers and rheumatoid arthritis—another autoimmune disease—but some lupus patients respond to the medication, too, the study authors said.

It's been unclear, though, why only certain lupus patients see benefits from rituximab, according to the researchers. Dr. Mauri said the new findings suggest a reason. People's response to rituximab may depend on whether they have normal activity in two genes related to interferon-alpha.

That, Dr. Mauri said, suggests that lupus patients should have gene testing before they're placed on rituximab. But, she stressed, "long-term studies—where patients get tested before, during and after treatment—are needed to prove that hypothesis unequivocally."

Expert Comment

A rheumatologist who was not involved in the study agreed. "At this point, more work is needed, including looking at feasibility and cost issues," said Rosalind Ramsey-Goldman, MD, a professor of medicine at Northwestern University Feinberg School of Medicine, in Chicago.

Dr. Ramsey-Goldman also agreed that the findings could eventually lead to new therapies, or point researchers in the direction of existing drugs for other conditions that could be "repurposed" to fight lupus.

And not all lupus patients would have this particular abnormality, according to Dr. Ramsey-Goldman. "SLE is probably a syndrome with multiple different immune system abnormalities," she said.

In general, Dr. Ramsey-Goldman explained, lupus is thought to arise from a combination of genetic susceptibility to autoimmune diseases and certain environmental factors.

Researchers still don't know what those factors are. But the suspects include certain infections, such as the Epstein-Barr virus, and on-the-job exposure to silica dust, according to the Lupus Foundation of America.

The Lupus Foundation of America has more on lupus risk factors at *lupus.org*.

Got MS? Parkinson's? Had a Stroke? Ballroom Dancing Can Help

Alexander Ng, PhD, associate professor, Program in Exercise Science, Marquette University, Milwaukee. His study, "Dancing with MS: Benefits of Ballroom or Recreational Social Dance for Persons with MS," was presented at the Consortium of Multiple Sclerosis Centers 2015 Annual Meeting.

W hen you have a chronic condition, you may not feel like dancing the night away. But dancing with a partner actually may be the best thing you can do for body and mind. Studies show that partnered dancing offers tremendous benefits to people with Parkinson's disease, Alzheimer's and other forms of dementia, and those recovering from a stroke.

Here's a new condition to add to the list—multiple sclerosis (MS). The progressive chronic central nervous system disease, which can alternate between flare-ups and periods of remission, can cause fatigue, muscle weakness and balance problems. It often affects the ability to walk unaided.

Whether it's the waltz, fox-trot or salsa, partnered dancing is a perfect activity for people with MS. "If you're with a partner, you might be able to do movements that you wouldn't ordinarily be able to do if you have issues with balance or impaired movement," says study author Alexander Ng, PhD, a professor of exercise science—and a recreational ballroom dancer himself. The partner offers physical support and can be somewhat of a coach, encouraging the patient to push himself or herself.

To test the theory, Dr. Ng included 12 people with MS who were able to walk at least 25 feet on their own and stand for at least five minutes without assistance. Some had no noticeable movement problems at all, while others needed the help of a cane or walker to get around. Six participated in hour-long dance classes…twice a week…for six out of eight weeks (to give participants flexibility around summer vacations). The other six people, the control group, didn't dance but received the same routine medical care as the dancers. Dances included the waltz, fox-trot, rumba and swing. (In the next study now in progress, they will also be including salsa, tango and merengue.) Before and after the dance program, both groups underwent a battery of tests such as walking unaided for 25 feet, getting up from a chair and walking three yards and then sitting down quickly (a measure of mobility), and tests for walking balance, which predicts the risk of falling.

The results: Dancers had higher scores on those tests for balance, mobility and endurance. They also had improvements in self-reported fatigue and depression (which tend to afflict people with MS) as well as cognitive benefits related to the ability to stay focused, while the control group did not.

It's a small, preliminary study, although another small study has found similar benefits when people with MS learn salsa dancing. As it turns out, there is a good body of research backing up partnered dancing for chronic conditions.

How Social Dancing Works as Therapy

At a minimum, dancing is aerobic exercise, which has been demonstrated to improve both physical and cognitive function in people with neurological disorders. Dance is also a complex activity that uses a combination of physical and mental tasks. Physically, dance requires balance, flexibility, speed and coordination—all skills that diminish in people with MS. And it calls on brain power—you have to remember and repeat steps, work with a partner and coordinate your movements together. Plus, it's social, which engages yet another part of the brain, and, last but not least, it's joyful. "When you're focused on dancing," says Dr. Ng, "troubles that may otherwise occupy your brain are shunted aside, so that you finish mentally refreshed."

Indeed, neuroimaging studies have shown that frequent dancing increases activity throughout the brain. When you're in the groove, it seems, your whole brain just lights up.

The strongest evidence for the benefits of partner dancing is in Parkinson's disease, another neurological condition in which movement is affected. Partner dancing actually echoes many of the key elements recommended in physical therapy for Parkinson's, such as responding to cues, learning new ways to move and engaging in balance exercises.

Studies show that partnered dancing helps people with Parkinson's develop a better gait while walking, have less rigidity in their movements, improve their ability to use their arms and hands and, in general, helps with functional mobility. One non-profit organization, Dance for Parkinson's (*danceforparkinsons.org*) offers resources in more than 100 communities in 13 countries.

Perhaps its strongest appeal is that it's fun, creative and social. Says Dr. Ng, "People don't tend to view dance as exercise or physical therapy…so they're more likely to want to do it." Nor do you need to find special classes for people with MS or other chronic conditions. While it's a good idea to get lessons in ballroom dancing if you're unfamiliar with the steps, it's not a requirement.

Dancing for the Rest of Us

Partner dancing is great for healthy aging for everyone, actually. Healthy older adults who are involved in amateur dancing score better on a list of motor and cognitive skills than their nondancing counterparts. Once you get good at it, you may even want to consider competitive ballroom dancing.

Bonus: It's said to make women feel more beautiful.

Surgery Best for Hashimoto's

People suffering from the autoimmune disorder known as Hashimoto's thyroiditis sometimes become so overwhelmed with fatigue, joint and muscle pain, and stiffness that they are unable to function. But preliminary results from a new seven-year study suggest that removing the thyroid could bring about vast improvements for patients.

Why: Thyroid removal appears to normalize production of antibodies that attack the thyroid.

If you have Hashimoto's: Ask your doctor if surgery (which may be covered by insurance) is an option. Thyroid-replacement medication must be taken indefinitely.

Ivar Guldvog, MD, researcher, Telemark Hospital Trust, Porsgrunn, Norway.

Hidden Parathyroid Disease Can Weaken Bones, Cause Kidney Stones and Brain Fog

Shonni J. Silverberg, MD, professor of medicine, division of endocrinology, Columbia University College of Physicians and Surgeons, New York City.

You get a painful kidney stone and get treated, and your doctor tells you to drink more water to prevent another one.

You break a bone, and it turns out that you have osteoporosis, so your doctor talks to you about diet, exercise and prescriptions.

You're feeling nauseous, don't feel like eating and are experiencing constipation and diarrhea. Your doctor suggests various tests to see if you have a gastrointestinal condition.

You have trouble concentrating, find that your memory isn't as good as it used to be and, in general, feel like you're experiencing brain fog. Your doctor asks if you've been sleeping well lately.

But what if all these symptoms were caused by a little-known disease...one that's entirely curable with surgery?

It's called primary hyperparathyroidism, a disease of the parathyroid glands, and it can cause havoc to the bones, kidneys and even the brains of sufferers.

A Disease With Terrible Symptoms...or No Symptoms At All

In a sense, you're lucky if you have symptoms. Some people have no symptoms at all even as the disease is causing serious harm. Fortunately, a common blood test for calcium levels that your regular doctor may routinely order can pick up the earliest signs. That's the first step to identifying the condition.

Unless you have symptoms, however, your doctor may not suggest surgery right away. Some physicians recommend watchful waiting for asymptomatic patients. But waiting while the disease may be damaging your body is controversial, even among experts.

Fortunately, the most current guidelines make it clear exactly who should get treated right away. Here's what you need to know.

A Tiny Gland Can Turn Your Whole System Upside Down

About one in 1,000 Americans have primary hyperparathyroidism, three times as many women as men. It's becomes increasingly more common over age 60. (Primary means it's not caused by another disease.)

A little background: Primary hyperparathyroidism is not a problem with the thyroid gland. Rather, it affects the tiny pea-size parathyroid glands on or near the thyroid. There are four of them, but usually only one is overactive, signaling excessive release of parathyroid hormone. That hormone's purpose is to maintain the right level of calcium in the blood, and when it's overactive, it signals the body to pull too much calcium from the bones into the bloodstream. That can weaken bones and lead to osteoporosis and fractures...cause kidney stones...and create neurological issues that affect concentration and memory and lead to depression.

Until the 1970s, people with primary hyperparathyroidism would be diagnosed when they went to their doctors with serious complaints—bone pain, broken bones, abdominal pain and kidney stones. (Other symptoms of severe disease may include nausea, vomiting, loss of appetite, constipation and an increased need to urinate.) Since that time, the disease is generally caught earlier through calcium tests, which are now part of the routine blood test you get during an annual physical.

If you have any of the symptoms or conditions mentioned above and you haven't had a checkup recently, ask your doctor for a blood test. If the result shows a high calcium level in your blood, your parathyroid hormone level will be tested...and if it is high, you'll likely be diagnosed with parathyroid disease. It's usually caused by a noncancerous tumor on one of the glands.

227

Although medication is sometimes prescribed to manage the disease, there are no medications that can cure it or treat all of its effects. The only way to cure it is through surgical removal of the overactive gland or glands. Within the first year, your bones become stronger, kidney stones wane and you may find that the brain fog and mood issues get better, too.

But what if you get the diagnosis after a regular checkup but don't have any symptoms? Should you still get your diseased parathyroid gland removed?

The Surgery Decision

Most people who show up at the endocrinologist with primary hyperparathyroid disease don't have any obvious symptoms, says Shonni J. Silverberg, MD, professor of medicine in endocrinology at Columbia University College of Physicians and Surgeons. When the calcium test was added to routine blood tests in the 1970s, patients began to be diagnosed when they were asymptomatic. The number of people diagnosed with the disease rose by a factor of four to five times.

Experts disagree about what to do if you don't have symptoms. Some recommend waiting because not everyone does develop clinical problems, and the disease progresses at different rates in different people...and more slowly in older adults. Other experts are concerned that those who don't receive surgery are needlessly putting themselves at risk for complications down the road.

Recently updated guidelines from an international group of experts can make that decision easier. Unless you are too frail for surgery, even if you have no clear symptoms you should have surgery if you are diagnosed with primary hyperparathyroidism and have any of these factors...

•**Very high blood calcium levels.** A normal blood calcium level for an adult ranges from 8.5 milligrams per deciliter (mg/dL) to 10.2 mg/dL, although there are slight variations based on different labs. If your calcium level is 1 mg/dL above the normal range, it's not just slightly but significantly elevated.

•**Silent kidney stones.** If you have kidney stones, you should have the surgery. When they're painful, you'll know you have them. But the new guidelines acknowledge that some people may have "silent" stones, meaning that they're there but not causing any symptoms. One study found that 15% of patients had kidney stones that were not causing symptoms. An ultrasound or other imaging test is recommended to detect any silent stones, and if any are found, you would be a candidate for parathyroid surgery.

•**Kidney trouble.** If your kidneys are not working well (impaired kidney function) for any reason, that's another reason to have surgery. This can be detected by a routine blood test as well.

•**Osteoporosis or fractures.** Patients with osteoporosis have low bone density and are at risk for fracture. Primary hyperparathyroidism can affect your bones, making them weaker. If you have low bone density, you should have surgery. Your physician can use a bone densitometry machine to noninvasively measure the density of your bones. The new guidelines now also recommend imaging of the spine to look for compression fractures, which can go undiagnosed but indicate that the bones are already fragile enough to have fractured...and support the need for surgery.

•**Early onset.** If you're under 50, you should have surgery because you are likely to develop symptoms in your lifetime.

Unlike many illnesses, primary hyperparathyroidism can be cured with surgery more than 95% of the time, so experts tend to recommend it. In most cases, you can go home the same day that you have the surgery, although it takes between one and three weeks to heal fully. Most of the time, you won't need any medication or further treatment (since you'll still have some working parathyroid glands), although you will have to have your blood calcium levels checked regularly and may need to take calcium/vitamin D supplements.

If you do opt for surgery, finding an experienced surgeon is key. The area is delicate and sometimes the glands are hard to find (or more than one is involved), so surgeons need to know how to respond in those circumstances. In general, a surgeon should do more than 50 parathyroid operations a year to be considered an expert. Don't be shy or embarrassed to ask how many of a certain type of operation a surgeon has done and if his/her complication rate is above the average, which is less than 1% for an experienced parathyroid surgeon.

Tingling Hands and Feet? It Could Be a Sign of Celiac Disease

Study titled "Risk of Neuropathy Among 28,232 Patients With Biopsy-Verified Celiac Disease" by researchers in the department of medical epidemiology and biostatistics, Karolinska Institutet, Stockholm, Sweden, published in *JAMA Neurology*.

If you have peripheral neuropathy, a form of nerve damage that affects your extremities, your doctor may test you for diabetes. It's a common cause. But now research suggests something else to look for as well—celiac disease, the autoimmune disease marked by the body's inability to digest gluten, the protein found in wheat, barley and rye.

If the new finding leads more doctors to test their neuropathy patients for celiac disease, that's a good thing, since 80% of the 2.4 million Americans with celiac disease don't even know they have the disease, according to population studies.

Here's what you need to know about the neuropathy/celiac connection.

A New Symptom of Celiac Disease Emerges

Earlier studies had suggested a neuropathy/celiac link, but they were iffy. The new research makes the connection stronger. Swedish researchers identified 28,000 people who were diagnosed with celiac disease and com-

pared them with 140,000 subjects who didn't have celiac disease. At the beginning of the study, which lasted about 10 years, none of the subjects had been diagnosed with peripheral neuropathy.

Here's what the researchers found...

• **People with celiac disease were five times more likely to be diagnosed with peripheral neuropathy over the course of the study, compared to people without celiac.** The percentages were small—less than a 1% chance of being diagnosed with neuropathy if you have celiac, but it translates into tens of thousands of Americans.

• **In a separate analysis, the researchers followed people who were diagnosed with peripheral neuropathy over the course of the study but weren't originally known to have celiac disease.** It turns out that they were 80% more likely to end up being diagnosed with celiac than people who didn't have neuropathy.

The new finding suggests that peripheral neuropathy may be an early warning signal for celiac disease. Researchers aren't sure exactly how the two diseases are connected, but they note that celiac is an autoimmune disease, and many autoimmune diseases are linked to nerve damage. That damage may be related to the systemic inflammation that the autoimmune response evokes. (This study doesn't say anything at all about non-celiac gluten sensitivity.)

The good news is that diagnosing and treating celiac disease may help forestall peripheral neuropathy. There is evidence that when people with celiac and peripheral neuropathy go on a gluten-free diet—the only effective treatment for celiac—the neuropathy may stop getting worse.

The bigger picture is that anything that helps diagnose people with celiac disease earlier is incredibly important. Undiagnosed, the disease can cause malnourishment, anemia, infertility, osteoporosis, heart problems and more. The earlier you get diagnosed and go on a gluten-free diet, which stops the disease from progressing, the less damage to your health.

Processed Foods Are Linked to Autoimmune Disease

Long-term exposure to the additives in processed foods—including glucose, sodium and fat solvents—is associated with a weakening of the intestine's resistance to bacteria and toxins. This weakening can contribute to the development of autoimmune diseases, such as type 1 diabetes, celiac disease, lupus and multiple sclerosis. This does not prove cause and effect, but you should consider eliminating processed foods from your diet, especially if you have an autoimmune disease or a family history of one.

Study by researchers at Technion-Israel Institute of Technology, Haifa, Israel, published in *Autoimmune Reviews*.

What You Should Do Now

The new finding means that anyone with either condition—or suspicious symptoms—should get tested...

•**If you have peripheral neuropathy,** ask your doctor to test you for celiac disease. That's the recommendation of the authors of the study.

•**If you suspect you have celiac disease**—common symptoms include bloating and gastrointestinal distress after eating bread or pasta—don't just stop eating foods containing gluten, because you can't be properly diagnosed unless you have been eating gluten. Do go to your doctor for a proper diagnosis.

•**A diagnosis requires a blood test,** which if positive is confirmed by an endoscopic procedure in which a tiny sample of the lining of the small intestine is removed and studied. That's how the people in the new Swedish study were diagnosed—and it's the only way to really know.

•**If you do have celiac disease,** you'll need to be on a completely gluten-free diet for life.

Chapter 12

EMOTIONAL HEALTH AND WELL-BEING

How to Make Positive Thinking Work for You

We're often told to think positive. Whether we want to lose weight…quit smoking…negotiate a raise or promotion…achieve great wealth…or get elected president, we're assured that the key is to ignore self-doubt, banish pessimism and believe that we can do it.

But positive thinking leads to productive action only if we know how to handle it. If we don't, pie-in-the-sky daydreams and unbridled optimism are more likely to lead to stagnancy than success. For example, a recent study found that people were less likely to make a substantial donation to a charity if they first fantasized that the problem the charity addresses had been solved. Indulging in the positive-thinking fantasy gave their minds the same positive feelings that they would have experienced if they actually had helped solve the problem, robbing them of the drive to take action.

So how do you employ positive thinking as a powerful force? The key is to use it as part of the following four-step strategy, which has been shown to actually increase our odds of taking productive action and achieving a goal…

• **Identify a goal.** Choose something you would like to achieve, whether you call it a "goal" or a "wish." This could be a short-term goal—something you could accomplish today—or a long-term goal that will take much longer. Your goal should be something that you believe you can realistically accomplish but that is somewhat challenging to you. Boil your goal down to a phrase of just three to six words.

Examples: "Book a trip" or "Lose five pounds."

• **Picture the best outcome.** Now imagine what it would be like if your wish came true in the very best possible way. How would you feel? How would your life change?

Let yourself mentally experience this imagined outcome. Revel in it for a few minutes. This helps link the wish to pleasurable feelings in your mind—indulging in fantasies can feel wonderful. Your blood pressure actually might drop, enveloping you in a sense of calm and contentment.

Gabriele Oettingen, PhD, professor of psychology at New York University, New York City, and University of Hamburg in Germany. She is author of *Rethinking Positive Thinking: Inside the New Science of Motivation.* WOOPMyLife.org

Dreamers tend not to progress beyond this stage, but two crucial steps remain to maximize your odds of making your wish come true.

• **Picture your greatest internal obstacle.** As soon as you stop fantasizing about the best possible outcome of your wish, ask yourself, *What one thing in me is most holding me back from making this wish come true?*

The goal here is to uncover your main internal obstacle, not an external one. If you see an external force as your main hindrance, there's a good chance that the problem will seem insurmountable. If you see something within yourself as the main problem, there's a good chance you will be able to develop a solution.

Example: If your wish is to get a promotion at work, the first obstacle that comes to mind might be, *My boss is a fool who does not appreciate me.* This is not the obstacle you need to identify—a foolish boss is an external problem. Make this obstacle internal by rephrasing it as, *I feel resentment toward my boss that makes it hard for me to earn his respect.*

Your internal obstacle might be instantly obvious, or it might take time to figure out. If it proves elusive, seek it through quiet, private contemplation. Do not ask other people for their input—your odds of understanding and overcoming the obstacle are much higher if you discover it yourself. If you're not certain whether you have identified the critical internal obstacle, you probably haven't—there's usually a "That's it!" moment of revelation when you have discovered it.

Helpful: People (especially women) often initially conclude that their main obstacle is, *I don't have time to pursue the goal.* You may want to dig deeper into why you can't seem to find the time. For example, you might realize that you cannot find time to pursue your wish because you devote lots of time to helping other people pursue their wishes…and that you do this because you fear not being needed. That fear is a major obstacle. Someone else might realize that she is not finding

time for a project because she is afraid of failing.

Boil your obstacle down to three to six words, then spend some time thinking about it. Picture how this obstacle stands in your way, stopping you from reaching your goal.

This reduces the odds that your mind will be satisfied with mere fantasy and helps you do what it takes to make the wish a reality.

Once you have identified and pictured your obstacle, you might realize that you need to modify or even switch your goal because the obstacle is so formidable that you can't overcome it—or the goal is just not worth pursuing.

Example: Your wish is to get up each morning and exercise. Your obstacle is that you feel distracted by everything you have to do during the day. Perhaps it makes sense to change your initial wish to "exercise in the evenings."

• **Develop a plan to overcome your obstacle.** This plan should fit a simple if/then format—If [obstacle X occurs], then I will [take action Y].

Example: If I feel insecure when someone questions my proposal, then I will remind myself that I am just as knowledgeable on this topic as anyone.

Developing a plan in advance to overcome your internal obstacle will not just help you overcome this obstacle…it may improve your odds of overcoming any obstacle that appears. The process of obstacle identification and if/then planning described above trains the mind to look for and get past obstacles, rather than get stopped by them on a nonconscious level.

Helpful: Find a quiet moment each day to identify your goal, your best outcome, your central internal obstacle and your if/then plan. By practicing this procedure every day, you will be much more successful in understanding your wishes and attaining your goals.

Stop Hating Your Body!

Sabine Wilhelm, PhD, chief of psychology and director of the OCD and Related Disorders Program at Massachusetts General Hospital, and professor at Harvard Medical School, both in Boston. She is author of *Feeling Good About the Way You Look: A Program for Overcoming Body Image Problems.*

When you look in the mirror, are you pleased with what you see? Many of us are aware of ways that we could look better but don't dwell too much on those imperfections.

For people with body dysmorphic disorder (BDD), their negative self-assessment can be crippling. They are tormented by one or more nonexistent or relatively minor "defects" in the face or body. As many as 5 million Americans—men and women—suffer from this disorder. Sadly, the shame that they harbor over their bodies and the belief that only surgery or medical treatment can repair their flaws too often prevents them from getting the psychological help that they need.

Latest development: A new form of therapy is now giving sufferers better odds than ever before of beating this disorder.

A Life-Altering Problem

For a person with BDD, thoughts about having a pointy nose, splotchy skin or some other perceived body flaw become a life-altering preoccupation. She is unconvinced by reassurances from friends, family members and doctors that the imperfection is minor at worst. In other cases, family and friends may not even be aware that their loved one has BDD. The sufferer becomes so excessively concerned with this perceived flaw, however, that it can prevent her from concentrating at work, socializing, developing intimate relationships or otherwise living a normal life.*

Men and women suffer nearly equally from BDD (slightly more women), but their preoc-

*To see if you may have BDD, go to The Body Dysmorphic Disorder Foundation's website, *BDDFoundation.org/ helping-you/questionnaires*. To find a therapist, go to the International OCD Foundation's website, *IOCDF.org*.

cupations are different. For women, concerns typically center on facial features, skin, stomach, weight, breasts, buttocks, thighs, legs, hips and excessive body hair. Men tend to obsess about their genitals, scrawny or flabby physique and thinning hair.

Three-fourths of people with BDD seek unnecessary cosmetic procedures, including surgery (which brings only temporary relief at best). Depression, anxiety and substance abuse are common among BDD sufferers, and their suicide rate is 45 times higher than that of the general population.

What Causes BDD?

Just why BDD develops is not clear, but the following factors appear to play a role...

• **Biological.** Recent studies have found that the brains of those with the disorder have abnormally high clusters of nerve connections that may affect how the brain processes visual information and connects it with emotion.

Important new finding: In a recent study, researchers at UCLA found similar activity patterns in the visual cortex of people with BDD and those with anorexia nervosa—an eating disorder also characterized by distorted body image.

• **Genetics.** Some evidence supports a role for genetics—the condition is more common among relatives of people with obsessive-compulsive disorder, which has some similarities to BDD.

• **Environmental.** If a child was a victim of abuse or relentless teasing, this can foster highly negative beliefs about one's looks. Growing up in a family or culture that focuses heavily on appearance may also make matters worse for a person who has a biological predisposition toward BDD.

Best Treatment Options

Psychotherapy and/or medication can significantly improve BDD.

Cognitive behavioral therapy (CBT) has been studied and seems to work well for this disorder. The idea is to help the person with

BDD identify specific feelings, thoughts and actions that cause him distress and fuel his excessive behaviors.

For example, learning to look objectively at one's beliefs surrounding appearance ("If I don't have a perfect nose, no one will ever love me") is a central part of CBT. So is "exposure and response prevention"—with this approach, patients practice refraining from rituals, such as repeatedly checking mirrors. It usually takes 22 sessions or so to improve symptoms.

Recent development: A new type of treatment strategy known as perceptual retraining also appears to be effective for BDD sufferers. A recent study showed that BDD symptoms decreased by at least 30% in most patients whose treatment included perceptual retraining. This therapy is based on research that has tracked the eye movements of people with BDD to understand how they fixate on their supposed flaws.

Perceptual retraining is done during office visits with a therapist and then practiced at home. With this therapy, a person who has BDD can learn to expand his attention from perceived imperfections to the big picture—for example, "Maybe my eyes are not as big as I would like them to be, but this does not mean that I shouldn't leave the house." This therapy may also help BDD sufferers identify similar patterns in social situations (obsessing that another person's hair looks better than theirs, for example) and change to a broader perspective.

Medication is also often needed. Selective serotonin reuptake inhibitor (SSRI) antidepressants, such as *citalopram* (Celexa) or *fluoxetine* (Prozac), are used most frequently. But to be effective for BDD, a higher dose than what would be used for depression may be required, and it may take longer to work—12 weeks instead of six, for example. Some people with BDD may have a neurotransmitter imbalance in the brain, which is relieved by an SSRI.

However, getting help—whatever form that may take—is the first step to overcoming the agony of living with BDD.

Research Reveals How to Avoid Bipolar Disorder Even If You Carry the Genes

Mount Sinai Hospital, news release.

Naturally occurring brain wiring changes might help prevent bipolar disorder in people who have a high genetic risk for the mental illness, a new study suggests.

The discovery about these brain wiring changes could help efforts to develop better treatments for the disorder, according to Mount Sinai Hospital researchers in New York City.

People with bipolar disorder experience severe swings in mood, energy and activity levels, and the ability to perform daily tasks. Genetics are a major risk factor, and people with a parent or sibling with bipolar disorder are much more likely to develop it than those with no family history of the mental illness.

Researchers used functional MRI to monitor the brains of bipolar disorder patients, their siblings who did not have the illness (resilient siblings) and unrelated healthy volunteers. The bipolar disorder patients and their resilient siblings had similar abnormalities in brain wiring that handles emotional processing, but the resilient siblings had additional changes in that wiring.

"The ability of the siblings to rewire their brain networks means they have adaptive neuroplasticity that may help them avoid the disease even though they still carry the genetic scar of bipolar disorder when they process emotional information," study lead author Sophia Frangou, MD, PhD, a professor of psychiatry, said in a Mount Sinai news release.

The study was published online in the journal *Translational Psychiatry.*

"A family history remains the greatest risk factor for developing bipolar disorder and while we often focus on risk, we may forget that the majority of those who fall into this category remain well," Dr. Frangou said.

"Looking for biological mechanisms that can protect against illness opens up a completely new direction for developing new treatments. Our research should give people hope that even though mental illness runs in families, it is possible to beat the odds at the genetic lottery," she concluded.

The U.S. National Institute of Mental Health has more about bipolar disorder at *http://www.nimh.nih.gov/health/topics/bipolar-disorder/index.shtml.*

Surprising Results: Light Beats Medication for Major Depression

Health Insider research.

Bright light therapy—the use of special fluorescent bulbs that are many times brighter than standard illumination—brings some of the power of sunlight indoors to treat mood disorders. It's an attractive nondrug approach with few, if any, side effects that's been shown to be effective for the treatment of seasonal affective disorder (SAD), the kind of depression that tends to arise in the winter and often resolves come spring or summer. And bright light therapy has also been tried for major depression, the more common form of depression that can strike at any time of the year.

Two recent studies provide new insights into how best to treat both conditions.

Light Beats Prozac for Major Depression

While earlier studies have found that bright lights can treat major depression, this larger randomized clinical trial compared the drug approach and the light approach alone and in combination. In the study, 122 patients (ages 19 to 60) with major depression got one of these four treatments for eight weeks—30 minutes a day of bright lights…20 milligrams of *fluoxetine* (Prozac) daily…a placebo…or bright light therapy plus Prozac. The researchers measured response based on a standard depression scale.

Results…

•**Everyone's depression symptoms improved.** Those who got just a placebo improved 6.5 points on a 60-point depression scale.

•**Those taking Prozac improved 8.8 points**—just a little better and not statistically significant.

•**Those exposed to just bright light therapy improved 13.4 points.** That's a major difference from the Prozac—and statistically significant.

•**The best results?** Those who had both Prozac and bright light therapy. They improved 16.9 points on the scale.

Light Fades for SAD

Bright light therapy is an established effective treatment for SAD, and a different new study confirms this—but with a twist. The researchers compared giving people with SAD either six weeks of daily light therapy (30 minutes in the morning) or six weeks of twice-weekly sessions of cognitive behavioral therapy (CBT). The CBT was tailored to SAD, helping the participants challenge their negative thoughts about dark winter months and to resist behaviors, such as social isolation, that made their moods worse. Each group was encouraged to continue with their respective therapies after the active phase of the study was over.

Both groups got much better in the first year. But in the second year, more of the light therapy subjects tended to relapse into SAD—46%. By contrast, only 27% of the CBT group relapsed.

Why the difference? One reason may simply be the effort that it takes to use a light box every morning. Indeed, more of the bright light subjects had stopped using the therapy compared with CBT users. Cognitive behavioral therapy, on the other hand, is a set of skills that you learn and which become easier to use over time. In other words, bright light therapy is an effective if time-consuming treatment, while CBT not only treats symptoms but can prevent SAD from coming back.

Should You Try Bright Light Therapy?

If you experience either major depression or SAD, these studies show that using this non-drug approach can be a very effective way to improve your depressive symptoms without side effects. It's worth discussing with your doctor or therapist.

But the latter study also suggests that if you are looking for long-term relief from SAD, don't neglect cognitive behavioral therapy to not only treat SAD but also help prevent it. To learn more about CBT and find a certified cognitive behavioral therapist in your area, visit the National Association of Cognitive-Behavioral Therapists (*http://www.nacbt. org/searchfortherapists.ASP*). These days, CBT is so popular you can even get it on an app on your smartphone (see page 253 for more information).

Depression and Anxiety Linked to Lower Wages for Women

Jonathan Platt, PhD student, department of epidemiology, Columbia University Mailman School of Public Health, New York City.

Katherine Keyes, MPH, PhD, assistant professor of epidemiology, Columbia University Mailman School of Public Health, New York City.

Mailman School of Public Health, Columbia University, news release.

The wage gap between American women and men might be one reason why women have higher rates of depression and anxiety, a new study suggests.

Women with lower incomes than men with similar levels of education and experience were about 2.5 times more likely to have ma-

jor depression than men. But, women who had incomes similar to their male counterparts didn't have a greater risk of depression than men, the research revealed.

"Our results show that some of the gender disparities in depression and anxiety may be due to the effects of structural gender inequality in the workforce and beyond," said study author Jonathan Platt, a PhD student at the Columbia University Mailman School of Public Health's department of epidemiology.

"The social processes that sort women into certain jobs, compensate them less than equivalent male counterparts and create gender disparities in domestic labor have material and psychosocial consequences," he said.

Study Details

The researchers looked at data gathered from more than 22,000 working adults, aged 30 to 65. The information was collected between 2001 and 2002.

Overall, women were nearly twice as likely as men to have been diagnosed with depression in the past year, the study found.

In addition to finding that women who earned less than men were far more likely to be depressed, the investigators also found that women had more than double the risk of generalized anxiety disorder in the past year.

But, again, when the researchers broke the results down by earnings, they saw the gender wage gap made a difference. Women who earned less than men had about a four times higher risk of anxiety disorder than men. The risk for women whose incomes were similar to their male counterparts was greatly decreased, the study showed.

The study was published in journal *Social Science & Medicine*.

Implications

These findings suggest that women may be more likely to place the blame for their lower income on themselves, and not on gender discrimination, the study authors said.

"If women internalize these negative experiences as reflective of inferior merit, rather than the result of discrimination, they may be at increased risk for depression and anxiety disorders," Platt said.

According to Katherine Keyes, MPH, PhD, the study's senior author and an assistant professor of epidemiology at Columbia: "Our findings suggest that policies must go beyond prohibiting overt gender discrimination, like sexual harassment."

It's commonly believed that gender differences in depression and anxiety have biological roots, said Dr. Keyes.

But, she added, "these results suggest that such differences are much more socially constructed than previously thought…"

To learn more about depression, visit the U.S. National Institute of Mental Health website, *nimh.nih.gov* and search "depression."

Why a Mental Health Therapist Is Best If You're Depressed

Michael D. Banov, MD, medical director, Northwest Behavioral Medicine and Northwest Behavioral Research Center, Marietta, Georgia. Dr. Banov is the author of *Taking Antidepressants: Your Comprehensive Guide to Starting, Staying On, and Safely Quitting*.

Are we really a "Prozac Nation"—brain-tamed on Prozac, Paxil, Zoloft, Luvox or a dozen other antidepressant agents? The National Center for Health Statistics tells us that one in 10 Americans over the age of 12 is on an antidepressant. Even more astounding, that statistic is nearly one in four among women aged 40 to 60.

With numbers that high, clinical depression—the kind that is a debilitating emotional illness and not just a passing day of the blues—must be overdiagnosed. This was confirmed by researchers at the Johns Hopkins Bloomberg School of Public Health. Their study looked at 5,639 patients in whom depression was diagnosed. It found that only 38% of the patients had symptoms that met the criteria for a depression diagnosis as established by the American Psychiatric Association. In study participants who were 65 or older, a certain other emotional illness was misdiagnosed as depression 87% of the time. That's outrageous!

The problem, at least in part, might lie with who's diagnosing depression and, in turn, prescribing the glut of antidepressants. In fact, the vast majority of these prescriptions are written by primary-care doctors and not by psychiatrists.

Too Much or Too Little?

Michael Banov, MD, a behavioral medicine and psychiatry specialist and author of the book *Taking Antidepressants: Your Comprehensive Guide to Starting, Staying On, and Safely Quitting*, doesn't see the situation in black and white. He believes that a number of people on antidepressants don't need them but request prescriptions—and get them—from doctors as quick fixes for complex problems. He also believes that many people who desperately need psychiatric care don't get appropriate help because of the stigma attached to it, ignorance about it, financial issues or other concerns. It's easy to seek help from a primary care doctor and get a prescription for a psychiatric drug. It's a lot more time, effort and money to receive a full mental health evaluation from a psychiatrist or behavioral health therapist.

Diagnosing depression is a specialized skill, according to Dr. Banov—not something that can be pulled off effectively in a 10-minute visit to the busy office of a general practitioner. As for psychiatric drugs, such as Prozac, Paxil and other antidepressants, they do have their place. They can be good tools to improve symptoms, in Dr. Banov's view. Ideally, drug therapy should be temporary and coupled with other strategies that become the main focus when drug therapy is completed.

These other strategies, of course, are also alternatives to antidepressants. Cognitive behavioral therapy and psychodynamic therapy have been proven to work. Lifestyle changes, including more exercise, less drinking and managing stress better, can help. And natural supplements and dietary changes are also effective.

A Tip for Older People

As mentioned above, the Johns Hopkins study showed that overprescription of antidepressants was especially a problem among the elderly. Dr. Banov said that antidepressants are often used to control older people who, for example, are suffering from dementia when they should be receiving more appropriate and meaningful care. Think about it—you may have a family member in a nursing home who is given an antidepressant because he or she is irritable and easily agitated. That person may really need more exercise and creative stimulation...or may have an underlying medical issue, such a thyroid problem or a nutritional deficiency, that is being overlooked.

On the other hand, older people who actually do have depression sometimes do not get the exact treatment they need because their symptoms are diagnosed as dementia, said Dr. Banov. For this very reason, said Dr. Banov, "a patient's care should be a partnership between the patient and doctor. And if at all possible, patients should educate themselves about depression, ask their doctors questions about treatment options and find out what the other alternatives are," he said.

Hormone Therapy Boosts Mood

Women taking oral hormones show improvements in depression and anxiety symptoms. Ask your doctor about hormone therapy—it usually is recommended only at the start of menopause for the shortest possible time at the lowest possible dose.

Study of nearly 700 women led by researchers at University of Wisconsin School of Medicine and Public Health, Madison, published in *PLOS Medicine*.

---

3 Shortcuts That Deliver the Stress-Relieving Effects of a Walk in the Woods

Health Insider research.

You're stressed...it's hard to concentrate...and you need a little nature to restore your spirits and refresh your mind. You know a nice long walk in the woods would do the trick.

That's not going to happen.

Here's what might help—three shortcuts that let you quickly experience the attention-restoring benefits of nature at work and at home...

• **Take a green micro-break.** In an Australian study, office workers were given a challenging task, accomplished it and then were asked to take a 40-second "micro-break" either looking at a bare concrete roof...or at a "green roof" that was covered with a flowering meadow. Then both groups repeated the task. Compared with the concrete watchers, the green-roof gazers were much more able to focus on the task the second time around—and made fewer errors. So if there's a window nearby that looks out on nature—even just a bit of nature transplanted by humans—take a look.

• **Put a plant on your desk—or four.** A Norwegian study tested volunteers given a demanding task. Some sat in an office setting that was bare, while others in one with four indoor plants, both "flowering" and "foliage." Those surrounded by plants performed better on tests that measure the ability to focus attention on a tough task.

• **Look at a nature video.** In a classic American study of volunteers who watched a high-stress video, those who then watched a nature-scene video had lower physiological stress levels than those who watched an urban-scene video. Visit *Youtube.com* and search "American Beautiful West."

Relaxation Pays

Study titled "Relaxation Response and Resiliency Training and Its Effect on Healthcare Resource Utilization" by researchers at Brigham & Women's Hospital and Massachusetts General Hospital, both in Boston, and other hospitals, published in *PLOS One*.

Meditation. Yoga. Stress relief. Social support.

You know they're good for you.

But now there's firm evidence that practicing these "wellness" skills can reduce your need for medical attention—and save you money.

Maybe lots of money.

So finds an analysis of more than 4,000 women (and men) who went through an eight-week program at Brigham & Women's Hospital in Boston called Relaxation Response Resiliency Program. Participants met for about three hours a week to learn relaxation techniques (through yoga, meditation and stress-reduction exercises) and resiliency building (through social support, cognitive-skills training and positive psychology).

How'd it all turn out? Fantastic. In the year after going through the program, the participants used 25% fewer medical services than a control group.

Average savings: $2,360 per patient per year.

Hearing Voices Doesn't Mean You're Crazy

Jan Dirk Blom, MD, PhD, head of the Outpatient Clinic for Uncommon Psychiatric Syndromes, Parnassia Group, The Hague, and assistant professor of psychiatry, University of Groningen, The Netherlands.

If you are the kind of person whose random thoughts literally sound like voices in your head—either you talking to yourself, a voice talking to you or a gaggle of voices in conversation with each other—you might start to wonder if you are "normal." You might even think you hear those voices with your ears, as if they were coming from outside of yourself. That sure seems like a call for help. After all, the early stages of some forms of dementia are associated with hallucinations—and hearing voices is a classic sign of schizophrenia. You may be surprised to know that the phenomenon is not all that uncommon—or necessarily abnormal. But some types of experiences are less "normal" than others.

Most people who admit to hearing voices are not crazy. In fact, 10% to 15% of the general population experience auditory hallucinations, ranging from simple sounds like hissing and ticking to dialogue among several voices.

One recent study of 153 women and men who reported regularly hearing voices found that it occurs across a wide range of psychiatric and mental health conditions, not just in people diagnosed with psychosis or dementia—and occurs in people who are otherwise perfectly normal. In the study, participants answered a survey of questions that allowed them to describe their unique experience of hearing voices (whether from within their minds or seemingly audibly) in detail. They were also asked whether they had ever had a psychiatric diagnosis and what the most recent diagnosis was. (The information on mental health diagnoses was corroborated with medical records.)

Seventeen percent of the study group were not mentally or emotionally ill, 16% had schizoaffective disorder (a combination of psychosis and either bipolar disorder or depression) and 14% had bipolar disorder. Other reported psychiatric diagnoses, represented to a lesser degree, included post-traumatic stress disorder, depression, anxiety disorder, obsessive-compulsive disorder and a few others. A little less than half (46%) of all the participants described the voices as auditory and about one-third described them as partly auditory and partly thoughtlike. Only 9% of the group described the voices they "heard" as exclusively thoughtlike.

What You Hear Matters

The nature of the voices people heard, either internally or externally, ranged widely. For some, voices commented on what was happening at the moment or were single or multiple voices in conversation that could interrupt or distract from real conversations. For others, the voices expressed commands that could be positive, neutral or negative. For example, one study participant reported that voices would tell her to do things such as take out the garbage or call a particular friend…whereas another participant reported that her voices were in the habit of screaming that she was damned and that God hated her. Another participant reported that the voices he heard could be "brutally sarcastic."

Although hearing voices often, understandably, elicited negative emotions (fear, anxiety, depression and stress), the experience could be emotionally uplifting as well. Slightly more than 30% of the study participants reported that their voices could, at least sometimes, elicit positive emotions. Notably, participants who did not have a psychiatric disorder were least likely to associate the voices they heard with fear or depression.

When Should You Act On What You Hear?

Besides psychiatric illnesses, hearing voices also can be triggered by stress, bereavement, sleep deprivation, a physical ailment (such as a brain tumor), use of marijuana or other illicit substance, and certain medications, such as antidepressants, or they can simply just occur, says Jan Dirk Blom, MD, PhD, assistant professor of psychiatry at the University of Groningen in The Netherlands. Dr. Blom was not involved in the study described above but is a top expert on auditory hallucinations. One theory for why they occur in some people is that parts of the brain associated with hearing and language are being overstimulated.

What separates normalcy from pathology in people who hear voices comes down to the ability to control the voices, the frequency of occurrence and the tone and content of the voices, says Dr. Blom.

Healthy people who hear voices internally or externally tend to have more control over them than do people who are mentally ill. That is, they can ignore or reasonably interpret them or turn them off. The phenomenon tends to occur less frequently in them than in the mentally or emotionally ill, and what is heard tends to be agreeable or neutral rather than negative. These characteristics can predict the lack of a psychotic disorder in up to 92% of voice-hearers, said Dr. Blom.

"Of course, when the experience of hearing voices is frequent and distressing and interferes with your daily functioning by, for example, causing difficulty concentrating or by giving commands that you know would be wrong to follow, chances are you need medical evaluation," says Dr. Blom. If you are troubled about hearing voices and your doctor has ruled out a physical cause, such as a medication side effect, Dr. Blom suggests finding a psychiatrist who specializes in psychotic disorders who can best assess whether you indeed have a psychotic or emotional disorder, another condition or merely have an odd quirk. Depending on the diagnosis, treatment (if needed) may include antipsychotic drugs or cognitive behavioral therapy.

If your voices don't cause discomfort and don't interfere with leading a normal life, the risks and side effects of drug treatment for auditory hallucinations might outweigh the benefits, says Dr. Blom. He mentioned that some very famous folks who influenced history for the better heard voices—Joan of Arc, Gandhi, Socrates, Charles Dickens and Sigmund Freud among several others.

Support for People Who Hear Voices

Self-help and peer-support groups for people who hear voices do exist, including the International Hearing Voices Network, an international group that provides a safe space for people to share their experiences and support one another (*hearingvoices.org*). Actor Anthony Hopkins, in fact, participates in the group! Sometimes all you need is just to be able to put an odd experience into context and know that you are not alone.

Natural Cures for Anger

Jamison Starbuck, ND, a naturopathic physician in family practice and a guest lecturer at the University of Montana, both in Missoula. She is past president of the American Association of Naturopathic Physicians and a contributing editor to *The Alternative Advisor: The Complete Guide to Natural Therapies and Alternative Treatments.*

When it comes to human emotions, explosive and out-of-control anger is one of the toughest. It's not only hard on relationships at home, work and/or school, it's also hard on the health of the angry person. Heart rate, blood pressure and the digestive system can all be affected. To curb anger, conventional doctors use both psychotherapy and prescription medications (such as antidepressants and tranquilizers). These approaches can help. But among the many patients I've treated for anger problems, lifestyle changes and natural medicine offer longer-lasting results. It's important to recognize that it's normal and healthy to feel and appropriately express anger, but when it becomes excessive, problems can develop.

If you or someone you love is struggling with anger, here's my advice…*

• **Watch your diet.** A good first step is to reduce known dietary nuisances such as caffeine, alcohol and high-sugar foods—all of which affect the brain and can interfere with your ability to cope with anger.

• **Review your hormone health.** Women can experience significantly worse anger when they are premenstrual or going through menopause. In men, anger often kicks up during middle age when their testosterone levels are waning. For both males and females, anger is common during puberty—another time when hormone levels are changing. If you suspect that your anger may be tied to your hormone health, ask your doctor about testing your testosterone, estrogen and progesterone levels. Both women and men have all three of these hormones, and for optimal emotional health, all three should be correctly balanced.

• **Check for allergens.** All kinds of allergies can wreak havoc with one's emotional stability. Whether you're allergic to inhalants (such as pollen, pet dander or dust) or to foods (such as dairy, wheat or eggs), these allergens can cause big problems. Sometimes, the only symptom of an allergy is emotional distress, irritability and/or volatile anger.

If you have frequent anger: Keep a diary of explosive events and the foods you ate and possible allergens in your environment during the 12-hour period prior to your angry feelings. Look for patterns. If you suspect a link, speak to your doctor about allergy testing. For food allergy testing, I recommend IgG blood testing…for inhaled allergens, IgE scratch testing.

• **Get more B vitamins.** Anger is often linked to fatigue and low blood sugar. Vitamins B-5 (pantothenic acid) and B-6 (pyridoxine), in particular, can help with both conditions. To ensure that your B vitamin levels are balanced, look for a B-complex supplement that includes B-5 and B-6.

• **Try botanical medicines. Gentler than pharmaceuticals,** herbal remedies can calm emotions without dulling the brain.

My favorite anger-fighting herbs: Passionflower and skullcap. Pick a product (tincture, capsule or tea) containing either one or both of these herbs. Individual sensitivities vary, so start with a low dose. Take it for several days to see whether your anger is improving. If it's not, slowly increase the dose, but do not exceed the manufacturer's recommended dose. Use during high-stress periods or any time that anger is a problem.

---

*If you have a chronic medical condition or take medication, talk to your doctor before trying any supplements.

Try This Little Trick for a Long, Happy Marriage

Karl Pillemer, PhD, gerontologist, Cornell University, author of *30 Lessons for Loving: Advice from the Wisest Americans on Love, Relationships, and Marriage.*

There's a surprising secret to a happy marriage—treat your relationship as if it were a lifetime date.

That bit of relationship genius came from Cornell University gerontologist Karl Pillemer, PhD, author of *30 Lessons for Loving: Advice from the Wisest Americans on Love, Relationships, and Marriage*. He learned it from a 70-year-old woman, Leigh. Leigh and her husband had each been married before and agreed to treat their marriage together as a lifetime date.

Here's why it works: When you go on dates, you do your best to be interesting, upbeat, attractive and attentive. You try to make the person you are with feel special.

When people have been married a long time, they take their partners for granted. We don't feel the need to make an effort, because, after all, we know they love us, so why do we need to? But you do need to, explained Dr. Pillemer. When you make an effort, you fuel the spark that makes a marriage thrive.

Another aspect of dating is that it's exciting because it offers an element of the unknown. Married couples who try new things...take spontaneous trips...and give surprise gifts... increase their odds of remaining happily married.

Treating a marriage like a date doesn't mean that there won't be trying times. The trick is to view the difficult days of a marriage like the time between dates—not as a problem with the relationship but as an unavoidable intermission from it. Then we look forward to when we can resume the date of our lifetime.

How Much Sex Makes Couples the Happiest?

How often should you have sex? Studies of more than 30,000 people show that couples who make love once a week report the highest level of happiness—more than those who have sex less frequently but no less than those who exceed a weekly tryst.

Explanation: Weekly sex is optimal to maintain an intimate connection between partners with busy lives.

Study titled "Sexual Frequency Predicts Greater Well-Being, but More Is Not Always Better," by Amy Muise, PhD, postdoctoral fellow, and other researchers in the department of psychology at University of Toronto Mississauga, Canada, published in *Social Psychological and Personality Science.*

Dating: The Surprising Way to Boost Your Health

Judith Sills, PhD, a Philadelphia-based clinical psychologist. A three-year National Science Foundation fellow, she is a contributing editor at *Psychology Today*. She is also the author of *Getting Naked Again: Dating, Romance, Sex, and Love When You've Been Divorced, Widowed, Dumped, or Distracted.*

If you're not in a committed relationship, maybe it's time to consider dating again. And if you're age 50 or older—the point at which most of us become much more focused on staying healthy—then it's an especially good time to give dating a chance.

While the prospect of dating as a mature adult can seem overwhelming or downright scary, here's some compelling motivation— the latest research indicates that being in a relationship can improve your health in a variety of ways.

And take heart: There are specific tips for daters who are 50+ that can make getting out there again much easier.

Health Benefits Galore

Plenty of singles age 50 or older say they don't need a relationship to be happy. But those who are in committed relationships seem to have significant health advantages over those who fly solo.

Case in point: An analysis of data from more than 300,000 adults found that those without strong relationships were 50% more likely to die from all causes over a seven-year period—a risk that's the equivalent to daily smoking! Additionally, men and women who live alone and have a heart attack are twice as likely to have a second heart attack within a few months.

The list goes on. Married people are less likely to get pneumonia than singles, and those who are married or live together in midlife are less likely to develop dementia.

How to Get Back Out There

If you have been out of the single world for a long time, you might not be sure that you want to get back in the dating game.

But one thing is certain: Humans have a deep need for intimacy and companionship.

And while some people are perfectly satisfied with their close friends and family, a healthy committed relationship generally offers a greater level of stability and support. After all, if your best friend moved to a different state, you wouldn't follow that person, but you likely would if it were your partner.

The advantage of later-life dating is that you've been through it all before. And you probably have some idea of what you're looking for. Also, while you may be a bit insecure in how you look as you age, you may have more confidence in your personality and social skills.

Advice for dating after age 50…

• **Get online.** The Internet is a fantastic way to meet people. The number of potential partners vastly exceeds those you'll meet any other way. If you're willing to put in the time—writing an interesting profile, putting up an attractive photo and wading through the possibilities—you will get dates. (They won't all be fabulous, but many will be fun and you'll start to meet people.)

There are hundreds of dating websites to choose from. The most popular sites, such as Match ($35/one month) and eHarmony ($59.95/one month), have the most members (and potential partners), but they tend to attract younger users.

Helpful: Try sites that target older adults, such as OurTime ($20/one month) or SeniorPeopleMeet ($20/one month). Monthly prices are lower if you sign up for a longer time. Plenty of Fish is a free dating site for all age groups.

• **Don't waste time.** A survey by the Pew Research Center found that one-third of those who connect online never take the next step and meet face-to-face. Unless your only goal is Internet flirting, pin down a time to meet. You don't want to rush it, of course, but don't wait too long. If you like the person after exchanging three or four e-mails, it's time for a phone call or a meeting (in a low-key public place like a coffee shop). If someone you're interested in doesn't ask you out first, take the plunge and do it yourself.

• **Set aside your preconceptions.** Dating sites have analyzed what their members want—or think they want. Women, for example, tend to respond to men of certain ages, or with particular jobs or education lev-

Fix an Unhappy Marriage

Researchers examined five years of data from married women and men, ages 57 to 85. People with spouses who were negative or critical were more likely to have heart health issues—women suffered more than men—than those with supportive partners. This effect worsened with age.

Theory: Relationship stress intensifies over time, and heart disease is harder to overcome in those who are older and more frail.

Study of nearly 1,200 married American women and men by researchers at Michigan State University, East Lansing, published in *Journal of Health and Social Behavior*.

els. Men tend to reach out to women who are blond. Give other types of people a chance!

•**Give yourself (and your date) some slack.** When dating, you will no doubt have some anxious and awkward moments. What do you do when every attempt at conversation withers and dies? Or when your date doesn't laugh at any of your jokes? Give yourself and your companion a break. First dates are hard, but it does get easier with practice.

Helpful: Forget the traditional dinner date. It's too much for a first meeting, particularly if the chemistry isn't there—or when you discover between the first and second courses that you do not seem to have a whole lot in common. Meeting for coffee, a drink or lunch is easier and less expensive—and you can quickly cut your losses when it just isn't clicking.

•**Keep your insecurities in check.** No, you're not the same person you were 30 years ago. You might have a few extra pounds or a few more wrinkles. Just don't let the nagging negative voice in your head—"I'm not good enough"…"He is way out of my league"…or "What if he doesn't ask me out again?"—ruin what could be a perfectly pleasant time.

Your date saw something in you before you met. Relax and enjoy yourself. Besides, everyone is insecure on first dates. The person sitting across from you is probably having his/her own insecure thoughts.

•**It's not a job interview.** An unfortunate first-date strategy is to ask a lot of questions. Granted, asking questions and showing interest will keep the conversation going. But it can also be intimidating—or simply off-putting.

Some women tell me that they "interview" potential partners to save time. They ask things like, "Are you looking for something serious?" "Do you own or rent?" "What kind of relationship do you have with your ex?" Men do their own interviewing but tend to take their cue from the workplace, posing questions such as, "So tell me…where would you like to be in five years?" None of this is friendly give-and-take—it feels more like interrogation.

My advice: Be a little less efficient. A date is a chance to get to know someone…to reveal a little about yourself…and have some fun. Keep it light.

•**Aim for a full stomach.** Think it's time to take a new relationship to the next level? A dinner date with great food could be the best way to do it. There may be some truth to the old cliché—the way to a man's (or woman's) heart is through the stomach. A study in the journal *Appetite* found that women who were shown romantic pictures after they'd eaten had more brain activation than women who looked at the same pictures on an empty stomach!

Talking About Problems Not Always Helpful

Charles Figley, PhD, founder of the Traumatology Institute (now at Tulane University).

Isn't opening up about our pain the only way we can come to terms with trauma and move on with our lives?

Not necessarily. One study, published in *The Journal of Nervous and Mental Diseases*, discovered that US Army veterans who repressed traumas rather than talking about

When a Friend Is Suffering…

What not to say to a friend who is suffering…

"I know how you feel"—you can't know exactly how someone else is feeling. "This is God's plan" can be enraging—"You think God wants me to suffer." "If you need anything, give me a call"—rather than putting the burden of effort on a person who already is burdened, ask when you can bring over dinner or help with the laundry.

Andrea Bonior, PhD, licensed clinical psychologist in private practice, Washington, DC, and author of *The Friendship Fix.*

them suffered no additional health problems and lived just as long as other vets. And the vets who repressed were less likely to exhibit symptoms of post-traumatic stress disorder.

"What people call repression is really a form of self-regulation," says Charles Figley, PhD, founder of the Traumatology Institute (now at Tulane University) and one of the co-authors of the army vet study. "It's the ability to compartmentalize information in a way that you can handle."

When people discuss traumas before they feel ready, it can lead to even deeper suffering, explains Dr. Figley. They might hear troubling words coming out of their mouths that they are not yet able to confront or refute. For example, a rape victim might tell herself that she was somehow to blame for the crime.

If you suffer from a trauma, you'll know if you are ready to open up about it, says Dr. Figley—it suddenly will feel safe to do so. Do not let anyone pressure you into talking if you don't want to. If a loved one suffers a trauma, make yourself available to discuss it, but do not push for this conversation or push this person into therapy.

Save a Loved One From Suicide

Thomas Joiner, PhD, director of the Laboratory for the Study and Prevention of Suicide-Related Conditions and Behaviors and author of *Why People Die by Suicide* and *Myths About Suicide*.

The instinct to live is hardwired in us. That's why suicidal tendencies can be so difficult—even impossible—to grasp for people who have never felt a desire to die. The more we do know, however, the better able we are to reach out to people who are at risk of dying by suicide. To better understand suicide, it's important to know the truth behind several long-standing myths...

MYTH: **Suicide is an act of anger or revenge.** Only 10% to 12% of suicides contain an element of anger or revenge. Unfortunately, these tend to draw media attention, painting all suicides with the same brush. In truth, the tendency to die by suicide can most often be attributed to two simultaneously occurring beliefs—the sense that one is a burden...and that one doesn't belong. People considering suicide often think of themselves as a liability for their families, along the lines of *They'd be better off without me.* When accompanied by a lack of belongingness—a sense of loneliness and social alienation—the result can be lethal.

MYTH: **Suicide is an easy escape, one that cowards use.** Suicide is very difficult to accomplish—only one death occurs for every 20 attempts. Combat soldiers and policemen, who require physical fearlessness in their work, for example, are at high suicide risk. When they experience feelings of alienation and being a burden, their bravery can turn deadly. Physicians and dentists, in particular, are also at high risk—they are so exposed to pain and injury every day that they can become inured to the natural human aversion to taking one's own life.

MYTH: **People often die by suicide on a whim.** When standing on top of a roof, many people experience a fleeting thought along the lines of *What if I jumped?* When driving a car around a sharp bend, a similar thought might occur—*What if I drove off the road?* It can feel like you had a sudden whim to end it all—but that's not what's happening.

That impulse is called the high-place phenomenon. It's considered to be an instinctual safety signal that causes one to pay greater attention and take precautions—for example, to back up from the rooftop. Moments later, though, your slower perceptual system kicks in and misattributes the safety signal as a kind of a death wish. It's nothing of the sort. Our studies have shown that the high-place phenomenon is, in fact, an urge to live, not die. By contrast, taking one's own life is usually preceded by detailed planning and resolve.

MYTH: **Unless you're depressed, you're not at risk for suicide.** While depression is a significant risk factor for suicide, it is not the only one. Mental disorders such as anorexia nervosa, schizophrenia and borderline personality disorder increase suicide risk. Additional risk factors include stressful life events (such as a death, divorce or job loss), access to firearms and historical factors, including a family history of suicide, previous attempts and childhood abuse. More than one in 10 suicides are related to chronic or terminal illness.

MYTH: Most people who die by suicide leave a note. Seventy-five percent of people who kill themselves don't leave a note or other message for loved ones. Unfortunately, that helps fuel the incorrect notion that the act was impulsive.

To understand why notes are so rare, remember that people who are considering suicide are typically in a state of misery and isolation, which makes it very hard to communicate. Those who do leave notes tend to provide factual instructions about day-to-day matters rather than an emotional missive.

MYTH: Suicidal behavior peaks around the end-of-year holidays. In fact, suicides tend to occur in the spring. That's true around the world. Why? The explanation that I favor comes back to the idea that suicide requires a great deal of resolve and focus. In the spring, all living things—human, animal, even plant—become more energetic. For most people that's a good thing, but a small percentage experience symptoms such as agitation, edginess and trouble sleeping. This clinical state of overarousal, combined with alienation and burdensomeness, is correlated with higher rates of suicides during the spring.

MYTH: There are more suicides in big cities than in rural areas. Not true. People who live in rural counties are 70% more likely to die by suicide than those who live in big, metropolitan areas. The reason may be that rural residents hold more physical occupations, which often go hand-in-hand with a higher level of everyday fearlessness. Another factor may be that they live far from their neighbors, resulting in social isolation.

The lack of easy access to doctors and other medical professionals may also contribute.

MYTH: If people want to die by suicide, we can't stop them. A landmark study found that 94% of people who were restrained from jumping off the Golden Gate Bridge in San Francisco were still alive decades later or had died from natural causes. This was true even though they had high-risk characteristics that suggest a determined mind-set—most were men (who are at greater risk than women)… had chosen a highly lethal method (jumping from a high structure)…and were rarely referred to mental health treatment after being restrained (unfortunate but not uncommon). Yet nearly all of them chose to keep on living. This suggests that intervention can save lives.

If you or a loved one is considering suicide or shows suicidal tendencies, there is help available! The suicide hot line 800-273-TALK is a great resource—callers speak with a trained crisis worker who listens to their problems and then provides information on mental health services in the caller's area.

Another good option: Reaching out to a primary care physician who can prescribe medication and/or recommend a mental health professional.

Better Suicide Prevention

According to recent research, of more than 5,000 men and women, those who participated in up to 10 sessions of psychosocial counseling (talk therapy) after attempting suicide had 27% fewer suicide attempts a year later than those who received no treatment.

To find a therapist: Go to the website of the American Foundation for Suicide Prevention, *AFSP.org*. Under the "Preventing Suicide" tab, click on "Find Help."

Annette Erlangsen, PhD, senior researcher, Mental Health Centre, University of Copenhagen, Denmark.

New Technique May Help People with Anorexia

King's College London, news release.

Brain stimulation may ease major symptoms of the eating disorder anorexia nervosa, a typically hard-to-treat condition, a new study suggests.

British researchers evaluated anorexia patients before and after they underwent repetitive transcranial magnetic stimulation (rTMS), a treatment approved for depression.

"With rTMS we targeted…an area of the brain thought to be involved in some of the self-regulation difficulties associated with anorexia," study first author Jessica McClelland, a postdoctoral researcher at King's College London, said in a school news release.

The treatment delivers magnetic pulses to specific areas of the brain. It feels like a gentle tapping sensation on the side of the head, McClelland explained. The treatment alters the activity of the nerve cells in the brain, she said.

"We found that one session of [brain stimulation] reduced the urge to restrict food intake, levels of feeling full and levels of feeling fat, as well as encouraging more prudent decision-making. Taken together, these findings suggest that brain stimulation may reduce symptoms of anorexia by improving cognitive control over compulsive features of the disorder," McClelland said.

The study was published in the journal *PLoS One*.

"Anorexia nervosa is thought to affect up to 4% of women in their lifetime. With increasing illness duration, anorexia becomes entrenched in the brain and increasingly difficult to treat. Our preliminary findings support the potential of novel brain-directed treatments for anorexia, which are desperately needed," study senior author Ulrike Schmidt, a professor from Kings College London, said in the news release.

You Can Change Memories

Did you know that bad memories can be changed to good ones? Scientists have identified the brain circuits that cause bad memories to turn good and have switched a lab mouse's particular bad memory into a good memory. This could lead to help for people with stress-related depression.

Study led by researchers at MIT, Boston, published in *Nature*.

Because of the promising findings, the researchers are testing brain stimulation to see if it offers longer-term benefits for people with anorexia nervosa, Schmidt added.

Up to 20% of anorexia patients die prematurely from the condition, the researchers said.

The U.S. National Institute of Mental Health has more about eating disorders at *http://www.nimh.nih.gov/health/publications/eating-disorders-new-trifold/index.shtml*.

Should You Be Screened for Depression?

If you're an adult over age 18, the answer is emphatically yes—at least once in your life. That's true even if you feel fine and have no known risk factors.

So recommends the US Preventive Services Task Force, an independent group that has great influence over the practice of medicine—and what insurance companies will cover.

Their latest advice is to screen everyone. Why? Depression is so widespread that it is the leading cause of disability in the US. It also shortens lives through suicide and makes it harder for people with health conditions to take care of themselves.

The Task Force also advised that doctors screen all women who are pregnant or have recently given birth for postpartum depression. That's new, too.

US Preventive Services Task Force, CNN, National Public Radio.

Can Early Menopause Trigger Depression?

Eleni Th Petridou, MD, MPH, PhD, professor, preventive medicine and epidemiology, National and Kapodistrian University of Athens, Greece.
JAMA Psychiatry, news release.

Premature menopause may increase a woman's later risk of depression, a new review suggests.

If further studies confirm the findings, doctors might try to identify women most likely to need psychiatric or hormonal treatment after their periods end, the researchers said.

In the United States, the average age of menopause is 51, according to the American College of Obstetricians and Gynecologists.

Study Findings

For the study, published in the journal *JAMA Psychiatry*, researchers analyzed the results of 14 studies that included nearly 68,000 older women.

Those whose menopause began when they were 40 and older had a lower risk of depression later in life than those with premature menopause, the study found.

Women who are older when menopause begins and have a longer reproductive life have greater exposure to the hormone estrogen, according to the study authors.

Implications

The findings suggest "a potentially protective effect of increasing duration of exposure to [natural] estrogens as assessed by age at menopause, as well as by the duration of the reproductive period," said Eleni Th Petridou, MD, MPH, PhD, of the National and Kapodistrian University of Athens, Greece, and colleagues.

"These findings could have a significant clinical effect by allowing for the identification of a group of women at higher risk for depression who may benefit from psychiatric

monitoring or estrogen-based therapies," the researchers concluded.

The U.S. Office on Women's Health has more about menopause at *womenshealth. gov/menopause*.

Antidepressants and NSAIDs Don't Mix

Antidepressants and NSAIDs don't mix, according to Byung-Joo Park, MD, PhD. Adults taking any type of antidepressant who also used nonsteroidal anti-inflammatory drugs (NSAIDs) such as *ibuprofen* (Motrin) were 30% more likely to suffer internal brain bleeding than adults who didn't take this drug combination, a study of more than 4 million people found.

Why: Both drugs slow blood clot formation.

If you take an antidepressant: Ask your doctor to monitor your blood-clotting ability if you also take an NSAID regularly...and adjust the dose or replace either drug if needed to reduce bleeding risk.

Byung-Joo Park, MD, PhD, professor of preventive medicine, Seoul National University, South Korea.

How to Quiet Your Mind for a Great Night's Sleep

Andrew Rubman, ND, medical director, Southbury Clinic for Traditional Medicines, Southbury, Connecticut. SouthburyClinic.com

You climb into bed, close your eyes... and your mind revs up. You start fretting...about money...health...people... undone tasks. You just can't relax. Or you fall asleep, only to wake up—worried. Maybe you're worried about not being able to fall asleep. It's anxiety, and it's a common cause of insomnia.

A relaxing routine before bedtime and a bedroom suited for sleeping are key parts of the solution, but sometimes you need extra help. One thing you want to avoid at all costs—dependence on sleeping pills, which can be addictive, lead to drowsiness and accidents the next day and, let's cut to the chase, are downright dangerous over the long term.

For help easing into a relaxed, deeper sleep, consider instead a supplement derived from green tea—L-theanine. It's becoming popular as a supplement, and it's showing up as an ingredient in "relaxation beverages" such as Just Chill and NeuroSleep.

To learn more, we spoke with naturopathic physician Andrew Rubman, ND, medical director of the Southbury Clinic for Traditional Medicines.

How L-Theanine Works In Your Brain

An amino acid found in tea, and in especially high levels in green tea, L-theanine increases alpha wave activity—the kind of brain waves associated with the most relaxed sleep state. This, in turn, increases the production of serotonin, dopamine and GABA (gamma aminobutyric acid), a trio of neurotransmitters that promote relaxed, positive moods.

While L-theanine has been studied as an antianxiety treatment, there are only a few clinical studies of its use for insomnia. In one, in boys with ADHD, a supplement containing 200 mg of L-theanine twice a day (400 mg total daily) for six weeks improved both sleep time and quality. In a Japanese study, adult men who took 200 mg a day for six days didn't sleep any longer—but they felt like they did. They also reported feeling more relaxed before bedtime, having fewer nightmares, and feeling less tired and more refreshed during the day.

It's a safe supplement, says Dr. Rubman. One key element is that it relaxes without causing grogginess...and there is no evidence that it can become addictive, as many sleeping pills can.

How to Use L-Theanine As a Sleep Aid

If you want to try L-theanine to help you sleep, Dr. Rubman suggests that you drink a cup of green tea as a soothing nightcap before bed rather than just taking the supplement...it's cheaper and may be as effective. A typical cup of green tea may have less than 50 mg of L-theanine, which is less than the 200 mg used in studies, but may help some people. Worried about the caffeine? Don't be, says Dr. Rubman—L-theanine inhibits the ability of caffeine to attach to receptors in the brain, so you'll be getting very little caffeine from one cup of the tea. (Green tea is already low in caffeine—about one-third as much as in regular tea—but you can also drink decaffeinated green tea, which has the same amount of theanine as regular green tea.) Make sure that you steep the tea for at least three minutes...10 is better...so that the L-theanine is extracted.

Try drinking green tea for a few nights, or a few weeks, and if it's not working for you, here's how to use an L-theanine supplement...

• **As with all supplements, consult with your doctor before taking it.** L-theanine may reduce blood pressure, for example, so if you're on blood pressure medication, you'll want to talk with your doctor before taking it.

• **If you decide to take it, try a dose of 200 mg for at least two weeks.** You can take it daily or just when you feel you need it or on nights when you don't have time to drink a cup of green tea.

• **If that dose doesn't work, you can safely take it as many as three times a day, for a total dosage of 600 mg a day.** Don't worry about taking it during the day. L-theanine may calm you, but it won't cause drowsiness.

• If this supplement doesn't work for you, consider other relaxing ones. Dr. Rubman often prescribes valerian root or 5-HTP to his patients. Try each one separately...on different days...so that you can figure out how each one affects you, and what works best.

Shut Down Before Bed

Tablet users may be losing sleep. The light from backlit electronic devices, including the iPad, iPhone, Kindle Fire and certain Nooks, disrupts the body's circadian clock and reduces rapid eye movement (REM) sleep. These devices emit short-wavelength enriched light, known as blue light, that suppresses melatonin in the body—the hormone that helps start the sleep process.

Best for nighttime readers: A printed book.

Two-week sleep-lab study by researchers at Brigham and Women's Hospital, Boston, published in *Proceedings of the National Academy of Sciences.*

Press Your Thumb Here for Blissful Sleep

Deborah Flanagan, certified reflexologist, founder of the Center for True Health in New York City and a member of the Reflexology Association of America.

If you have trouble sleeping, try this simple do-it-yourself reflexology move.

Reflexology involves applying mild pressure to specific spots on the hands and feet believed to correspond with different body organs. While there isn't good scientific evidence that reflexology can treat diseases such as asthma and diabetes (as some people claim), there are some small studies that find that it can help with insomnia…and there's no harm if it doesn't help.

Deborah Flanagan, a certified reflexologist and founder of the Center for True Health in New York City, offers a do-it-yourself approach…

• **Locate the middle of the "whorl" of your right thumbprint.** In reflexology, this corresponds to the pituitary gland, which helps regulate sleep.

• **Press the side of your left thumbnail into the center of the whorl and hold it for 45 seconds.**

• **Switch thumbs and hold for another 45 seconds.**

• **Do this two to three times per day.**

• **You can also try this "in the middle of the night**" if you wake up and have trouble getting back to sleep," says Flanagan.

To Sleep Better, Make Your Own Placebo

Article titled "The Placebo Effect: History, Biology, and Ethics," by Patrick Lemoine, MD, professor of psychiatry and director of clinical studies, University of Claude Bernard of Lyon, France, published in *Medscape.*

Ted. J. Kaptchuk, director, Program in Placebo Studies, Beth Israel Deaconess Medical Center, Boston.

Wouldn't it be great if you could just take a "sugar pill" to get to sleep?

Maybe you can. Recent research has shown that placebos—sugar or other non-active material given to patients in place of actual drugs—make good sleep medicine. About half of the effectiveness of prescription sleep medications comes from the placebo effect, research shows. The "real" drugs, meanwhile, may leave us groggy, memory-impaired and more accident-prone—and can lead to a drug dependency. They are widely overprescribed, especially amongst the elderly.

But if you know you're just taking a sugar pill, is it really a placebo? Don't you need to believe you're really taking a sleeping pill for the placebo effect to work?

One French doctor has devised a clever method that lets his patients use the power of the placebo to wean themselves from reliance on prescription or over-the-counter sleeping pills. *Here's how you can do it yourself…*

The Power of Placebos

First, a little background. The term placebo (Latin for "I shall please") has been used to refer to medicine for more than two centuries (Thomas Jefferson wrote about them), but most physicians believed these inert pills exerted no real physiological action—they simply allowed patients to fool themselves into feeling better.

Now we know better. The belief that you are taking medicine can unleash powerful, positive physical changes in your body. "A host of studies have shown that treatment with placebos elicits an array of physiological responses," says Harvard Medical School professor Ted J. Kaptchuk, who directs the Program in Placebo Studies at Beth Israel Deaconess Medical Center in Boston. "These include stimulating neurotransmitters such as the body's own opioids, cannabinoids, dopamine and serotonin, all of which can alleviate pain, depression, anxiety and fatigue. We have an entire pharmacy of substances within us—and placebos help trigger their action."

Your Recipe for Zzzs?

Patrick Lemoine, MD, a professor of psychiatry at the University of Claude Bernard of Lyon in France, finds that many of his patients have trouble letting go entirely even if they have cut back. For them he uses homemade placebos to wean his patients off prescription pills. "It's a bit like when a child learns to swim and refuses to let go of a floating device the instructor has gradually deflated," he writes.

His weaning technique entails transferring prescription sleep medication into empty capsules and doing the same with sugar, then mixing the drug capsules and sugar capsules together so that on any given night, you won't know whether you're taking a real or fake pill.

Below is a plan based on his recommendations for patients who are used to taking a sleeping pill every night.

Make sure to first ask your pharmacist whether your prescription sleeping tablets can be safely crushed and ingested in capsules...

• **First, gather your materials.** Buy a bag of at least 150 empty capsules—choose the opaque sort over the clear—at your drugstore or online. Next, you'll need sugar, or, if you'd rather not take in even a tiny amount of sugar, you can substitute cornstarch. Finally, you'll need something with which to crush your sleeping pills—a mortar-and-pestle or, if you prefer, a capsule-filling kit (easily found online).

• **Next, count out 30 empty capsules.** Insert one finely crushed sleeping pill into each of 25 of the capsules. Now put about the same amount granulated sugar or whatever placebo material you have chosen into each of the remaining five capsules.

• **Put all of the capsules in a jar or empty pill bottle,** and shake gently to mix them around.

• **For the next month, take one capsule from this bottle each night.** On any given night, you won't know whether you've taken the sleeping drug or a placebo. But you will know that on any given night, there's a very good chance that you are taking the sleeping drug, because 25 out of the 30 capsules contain the drug.

• **The second month,** fill 20 capsules with the sleep aid and 10 with the placebo.

• **The third month, make it even-steven**—15 drug-filled caps, 15 placebo-filled caps. For the fourth month, it's 10 drugs/20 placebos.

Fifth month: Five drugs/25 placebos. For the last month, one drug/29 placebos.

By the end of the process, if all goes well, you'll be sleeping like a baby with almost no help from drugs. You may want to wean yourself from sleep drugs in just a few months rather than the full six, and that's fine. What's described above is not a scientifically proven method, but just one doctor's approach that works for some of his patients, so feel free to adapt the approach as you see fit.

For example, there's no reason to start taking a pill every night if you're in the habit of taking sleeping pills only when you feel that you need them. In that case, mix up a batch of sleeping pills plus some number of placebos beforehand, and take one pill when you feel that you need a little help. And if you have trouble giving up the idea that you might be taking a sleeping pill, you could go back to the 5/25 or even the 1/29 formula.

You'll still be taking a lot fewer sleeping pills. (*Note*: If you're traveling, especially if you're flying, leave these pills at home. You won't be able to show that they are prescription medicines if you are asked.)

Another approach: Try a half dose of your standard sleeping pills, either cut in half (check with your pharmacist to see if yours can be cut in half safely) or mixed in with placebos as above. You can also use the placebo effect to make other types of prescriptions work better.

Finally, it's also possible that taking a placebo might work for you even if you know it's a placebo. "We've done several studies using 'open label' or 'honest' placebos (where the person taking them knew they were ingesting an inactive substance) with very good results," says Professor Kaptchuk.

In the end, learning to harness the power of placebos to get better sleep is really about activating your own abilities—and there are many paths you can take.

A Healthy Gut Is Linked to Happiness

Study titled "A Randomized Controlled Trial to Test the Effect of Multispecies Probiotics on Cognitive Reactivity to Sad Mood" by researchers at Leiden University, The Netherlands, published in *Brain, Behavior, and Immunity*.

Is a healthy stomach the key to happiness? It's beginning to seem that way. A healthy gut population of beneficial bacteria is increasingly being found to have not just physical but mental health benefits. In the latest study, researchers found that probiotics actually seem to chase away bad feelings.

What's particularly interesting about this recent study is that it focused on the kind of bad moods that are linked with an increased risk for depression—even in psychologically healthy people. And anything that can help with depression and that is also totally safe, well, that's exciting.

The Mind-Altering Power of Probiotics

In the placebo-controlled, randomized study, researchers at Leiden University in The Netherlands assigned 40 healthy adults without mood disorders to take either a daily probiotic supplement or a placebo supplement for four weeks. Each probiotic supplement contained a mixture of bacterial strains known to be important for a healthy human gut, including Bifidobacterium and Lactobacillus. The placebo was basically starch. Before and after the four-week pill period, participants answered survey questions to gauge their moods as well as vulnerability to depression and anxiety.

The result: Participants who took probiotic supplements were less prone to "rumination"—the tendency to dwell excessively on negative events or feelings—and had less aggressive feelings when they did feel sad. That's important, the study authors note, because a tendency to ruminate "is sufficient to turn mood fluctuations into depressive episodes." And aggressive thoughts are associated with depression and the risk for suicide.

Prevention in a Pill?

Does this study mean we can prevent depression by eating the right foods or taking the right supplements? We can't know yet. It's more than a stone's throw to go from improved moods to actual prevention of depression or anxiety disorders. Frankly, we're just beginning to understand the connection. In a way, that's what makes it so fascinating—and promising. We have more to learn before health professionals can use specific probiotics as a way to help people protect themselves from depression—or to treat it. But that may be the future.

Nor was this study designed to answer the "how" question—but the researchers do suggest possible mechanisms based on research. One theory is that healthy gut bacteria increase blood levels of tryptophan, an amino acid that boosts brain levels of the mood-boosting chemical serotonin (which often are too low in people with depression). A second theory is that healthy gut bacteria make it less likely that toxins in the gut will "leak" out and activate inflammatory pathways that play a role in depression. The third theory is that gut bacteria may directly improve gut/brain signaling in ways that enhance positive emotions.

Whatever the mechanisms, it seems clear now that a healthy gut is good for the mind as well as the body. We already know probiotics have been shown to prevent or treat infectious diarrhea, traveler's diarrhea, antibiotic-associated diarrhea, irritable bowel syndrome, yeast infections, eczema and other conditions. Now there may be a new benefit—more happiness and less risk for depression.

So go ahead and enjoy probiotic-rich foods such as yogurt and kefir, pickled vegetables such as kimchi and sauerkraut, tempeh and miso. If you choose to supplement, look for products that contain both Bifidobacterium and Lactobacillus acidophilus, which colonize the human gut and so may provide benefits even after you stop taking them, according to naturopathic doctor Andrew L. Rubman.

Whatever you do, don't just stop taking any medication that was prescribed by your doctor and start taking a probiotic supplement instead. If you have a mood problem that lasts more than two weeks, especially if it is interfering with your life, don't put off seeing your doctor.

Let Your Phone Be Your Therapist: 7 Psych Apps That Really Work

Kristen Mulcahy, PhD, psychologist and director, Cape & Islands Cognitive Behavioral Institute, Falmouth, Massachusetts.

Got anxiety? Depression? Obsessive-compulsive disorder? There's an app for that...and that...and that.

Of course, it's not that simple. These complex emotional disorders can be very challenging to treat well, and there is no substitute for a good relationship with a talented, experienced therapist.

But apps have a place. Many people have trouble sticking with therapy for a variety of reasons. Other people who are in therapy find it really useful to have easy ways to practice what they've learned between sessions. And some people who aren't in therapy still want a convenient, practical way to help manage bad moods, unwelcome thoughts and troublesome behavior patterns.

One category of psychological app is becoming increasingly popular with the public and even with many therapists. These are based on cognitive behavioral therapy (CBT), a kind of therapy that focuses on how our thoughts make us feel, how our feelings affect our thoughts and how both affect our behaviors. CBT helps people identify destructive thinking and learn how to restructure negative thought patterns, modify beliefs and change behaviors. Traditional CBT, in person with a therapist, has proven to be effective for depression, anxiety, insomnia, phobias, panic attacks, obsessive-compulsive disorder and many other conditions.

To discover CBT apps worth exploring, we spoke with psychologist Kristen Mulcahy, PhD, clinical director of the Cape & Islands Cognitive Behavioral Institute in Falmouth, Massachusetts. She's also an app developer herself. If you're already in therapy and you're interested in one of these apps, bring it up in your next session and discuss how it might be incorporated into your program.

Here are cognitive behavioral therapy apps for five different purposes...

For Redirecting Negative Thought Patterns

Thought Diary Pro allows users to write down their worrisome thoughts, along with the time, significance and consequences of those particular thoughts. The app helps you recognize "cognitive distortions" (thinking errors) and prompts you to change each one to more a more accurate—and productive—thought. An optional feature allows users who are in therapy to send their thought diaries via e-mail to their therapists. The app can also be used by people who are practicing CBT on their own. $4.99. Available on iTunes.

Cognitive Diary CBT Self Help, an app for Android devices, works similarly, allowing users to write down their troublesome thoughts, challenge them and review progress. Free. Available on Google Play.

For Improving Moods

Moodkit was designed by CBT experts. The activity tool suggests techniques to reduce negative thoughts. The thought checker helps identify situations or thoughts that cause distress, modify such thinking and evaluate the effect of those thoughts. A tracker helps you keep a record of your moods so you can monitor your progress, and a built-in journal lets you save your notes. $4.99. Available on iTunes. It can be used on its own or as an adjunct to professional treatment.

Depression CBT Self-Help Guide includes a screening test to monitor moods, a cognitive thought diary to learn how to challenge stressful thinking, articles on CBT and a tracking feature. Free. Available on Google Play.

For Getting Better Sleep

CBT works well for insomnia. The CBT-i Coach, developed by experts from Stanford University and the Veterans Administration,

helps you develop sleep routines and improve your sleep environment by creating a sleep prescription, maintaining a sleep diary and setting reminders. Such a structured program has been shown to improve sleep and alleviate insomnia. Although the app can be used on its own, it was designed to be used in addition to professional counseling and should not be used to replace therapy for those who need it. Free. Available on iTunes and Google Play.

For Anxiety

Mayo Clinic Anxiety Coach, designed by Mayo Clinic anxiety experts, can be used for people with specific phobias, general anxiety, social anxiety, panic disorder or obsessive-compulsive disorder. Users identify their fears and then create a list of tasks that, although anxiety-provoking, will help them overcome their fears. If you're fearful of meeting new people, for example, the app will suggest activities such as chatting with a store employee that you can add to your To Do list. Before tackling the activity, you'll rate your anxiety level, then role play the activity on the app—and re-rate your anxiety level. Then you'll try it in the real world, reporting your anxiety level after each try. Users can track their progress in the checkup section and learn more about anxiety, phobias and CBT. While the app can be used on its own, the developers caution that it does not replace professional therapy. $4.99. Available on iTunes.

For Obsessive-Compulsive Disorder

Dr. Mulcahy readily admits that she is biased in favor of an app for OCD called Live OCD Free...because she developed it and has a financial interest in it. The app is based on the "exposure and response prevention" treatment method for OCD, an anxiety disorder characterized by obsessive thoughts and compulsive behaviors. "Exposure and response prevention is well suited for an app because it is a very structured program," Dr.

Mulcahy says. It works to reduce obsessive-compulsive symptoms by helping users to gradually expose themselves to anxiety-provoking situations while resisting any compulsive behavior. For example, users create a hierarchy of anxiety-provoking "exposures," such as touching a doorknob or purposefully making things messy/uneven. It also helps users practice resisting the urge to engage in compulsive behaviors such as hand washing. With practice, it becomes easier to resist the compulsion and anxiety diminishes. Both the OCD Institute at McLean Hospital and Butler Hospital/Brown University are studying the app in clinical trials. There is a children's version as well. $79.99. Available on iTunes. The app can be used on its own or with a therapist.

When You Need a Therapist

Regardless of which smartphone app you try, if you don't get the results you need and you aren't seeing a therapist, start seeing one. *Here are some of the reputable organizations that may help you find a qualified therapist trained in CBT...*

- **Association for Behavioral and Cognitive Therapies**
- **Anxiety and Depression Association of America**
- **National Association of Cognitive-Behavioral Therapists**
- **Academy of Cognitive Therapy**

If insomnia is your primary issue, you can find a sleep professional on the website of the National Sleep Foundation *sleepfoundation.org*. You may want to ask whether he/she is trained in CBT for insomnia.

The Happy Spice: Vanilla

Want a quick mood boost? Go vanilla. People who ate vanilla-flavored yogurt had more positive moods, according to a new study, while those who ate fruit-flavored yogurts (strawberry, pineapple) experienced no emotional lift. Interestingly, the emotional responses to the different yogurts was unrelated to whether the subjects said they liked the tastes or not—that is, even if it's not your favorite flavor, vanilla might still make you feel happier. Earlier studies have found that the mere aroma of vanilla—even when it's barely noticeable—lowers the heart rate and eases anxiety.

Study titled "Are Implicit Emotion Measurements Evoked by Food Unrelated to Liking?" by researchers at Wageningen UR Food & Biobased Research, et al., Austria, and VTT Technical Research of Finland, published in *Food Research International*.

APPENDICES

Appendix I
NUTRITION AND FITNESS BREAKTHROUGHS

5 Reasons You Can't Lose Weight...

Fact: Most people can't lose weight and keep it off just by focusing on calories and exercise. Millions of Americans who exercise and diet still can't drop all the pounds they want to—or keep off the pounds that they manage to lose initially. Why not?

It's because weight loss (or the tendency to gain weight) depends on thousands of biochemical reactions that aren't affected just by exercise and calories. Most people need a multilevel approach to get their weight where they want it.

Here's what to do...

Prevent Insulin Surges

Research has shown that high insulin triggers food cravings, particularly cravings for high-carbohydrate (and calorie-rich) foods. And elevated insulin stimulates the liver to convert blood sugar into fat.

One cause of elevated insulin is a low-fiber diet—most Americans consume only about 15 grams a day, far less than the 30 to 50 grams that many experts recommend.

People who increase their fiber intake by eating more fruits, vegetables, legumes and other plant foods feel less hungry. They're less likely to load up on fattening, sugar-rich foods. More of their blood sugar is burned as energy—and less is stored as fat.

Bonus: Fiber can help reduce cholesterol and reduce the risk for heart disease, high blood pressure and diabetes.

My advice: Look for foods that contain at least 5 grams of fiber per serving. A single cup of lentils, for example, has about 15 grams of fiber. A large apple has about 5 grams, and a sweet potato has about 6 grams.

Many of my patients take advantage of high-fiber powders or drinks. These products typically contain 10 grams or more of fiber per serving—some contain as much as 30 grams. Supplementing with fiber can help if you're not getting enough from "real" foods. Make sure you choose a fiber supplement that does not have a lot of sugar added.

Important: Drink at least a few extra glasses of water a day when you're increasing fiber. Fiber absorbs water in the intestine and can lead to constipation if you don't stay hydrated.

Pamela Wartian Smith, MD, MPH, MS, codirector, Master's Program in Medical Sciences with a concentration in metabolic and nutritional medicine, Morsani College of Medicine, University of South Florida, Tampa. She is author of *Why You Can't Lose Weight: Why It's So Hard to Shed Pounds and What You Can Do About It.* CFHLL.com

Beware of Sleep-Deprivation Cravings

It's estimated that about 60 million American adults don't get a good night's sleep. Sleep deprivation causes the body to produce more ghrelin (an appetite-stimulating hormone) and less leptin (a hormone that suppresses hunger).

Research has shown that sleep loss tends to trigger cravings for "quick energy" foods such as sodas and snacks. Paradoxically, these are the same foods that ultimately can increase your overall fatigue.

My advice: In addition to better sleep hygiene—such as keeping regular hours, not watching TV or using a computer in bed and avoiding late-day caffeine—sip a cup of chamomile tea about an hour before going to bed. It's a natural tranquilizer that will help you fall asleep more quickly. Lemon balm tea has a similar effect.

Also helpful: Talk to your doctor about taking 100 mg to 200 mg of a magnesium supplement daily at bedtime. It's a "calming" mineral that helps the brain shut down at the end of the day.

Reduce Cortisol

Cortisol is a hormone that slows metabolism and causes more calories to be stored as fat. Cortisol also stimulates appetite and increases levels of neuropeptide Y, a substance that triggers carb cravings.

Chronic stress increases cortisol. People have gotten so accustomed to living in a high-stress world that they don't even notice they are stressed. But your body notices.

Warning: Elevated cortisol causes more of the body's fat to be stored in the abdomen. Abdominal fat increases the risk for heart disease and other serious conditions—and is harder to lose than other types of fat.

My advice: Ask your doctor for a saliva test for cortisol. It will indicate how much (or how little) stress you really have. I have found that people who test high get really motivated about taking life down a notch—with exercise, meditation, fun hobbies, etc.

The test typically costs between $50 and $150 or more and may be covered by insurance.

Lifestyle changes will help most people cope with stress more efficiently, but they don't work for everyone. You may need a nutritional supplement to reduce cortisol. I recommend combination products because they tend to work better than single-ingredient supplements. The active ingredients should include magnesium and the herbs ginseng, ashwaghanda and rhodiola. Ask at your pharmacy or health-food store for recommendations. Take the dose listed on the label.

Reduce Inflammation

If you're overweight, you can assume that you have ongoing inflammation in your body. Unlike the acute inflammation that accompanies wounds and infections, such chronic inflammation occurs when the body continues to produce inflammatory substances (such as cytokines) even in the absence of injuries or infections.

The body's adipose (fatty) tissue produces C-reactive protein and other chemicals that fuel inflammation. Chronic inflammation makes the body resistant to the appetite-suppressing effects of leptin. It also interferes with the breakdown of fat and causes fat cells to get larger.

Inflammation also has indirect effects on your weight. Suppose that you have rheumatoid arthritis, asthma or another inflammatory condition. You'll naturally be less active and more likely to gain weight.

My advice: Ask your doctor to test you for indicators of chronic inflammation. The tests might include CRP (C-reactive protein), ESR (erythrocyte sedimentation rate) or an inflammatory cytokine profile.

Also, eat less meat, fat and processed foods (which tend to be inflammatory) and more plant foods. A Mediterranean-type diet is probably ideal because it's high in anti-inflammatory compounds—from fish, vegetables, olive oil, etc.

Deal with Menopause

The average woman gains 12 to 15 pounds or more during menopause. This is partly due to an age-related drop in metabolism. In addition, the menopausal decline in estrogen causes the body to seek this hormone elsewhere—and fat cells are the primary source. The result is that your body works harder to convert calories into fat. The increase in fat slows your metabolism even more, which promotes even more weight gain.

My advice: Hormone therapy is an effective way to prevent menopause-associated weight gain. See a doctor who specializes in bioidentical natural hormone replacement. Bioidentical hormones don't appear to have the same health risks that have been linked to synthetic hormones.

Also important: Exercise for at least 30 minutes three to four days of the week—more if you can. A combination of aerobic exercise and strength training is ideal. Regular exercise helps counteract the drop in metabolism caused by menopause-related fluctuations of estrogen, progesterone and other hormones.

Balance Hormones to Lose Weight and Feel Great

Michael Aziz, MD, attending physician Lenox Hill Hospital and founder and director, Midtown Integrative Medicine, both in New York City. He is author of *The Perfect 10 Diet.*

Many of the most popular weight-loss plans these days are a variation on the popular low-fat or low-carb approaches. However, few people succeed on any of these eating plans. But there is a science-based diet that truly is effective.

It's called The Perfect 10 Diet Plan, named for the way it helps the body balance 10 hormones that are important for weight loss. Internist Michael Aziz, MD, founder and director of Midtown Integrative Medicine and attending physician at Lenox Hill Hospital, both in New York City, developed the program, which guides people in losing weight rapidly and comfortably while also optimizing long-term health. Thousands of people have successfully lost weight using this plan—and noticed an improvement in their health.

How the Diets Stack Up

We are a nation in "hormonal chaos," says Dr. Aziz, and flawed research was behind the initial popularity of low-fat diets. Few doctors understood the difference between good fats and bad, so dieters were urged to shun all fats and eat lots of carbohydrates instead. However, eating like this triggers excessive insulin, a hormone that stores fat…makes people hungry…and can start people down a path toward diabetes.

Other disadvantages: Dr. Aziz says that eating so many carbs also negatively impacts other hormones, including human growth hormone (HGH), which helps people stay youthful…leptin (an appetite-regulating hormone)…and the sex hormones (testosterone, estrogen and progesterone). All this leads to a sluggish metabolism that makes weight loss harder.

On the other hand, low-carb diets (including the popular Atkins diet) urge people to minimize carbohydrates and load up on fats in order to keep insulin in check. This helps you shed pounds but doesn't address the problems related to other hormones. Plus, it also overloads people with unhealthy amounts of protein—slowing thyroid function, which is crucial for weight control. Furthermore, Atkins and these other low-carb eating plans allow lots of nitrite-rich processed meats, including bacon and cold cuts, which are linked to several types of cancer.

In contrast, The Perfect 10 Diet Plan considers all 10 hormones that are key to weight loss and control, which are…

- **Insulin**
- **Leptin**
- **Human growth hormone (HGH)**
- **Thyroid hormones**

- **Cortisol (the "stress hormone")**
- **Glucagon (which controls blood sugar)**
- **Dehydroepiandrosterone (DHEA, which combats depression and fatigue)**
- **Testosterone**
- **Estrogen**
- **Progesterone**

Perfect 10 Foods

In his book, *The Perfect 10 Diet*, Dr. Aziz explains that calorie restriction is not the key to successful and lasting weight loss—rather the point is to avoid "diet" foods (he calls them "fake foods") that have chemical ingredients added. Instead choose whole foods that contribute to a healthy metabolism, helping with weight loss while also satisfying your hunger.

To follow the Perfect 10 Diet, you should base your daily caloric intake on a 40/40/20 formula—get 40% of your calories from carbohydrates...40% from fats...and 20% from protein. *You can select from the following foods...*

- **Vegetables**—you may have unlimited amounts of greens (including peas and beans) and other nonstarchy veggies, while starchy ones (such as potatoes and corn) are allowed only occasionally, in very small amounts.

- **Fruits**—especially berries and citrus fruits packed with vitamin C. Limit yourself to two servings a day since fruit is high in fructose, which is used only by the liver, leaving the excess stored as fat.

- **Proteins**—mostly seafood, poultry (including zinc-rich dark meat, important for the productions of sex hormones)...whole eggs...and if you like it, a serving of red meat once in a while.

- **Saturated fats**—you may have one serving per day of butter (one pat) and use coconut oil (one serving is one tablespoon) as needed both for cooking or to spread on vegetables. Dr. Aziz explains that many studies over the years have confirmed that saturated fats can be helpful because they boost production of sex hormones, thus contributing to more rapid weight loss.

Other allowable fats: Olives and olive oil...avocados and avocado oil...and nuts, all of which are rich in nutrients.

Forbidden Foods

The Perfect 10 Diet strictly forbids foods that act against good hormone balance. *In addition to those fake fats, you should avoid...*

- **Artificially "fat-free" and "low-fat foods" (including dairy).** Foods in this group are manipulated to have less fat than their unprocessed forms, and as a result, they usually have higher amounts of sugar that spike insulin release.

- **Soy protein isolates.** This food ingredient may sound healthful, but it is in fact highly processed and may disrupt hormonal balance due to increased concentrations and potential imbalances in isoflavones (antioxidants found in plants). Be on the alert for this ingredient in weight-loss shakes, protein bars, low-carb products and many other processed foods that are labeled "healthy."

Off to a Quick Start

To help you take off and then keep off excess pounds, the Perfect 10 Diet includes three stages...

- **Stage One gets you off to a rapid start.** Each day, you may have three meals plus one or two snacks from the accepted food list, but no grains of any sort or alcohol. Follow this for about three weeks.

- **Stage Two supports continuous weight loss but provides additional choices (whole grains and a bit of alcohol).** Once weight loss has begun in earnest and you have grown accustomed to following the diet regimen and exercising regularly, you may add one to three servings of whole grains per day, including whole-grain pasta, and an occasional glass of organic wine.

- **Stage Three is a weight-maintenance plan that also is an excellent choice for general good health,** says Dr. Aziz. Now you may add yet another whole-grain serving each day and even have an occasional sweet treat such as a piece of dark chocolate.

In summary, eating whole foods that nourish rather than challenge your body will result in naturally balanced hormones, which will help you lose weight and feel great. Since it is smart to continue to keep a close eye on your hormone balance, in his book Dr. Aziz also provides advice on what lab tests you should ask your doctor to perform at the start of your diet and periodically thereafter. He also includes recipes and other suggestions for making this way of eating satisfying and one that can be healthfully maintained as time goes on...the true measure of a successful diet for health!

Odd Secret to Staying Slim

Karen Larson, editor, *Bottom Line Personal*, with Marcia C. de Oliveira Otto, PhD.

I eat the same breakfast every morning— plain Greek yogurt with wild blueberries and a sprinkling of walnuts. That unvaried menu might strike you as unexciting, but it turns out my monotonous morning meals could be helping me keep off pounds.

Many people believe that it's perfectly fine to eat whatever they want as long as they don't eat too much of any treat—overindulgence is considered the enemy, not the unhealthy foods themselves. But a recent study cast serious doubt on this "everything in moderation" consumption philosophy. When researchers tracked the diets of more than 6,000 people, they found that after five years of follow-up, the waist circumferences of people who ate very varied diets increased at more than double the rate of the waistlines of people who ate the same foods frequently.

When the researchers dug deeper into the data, they discovered a potential explanation—people who eat a wide variety of foods tell themselves it's OK to have a piece of cake

as long as they have only a thin slice. Those people might be right, too—except that they make the same rationalization with a single scoop of ice cream...a few pieces of candy... a snack-size bag of chips...a small soda, etc.

In theory, the solution is to eat a diverse diet and skew it toward healthy items. But according to Marcia C. de Oliveira Otto, PhD, an assistant professor at The University of Texas Health Science Center and lead author of the study, the greater the difference among foods a person consumes regularly, the more difficult it becomes for that person to eat a healthy diet even if he/she truly tries to eat healthfully.

Otto's advice: Find a few healthy foods you really like, and stick with them.

How Alcohol Tells Your Brain to Eat More...and How to Fight Back

Study titled "The Aperitif Effect: Alcohol's Effects on the Brain's Response to Food Aromas in Women" by researchers at Indiana University School of Medicine, Indianapolis, and Purdue University, West Lafayette, Indiana, published in *Obesity Biology and Integrated Physiology*.

Ever wonder why food can seem irresistible when you're having a drink or two? So do brain scientists. Now they have a clue.

Researchers at the Indiana School of Medicine studied what happens in the brain when the "aperitif effect" kicks in—the scientifically well-known tendency to consume more calories if you've also been drinking...even moderately. For men, the extra calories are more than 400, while for women they are about 300. Some of those extra calories come from the booze itself, but about 40% come from eating more food.

The new research suggests that having a drink or two lets our brains do what comes naturally—pay attention to food.

How Alcohol Unleashes Animal Appetites

The study: After breakfast, 35 normal-weight women who were not vegetarians (you'll see why when you see what they got for lunch) were given an IV drip that contained either a saline solution on one day…or enough alcohol to make them mildly buzzed on another day. According to the study, the subjects reported "a clear subjective sense of alcohol exposure."

Why intravenous? To skip gut effects of alcohol and hone in on what's going on just in the brain. Why only women? To make sure that differences in food preferences were due to the alcohol, not gender differences. Future studies may look at men.

Then, the smell test: While hooked up to MRI brain scanners, the women took in the tantalizing aromas of food—Italian meat sauce, roast beef—and then the pleasant nonfood scent of a Douglas fir tree.

Next, lunch was served, either pasta with Italian meat sauce or noodles with shredded beef in gravy. The women were asked to rate their hunger…and were allowed to eat as much as they wanted.

Results: On the boozy day, they didn't think they were any hungrier than on the sober day. Hunger hormones actually went down (possibly due to calories in the alcohol). And yet…the women ate on average about 7% more food on the alcohol day.

Why? One clue lies in a part of the brain called the hypothalamus, which affects appetite and metabolism. On the sober day, brain images looked the same when the women smelled the food odors as when they smelled the fir tree odor. But when they had alcohol coursing through their veins, the hypothalamus lit up only for the food smells.

Why did the women lose interest in a pleasant outdoorsy smell when they were a little buzzed? Researchers speculate that the shift of attention toward food is a remnant of an evolutionary instinct. Alcohol reduces inhibitions so that our "animal instincts" kick in and we focus on what matters for survival…such as food.

How to Make the Aperitif Effect Help You

Now that you know for sure that alcohol makes you super-receptive to food, if you're watching what you eat, pay closer attention to what and when you drink. For example, if you're going to a party, eat a filling, nutritious snack beforehand (before you drink any alcohol), intersperse a low-alcohol drink with a nonalcoholic one and pay special attention to the tendency to overeat. Ditto for having a cocktail at a restaurant. To make sure that it doesn't lead to overeating the bread and butter that magically appears at your table, why not ask the server to take the bread back?

But you don't always need to fight biology. Sometimes, it's just fine to enjoy a glass of wine or a frosty mug of beer, and bask in the knowledge that it's helping you relish your meal a little more keenly. That's healthy, too.

Why a Big Belly Is Worse Than Being Obese

Study titled "Normal-Weight Central Obesity: Implications for Total and Cardiovascular Mortality" by researchers at Mayo Clinic, Rochester, Minnesota, St. Anne's University Hospital Brno, Czech Republic, and University of Ottawa Heart Institute, Ontario, published in *Annals of Internal Medicine*.

Surprisingly, a normal-weight woman who has a big stomach is more likely to die early from heart disease than an overweight or even obese woman who has a flat stomach.

You could call it the Big Belly Paradox.

Bellies Matter More Than Weight

Mayo Clinic researchers examined data on about 15,000 adult men and women who were followed over 14 years. They had data not only on overweight/obesity as measured by the body mass index (BMI), but also waist-to-hip ratio, which measures how big your stomach is compared with your waist.

The healthiest combo, of course, was a normal weight and a flat stomach. But it's also possible for a normal weight woman (or man) to have a paunch—and some folks who are heavy carry their excess weight more on their backsides than on their bellies. *Here's where the results get interesting...*

• **For women,** those with normal weights but big stomachs were 40% more likely to die than overweight woman with flat stomachs—and 32% more likely to die than obese women with flat stomachs.

• **Normal-weight men** with big stomachs had twice the mortality risk of men who were overweight or obese but had flat stomachs.

What's so bad about big bellies? A waist-to-hip ratio that's 0.85 or higher (for women) or 0.90 or higher (for men) is a sign of "central obesity"—the kind of fat that's inside the abdomen and other internal organs rather than just under the skin. This "visceral" fat accumulates around the pancreas, heart and other organs that aren't designed to store fat. That can lead to excess insulin, high blood sugar, high cholesterol and problems in the functioning of the heart. The result is an increased risk for heart disease, diabetes and other metabolic diseases.

Researchers used to think the big belly was primarily a problem only if you were already overweight or obese. The new research suggests that a big belly is a serious problem whatever your weight.

To be sure, having a high waist-to-hip ratio is more likely if you are overweight or obese. Only 3% of women and 11% of men who were normal weight had central obesity, for example, compared to rates among the overweight of 12% (women) and 37% (men).

But it's clear that this is a risk factor that everyone who wants to live a long, healthy life should pay attention to. Here's how to find out where you stand.

How to Measure Your Waist-to-hip Ratio

While medical facilities have sophisticated methods of measuring central obesity precisely, measuring your waist-to-hip ratio is proven to be accurate, and it's something you can do yourself...

• **First, find your true waist**—it's not necessarily where your belt falls. Locate your hip bone on one side, and then move upward until you can feel the bones of your bottom rib. Halfway between your hip and that first rib bone is your waist. For most people, it's where the belly button is.

• **Measure your waist with a tape measure.**

• **Measure your hip with a tape measure.**

• **Divide the waist measure by the hip measure.** For example, if your waist is 28 and your hip is 36, you'd divide 28/36 to get a ratio of 0.78.

Here's a shortcut: For most women, a waist of 35 inches or above is a good quick indicator of central obesity, according to the American Heart Association.

If you do have a big belly, you know what to do—lose weight. The good news is that belly fat is the easiest to lose. It's the first to come off when change your diet and exercise habits...for the better.

"Virtual" Alternative to Weight-Loss Surgery

Jennie J. Kramer, MSW, LCSW, founder and executive director, Metro Behavioral Health Associates Eating Disorder Treatment Centers, New York City and Scarsdale, New York. Kramer also is the coauthor, with Marjorie Nolan Cohn, of *Overcoming Binge Eating for Dummies.* mbhany.com

Real bariatric surgery involves stapling off or removing part of the stomach...or cinching a plastic gastric band around the stomach. Either way, the amount of food that can be consumed is drastically reduced and rapid weight loss typically occurs. However, surgery carries significant risks, including the possibility of cardiac problems, pneumonia, bowel obstructions, bleeding, infection and even death. Also, certain foods must be permanently avoided after surgery because they would cause serious cramping, diarrhea or other upsets.

Safer alternative: The "virtual surgery" called gastric band hypnosis (GBH) carries none of those risks, according to Jennie J. Kramer, MSW, LCSW, founder and executive director of Metro Behavioral Associates Eating Disorder Treatment Centers in New York City and Scarsdale, New York, whose center provides GBH in conjunction with psychotherapy and nutritional counseling. With GBH, surgery takes place only within the "theater of the mind," not in an actual operating room, Kramer said. In essence, during hypnosis, the person's brain is retrained to believe that the stomach has undergone surgery to make it smaller—so that afterward, he feels satisfied with much smaller amounts of food and thus loses weight. "And since there is no cutting, there is no anesthesia, no pain, no scarring, no recovery time and no risk," Kramer said.

The GBH experience: After an initial consultation, the GBH protocol typically consists of four weekly hypnosis sessions, each lasting 60 to 75 minutes. The virtual "surgery" is done during the first session. The patient reclines comfortably and is hypnotized so that he is in a fully conscious yet deeply relaxed state.

Then the practitioner mentally guides the patient by describing each phase of the procedure...donning a hospital gown, signing a consent form, being wheeled into the surgical prep area, receiving anesthesia, having the gastric band applied around the stomach, closing the incision and being wheeled into the recovery room. To make the experience seem more real, the patient listens to hospital sounds (doctors and nurses talking, monitors beeping, etc.) through headphones. Some practitioners also may arrange for the patient to smell an appropriate aroma (such as an antiseptic) and/or feel a scratch on the back of the hand when "anesthesia" is administered. When the virtual procedure is finished, the patient is brought back out of the hypnotic state.

Why might this work? "The subconscious mind, which is where hypnosis takes effect, is very susceptible to positive suggestions and does not really differentiate between fantasy and reality," Kramer said. "So if your subconscious mind believes that you have had actual gastric banding surgery, your body—including your appetite and satiety cues—responds as if you'd really had the surgery."

Effective, but Not Magic

The patient's work doesn't end when the hypnosis component of the therapy is finished—because he still has to make permanent changes in his diet. "Let me be clear that GBH is no more a miracle than bariatric surgery. GBH can fail in exactly the same way that surgery can fail if the proper supports are not in place and the underlying causes of food addiction are not addressed," Kramer said. "You have to look at the patterns in your life to find out how your relationship to food got so distorted, then develop a healthier and sustainable relationship with food. That way, GBH can be a kick-start that sets you on the road to losing weight and keeping it off."

To that end, Kramer said, a complete GBH program includes not only the virtual surgery element, but also additional hypnotherapy and counseling during which patients explore the issues that underlie their weight problems and that trigger their overeating.

During the second, third and fourth hypnosis sessions, which take place a week apart, the hypnotherapist addresses the emotional aspects of overeating. For example, Kramer said, the patient might be asked to recall past incidents related to eating...or to summon up an image of himself as a child, then have a kind and gentle conversation about food with that child. Another exercise might involve imagining a beautiful, safe, comfortable place—one to which he can return, in his own mind, whenever he needs help coping with cravings, anxiety or stress. The patient also works on these emotional issues at home every day, guided by CDs and workbooks provided by the hypnotherapist.

Following that, patients participate in six monthly sessions of individual and/or group therapy that reinforce positive lifestyle changes as the excess weight is being lost. Kramer also recommends participating in a relevant 12-step group such as Overeaters Anonymous and receiving nutritional counseling as further insurance against going back to old unhealthy eating patterns after GBH.

Practical Matters

How effective is GBH? Numerous studies have shown that hypnosis is an effective means of bringing about weight loss, and that when used in combination with psychotherapy, hypnotherapy is more effective than psychotherapy alone. But the question about GBH specifically is still under investigation because no randomized clinical trials have yet been published on the technique. "Currently, a trial is being conducted under the auspices of the National Health Service of Great Britain, and the results thus far are quite compelling," Kramer said.

Who is a candidate for GBH? Due to its risks, actual bariatric surgery generally is limited to people who are morbidly obese, with a body mass index (BMI) of 40 or higher...or to obese people with a BMI of 35 to 40 who also have a serious weight-related health problem, such as type 2 diabetes, high blood pressure or severe sleep apnea. But because gastric band hypnosis is virtual and completely safe, it is an option not only for obese people, but also for those who are merely overweight.

Finding a practitioner: Many hypnotists work with patients who want to lose weight, but you may have to hunt some to find one who's trained in GBH. One option is to visit the website of the program's British originator, Sheila Granger (*SheilaGranger.com*), which lists practitioners who have trained directly with Granger. Or check with established professional organizations such as the National

Guild of Hypnotists and the International Association of Counselors and Therapists to find hypnotherapists near you, then contact them to ask whether they practice GBH. Note that techniques similar to GBH are known by other names, including virtual gastric band (VGB) and various trademarked terms.

The cost: Actual weight-loss surgery typically costs $20,000 to $35,000. Though GBH is far less expensive than surgery, it's not cheap, typically running $1,000 to $1,500 for the first four sessions, plus about $200 for each of the six subsequent monthly sessions, for a total of about $2,200 to $2,700. Unfortunately, health insurance generally does not cover these costs. However, hypnosis for medical reasons is an allowable expense for health-care flexible spending accounts and health savings accounts—and if it allows you to get your weight down for good, it could be an excellent investment in your health and well-being.

Safer, Cheaper Weight-Loss Surgery

Barham Abu Dayyeh, MD, MPH, assistant professor, medicine, and gastroenterologist, Mayo Clinic, Rochester, Minnesota.
Subhash Kini, MD, associate professor, surgery, Mt. Sinai Medical Center, New York City.
Clinical Gastroenterology and Hepatology.

A new type of weight-loss procedure offers an alternative to traditional bariatric surgery for people who are mildly to moderately obese, researchers report.

The procedure is called endoscopic sleeve gastroplasty, and it involves using an endoscope—a flexible tube inserted through the mouth—rather than making an incision in the body. When the endoscope reaches the stomach, the surgeon places sutures in the stomach, making it smaller and changing its shape.

A small study found that the procedure resulted in a loss of about 50 percent of excess weight when measured six, nine and 12 months after the procedure.

"We're able to go inside the stomach to its connection to the esophagus," said study author Dr. Barham Abu Dayyeh, a gastroenterologist at the Mayo Clinic in Rochester, Minnesota. From there, the surgeons use suturing equipment to create a banana-sized sleeve that serves as a mini-stomach.

"It delays the emptying of the stomach, and food sits in it for longer periods of time. Patients will be able to follow a low-calorie diet, fewer than 1,000 calories a day, without being hungry all the time," he said.

"We're not cutting or removing any part of the stomach or digestive tract," Abu Dayyeh explained. "There's a low risk of having any nutrition deficiencies, because you're leaving the gastrointestinal tract and stomach alone," he added.

Although the procedure still needs to undergo further research, Abu Dayyeh believes it has potential. "It's a whole paradigm shift," he said. "This technique offers more effective weight loss at lower risk and cost."

Not everyone is convinced, however.

Dr. Subhash Kini, a weight-loss surgeon and associate professor at Mt. Sinai Medical Center in New York City, is skeptical. He said surgeons have tried similar approaches using incisions, and they haven't worked well. In addition, he said, the length of the new study was short, and it didn't take into account the fact that weight-loss surgeries tend to fail at two years and beyond.

The findings were published recently in the journal *Clinical Gastroenterology and Hepatology*. Two of the study authors disclosed potential conflicts of interest. Abu Dayyeh is a consultant for a company called Apollo Endosurgery, which provided partial funding for the study and has supported his research. Study coauthor Dr. Christopher Gostout is Apollo Endosurgery's chief medical officer and holds a stake in the firm.

Currently, more than a third of people in the United States are obese, according to the U.S. Centers for Disease Control and Prevention. Beyond just being a cosmetic problem, obesity can lead to serious health risks including type 2 diabetes, certain types of cancer, high blood pressure, high cholesterol, heart disease and stroke, the CDC says.

Weight-loss surgery (also called bariatric surgery), which limits the amount of food a person can eat, is one option for people with a body mass index above 40, according to the American Society of Metabolic and Bariatric Surgery. Body mass index is a rough estimate of a person's fat based on height and weight measurements.

Weight-loss surgery may also be recommended for people with a BMI of 35 or above if they have other health risks, such as type 2 diabetes, the society says.

But many people with a BMI under 40 don't qualify for weight-loss surgery under current guidelines, said Abu Dayyeh. "The only thing that's left for them is medications or lifestyle modifications," he said.

Even people who do qualify for weight-loss surgery may choose against it because of the costs and risks, Abu Dayyeh said.

For the new study, researchers tested the new technique on 25 obese people with an average body mass index of 36. The average age of the study volunteers was 48. Only three of the subjects were men.

After the procedure, the study volunteers lost between 45 percent and 53 percent of their excess weight.

Weight information was only available for eight patients at the 20-month mark. At that time, five had maintained their weight loss, but three of the patients had regained all of the lost weight, the study reported.

Three patients had serious side effects after the procedure, including a collapsed lung and a blood clot in the lung. But all recovered, according to the study. The researchers said they adjusted the technique after these cases and didn't encounter any more serious side effects.

The cost of the procedure is about $10,000 to $15,000, roughly a third of the cost of other weight-control procedures, Abu Dayyeh said.

What about availability of the procedure?

Want to Feel Less Hungry? Cut Back on Red Meat

Too much dietary iron—common in diets that are heavy in red meat—stimulates the hormone leptin and boosts appetite, finds a new study from Wake Forest.

Study titled "Adipocyte Iron Regulates Leptin and Food Intake" by researchers at Wake Forest Baptist Medical Center, Salem, North Carolina, published in *Journal of Clinical Investigation*.

Abu Dayyeh said it's now being offered at centers in the United States and worldwide. More study is needed, he said, and the researchers have just submitted a new analysis of the technique in about 270 patients.

The Sounds You Make Eating May Be a Diet Aid

Brigham Young University, news release.

If you want to cut back on how much you eat, it might be a good idea to keep things quiet during meals, researchers suggest.

In a series of experiments, they found that people tend to eat less if they're more conscious of the chewing, chomping and crunching sounds they make while eating—and that loud TV or music can mask those sounds.

For example, study participants wore headphones that played either loud or quiet noise while they ate pretzels. Those exposed to loud noise ate four pretzels, while those in the quiet noise group ate 2.75 pretzels.

"The effects many not seem huge—one less pretzel—but over the course of a week, month or year, it could really add up," said study coauthor Ryan Elder, assistant professor of marketing in the Marriott School of Management at Brigham Young University, in Provo, Utah.

The study was published recently in the journal *Food Quality and Preference*.

The 30-Second Food-Craving Cure

Dawn Jackson Blatner, RDN, a registered dietitian nutritionist, certified specialist in sports dietetics and nutrition consultant for the Chicago Cubs, based in Chicago, and author of *The Flexitarian Diet*.

Got a bout of late-night cravings? The quick and easy solution is at your fingertips...

What to do: Tap your head! With either index finger, tap your forehead for 30 seconds.

What it does: This simple motion will reduce the intensity of your food cravings. In a study of 55 obese people at Mount Sinai-St. Luke's Weight Loss Program in New York City, it was the most successful "distraction" tactic...better than tapping your toes, tapping your ear or staring at a blank wall (the control group). All worked, but forehead tapping was the most effective.

How it works: No one knows for sure. But it's possible that simply distracting yourself can be a brief time-out that lets your emotional urges calm down...plus, forehead tapping might stimulate an acupressure region that reduces stress hormone levels.

The Whole30 Diet: Help or Hype?

Katherine Zeratsky, RD, LD, registered dietitian, Mayo Clinic, Rochester, Minnesota.

New diets used to just help you lose pounds. Now they promise to transform your very being. One of the newest ones boasts transformation and simplicity. No counting of calories or grams or points, no weighing portions or yourself, just eating simple wholesome foods that harken back to our hunter-gatherer days. After a few short weeks, according to Dallas and Melissa

Hartwig, the husband-and-wife team who created this diet—he's a physical therapist, she's a certified sports nutritionist—your life will change.

But will it really? And for the better?

For the Next 30 Days, No Ice Cream and No Tofu for You!

Like the popular Paleo diet, which it resembles in some ways, the Whole30 diet program emphasizes "real" food inspired by the hunter-gatherer life that existed before agriculture. *The program, which you are supposed to follow for 30 days, includes two food categories…*

• **Foods You Can Eat**—Seafood, poultry, red meat, eggs, oils, vegetables, fruits, nuts, seeds

• **Foods You Can't Eat**—Dairy, grains, legumes, alcohol, added sugar, additives (MSG, sulfites, corn starch, lecithin, carrageenan)

So…no yogurt or peanut butter (peanuts are legumes, not nuts) or bread or gluten-free quinoa (technically a seed but not allowed anyway) or soymilk or commercial ketchup (added sugar). Almond milk? Probably not… it likely contains carrageenan. Canned tuna? Check the label—the broth may be made with soy. *There are a few exceptions to the rules…*

• **No dairy but clarified butter (ghee) is allowed.**

• **No added sugar, and fruit juice (often high in sugar) is "not recommended"**—but you can buy foods that use fruit juice as a sweetener.

• **Green beans, although technically legumes, squeak through.**

Otherwise, the diet stresses complete elimination of foods on the "no" list for the full 30 days. If you slip and have a sip of coffee lightened with milk or sweetened with stevia, the timer resets and you're sent back to day one.

Why so strict about slipping up? The Hartwigs claim that dairy, legumes and grains (not to mention sugar and additives) are psychologically unhealthy, hormone-unbalancing, gut-disrupting and inflammatory. After 30 days of strict abstention from these classes of foods, they claim, you'll have "reset" your body so that your metabolism works better and you are no longer subject to systemic inflammation. Testimonials on the site, including those from health professionals, state that the program helps with conditions as varied as asthma, high blood pressure, high cholesterol, diabetes, chronic pain, chronic fatigue, fibromyalgia, depression, anxiety, insomnia… and, of course, weight loss.

After 30 days, you can let a few eliminated foods back into your life, but if you find yourself eating more "dirty" than "clean," according to the website, go back to the Whole30…even if only for a week.

Don't Be Surprised If This Unbalanced Diet Makes You Feel Better

To get an independent view of this program, we went to our own source, Katherine Zeratsky, RD, LD, a registered dietitian and nutrition educator at the Mayo Clinic in Rochester, Minnesota. *Here's what we found…*

• **Whole30 is scientifically unsubstantiated.** There simply are no studies in published journals on this particular diet. None.

• **You might well feel better on it.** "If people who weren't eating well started eating more nutritious foods, like more fruits and vegetables, and less processed foods, they would start feeling better," said Zeratsky.

• **But if you did feel better on it, you shouldn't jump to conclusions.** That pep in your step wouldn't necessarily mean that your body reacts badly to beans…or grains… or dairy. "You shouldn't be quick to assume that you had an allergy or sensitivity to those eliminated foods," she said. You may feel better because you're taking in, say, less sugar.

• **Your blood pressure might go down.** All those fresh fruits and vegetables, and no processed and packaged foods, means a lot less sodium and plenty of potassium. That plus weight loss is a good formula for lowering blood pressure.

• **It might be nutritionally unbalanced.** Without dairy or fortified foods like tofu, calcium intake will likely be low. If you're a vegetarian or a vegan, you'll need to avoid meat/poultry/seafood and beans and lentils, which makes it hard to get enough iron.

• **It's probably safe for healthy people—for 30 days.** "A generally well-nourished person is probably not going to become malnourished in that period of time," said Zeratsky. "Everybody doesn't need to have 100% of each nutrient every day."

The real question is what happens next. If you really think you have a sensitivity or allergy to a food or food group, work with a health professional, who may put you on a carefully monitored, more comprehensive food-elimination diet—in which case, you might discover that you have trouble with some food that is on the Whole30 "yes" list! You'd never learn that from the Whole30 diet.

Finally, there's that pesky problem of eating healthfully as a sustainable lifestyle. If this diet helps you discover that you can live without, say, a nightly dessert or afternoon vending machine temptation, wonderful. But the big test comes when you take off the training wheels and have to ride the bicycle on your own.

"Paleo" Diet Helps Women's Hearts and Waistlines Even Without Cutting Calories

Caroline Blomquist, doctoral student, department of public health and clinical medicine, Umea University, Sweden.

Caroline Apovian, MD, director, Nutrition and Weight Management Center, Boston Medical Center.

Connie Diekman, MEd, RD, director, university nutrition, Washington University in St. Louis, and former president, Academy of Nutrition and Dietetics.

Endocrine Society annual meeting.

The so-called Paleo diet may help older women lose weight and lower their future risk of diabetes and heart disease, a new study has found.

Women experienced these benefits by sticking to the guidelines of the Paleo diet, even though they were not required to restrict their calorie intake, the researchers said.

About the Paleo Diet

A Paleo diet requires people to eat foods similar to those available to humans during the Paleolithic period, which dates from 10,000 to 2.5 million years ago, according to the Mayo Clinic. The diet typically includes foods that could be obtained by hunting and gathering—lean meats, fish, fruits, vegetables, nuts and seeds—and limits foods that became common with the advent of farming, such as dairy products, grains and legumes.

The Study

In this study, Blomquist and her colleagues had 35 postmenopausal women who were obese but had normal blood sugar levels follow a Paleo diet for two years.

The group aimed to consume 30% of their daily energy intake from protein, 30% from carbohydrates, and 40% from fats mainly made up of "good" unsaturated fats.

The diet used in the study included lean meat, fish, eggs, vegetables, fruits, nuts and berries, with rapeseed, olive oils and avocado as additional fat sources. It excluded dairy products, cereals, added salt and refined fats and sugar.

A "control group" of 35 postmenopausal women were asked to follow a low-fat diet consisting of 15% protein, 30% fat and 55% carbohydrates.

After two years, the women eating the Paleo diet reported they had decreased their intake of "bad" saturated fats by 19%, while increasing by their intake of monounsaturated fats by 47% and their intake of polyunsaturated fats by 71%. In comparison, the women on the low-fat diet reported no significant changes in their intake of fats.

Specific fatty acids associated with insulin resistance were significantly lower in the women eating Paleo-type foods compared with those on the prudent control diet.

Both diets, however, resulted in similar—and significant—weight loss, the researchers said.

Implications

The study results indicate that the Paleo diet could prove an effective means of battling the obesity epidemic, said lead study author Caroline Blomquist, a doctoral student at Umea University in Sweden.

Expert Commentary

"I'm not sure I would say this is a Paleo diet," said Caroline Apovian, MD, director of the Nutrition and Weight Management Center at Boston Medical Center. "This is more of a cross between a Paleo diet and a Mediterranean diet."

Still, Dr. Apovian said it makes sense that the Paleo diet could provide some health benefits.

"You're basically eliminating all processed and simple carbohydrates, which we know is one of the exacerbations or causes of overweight, obesity and insulin resistance," Dr. Apovian said.

But the diet could cause some deficiencies in crucial nutrients, said nutritionist Connie Diekman, MEd, RD. She is director of university nutrition for Washington University in St. Louis and a former president of the Academy of Nutrition and Dietetics.

Eliminating all dairy could put calcium, vitamin D and potassium intakes at risk, while cutting back on legumes and whole grains could cause deficiencies in fiber, manganese, magnesium and selenium, said Diekman.

"Avoiding beans and grain foods also makes meeting nutrient needs harder," she said. "The beauty of including all food groups is that, when consumed in proper portions, we can more easily meet nutrient needs. When a food group is skipped, nutrient balance can be impacted."

It also can be difficult for a person to follow a lifestyle diet like Paleo, Diekman added.

"The best advice I would give is to find an eating plan that does two things—includes the foods that you enjoy and meets your nutrient needs—and then learn about proper portions," she said.

For more on the Paleo diet, visit the website of the Academy of Nutrition and Dietetics, *eatright.org*, and search "Paleo diet."

Eat This Plus That!

Tonia Reinhard, MS, RD, registered dietitian and professor at Wayne State University, Detroit. She is author of *Superfoods: The Healthiest Foods on the Planet and Superjuicing: More Than 100 Nutritious Vegetable and Fruit Recipes.*

Well-chosen food pairings do more than just excite your taste buds. Consuming certain food combos or food and drink combos creates a synergy that increases the absorption of important nutrients and phytochemicals.

Here are four supercharged combinations…

Fish + Wine

The American Heart Association recommends eating fish at least twice a week. The omega-3 fatty acids in fish have been shown to reduce triglycerides, irregular heartbeats and blood pressure and slow the growth of arterial plaques. It turns out that wine can boost those omega-3 levels.

A large European study looked at the dietary habits and alcohol consumption of more than 1,600 people. The participants underwent comprehensive medical exams and gave blood samples that were used to measure omega-3 levels. Their amount of "marine food intake," defined as the total intake of fish, shellfish, cuttlefish, squid, octopus, shrimp and crab, was also measured.

The researchers found that people who drank moderate amounts of alcohol (one daily drink for women and two for men) had higher concentrations of omega-3s than nondrinkers, despite consuming similar amounts of marine food. Wine drinkers had the biggest gains, but people who drank beer or spirits (such as Scotch) also showed an increase in omega-3s.

Important caveat: The study found that heavy drinkers had lower amounts of omega-3s.

Lemon + Tea

Both black and green teas contain catechins, a group of antioxidants that are surprisingly good for cardiovascular health. A study published in *Stroke*, which looked at more than 83,000 Japanese adults, found that those who drank two to three cups of green tea daily were 14% less likely to have a stroke than those who rarely drank tea.

Tea has been found to reduce cholesterol and reduce the risk for cancer, diabetes and heart disease. But there's a catch—the catechins in tea aren't very durable. They tend to break down during digestion, leaving behind less than 20% of the active compounds.

Tasty solution: Add a squeeze of lemon to your tea. A laboratory study published in *Molecular Nutrition & Food Research* found that combining lemon juice with tea allowed 80% of the catechins to "survive" post-digestion. Orange, lime and grapefruit juices also stabilized the compounds, although not as much as the lemon.

If you prefer bottled to brewed tea, you'll get a similar effect by picking a product that includes vitamin C—listed as ascorbic acid on the label.

Citrus + Iron-Rich Foods

Low iron is common in people who take acid-suppressing drugs for GERD and in people who have gastrointestinal problems in which inflammation and bleeding occur (such as inflammatory bowel disease and bleeding ulcers).

Many foods contain iron. Iron-rich animal foods include beef, liver, oysters and sardines. Iron-rich plant foods include dark leafy greens such as spinach, kale and collard greens…beans…lentils…whole grains… and nuts. But iron is not the easiest mineral to absorb. The body can absorb only 2% to 20% of the non-heme iron in plant foods. The absorption of the heme iron from meats and fish/shellfish is better but still not great— typically between 15% and 35%. And certain supplements such as calcium can interfere with iron absorption.

How can you boost absorption of iron? By eating citrus fruits or other vitamin C–rich foods such as strawberries and yellow and red peppers with heme or non-heme foods.

Examples: Add orange slices to your kale salad…or yellow peppers to your beef stew. One study found that consuming as little as 63 mg of vitamin C (a little more than the amount in one orange) nearly tripled the absorption of non-heme iron.

Fat + Salad

Salads are rich in carotenoids—antioxidants such as lutein, lycopene and beta-carotene that reduce your risk for cancer and heart disease, preserve bone density and prevent macular degeneration. A fat-based salad dressing can maximize the absorption of these carotenoids (so avoid fat-free salad dressings). Researchers at Purdue University served participants salads with dressings made from a monounsaturated fat (canola oil)…a polyunsaturated fat (soybean oil)…or a saturated fat (butter). All the fats boosted absorption of the carotenoids, but the monounsaturated fat required the least amount of fat to get the most carotenoid absorption. Another monounsaturated fat often found in salad dressings is olive oil.

You can get similar benefits by adding hard-boiled eggs to your salad. The fat from the yolks will increase your absorption of carotenoids. In a Purdue University study published in *The American Journal of Nutrition*, participants who ate a salad with one-and-a-half eggs had double the carotenoid absorption of people who had a salad with no eggs.

Whole Grains Protect Your Health

Julie Miller Jones, PhD, CNS, LN, certified nutrition specialist and licensed nutritionist, and distinguished scholar and professor emerita of food and nutrition, St. Catherine University, St. Paul. She regularly writes and lectures about whole grains and dietary fiber.

You know that you're supposed to eat whole grains, but many people just don't like whole-wheat pasta...or whole-wheat anything. To make sure you're eating enough whole grains, offer your taste buds more variety.

Here's what some recent studies found...

•**People who ate three or more servings of whole grains and less than one serving of refined grains (white bread, cookies, etc.) daily averaged 10% less belly fat**—linked to cardiovascular disease and diabetes—compared with people who ate the fewest whole grains and the most refined grains.

•**People who consumed the most fiber,** primarily from whole grains, were 22% less likely to die during a nine-year study than those who ate the least fiber. Fiber's protective effect was particularly pronounced in women.

•**Two recent analyses from John Hopkins** showed that those eating the most dietary fiber had a lower risk for death from any cause than those eating the least. For every additional 10 grams of dietary fiber, there was a 10% reduction in risk for death from any cause.

•**In a Harvard study,** compared with people who rarely ate whole grains, those who ate the equivalent of one bowl of oatmeal daily had a 9% reduced risk for early death...and for each additional daily ounce of whole grains, that risk was reduced by another 5%.

The problem is, fewer than 5% of Americans consume the USDA-recommended minimum of about three ounces of whole grains per day. What's the big deal? Whole grain contains the entire edible part of a grain (a.k.a., "seed")—including the germ (technically the sprout of a new plant)...endosperm (the seed's energy storehouse)...and nutrient-rich bran (the seed's outer layer). Refined grains, on the other hand, are stripped of their bran and germ layers during milling.

Enriched refined grains, however, can have a place in a healthy diet—minerals contained in the grains can be better absorbed from an enriched product than one with a lot of fiber and bran. And if a whole-grain pasta or bread that is partly enriched refined grains is more appealing, at least it gets you to eat some whole grains. But, the greater the variety of whole grains you eat, the better. Each whole grain brings different nutrients, fibers and phytonutrients to the table, so it is worth exploring and enjoying various types.

Lesser known but delicious whole grains can be found in supermarkets, health-food stores and online. Check out these...

Amaranth provides protein, calcium, iron, phosphorus, potassium and many other nutrients. It's also free of gluten, a protein in wheat, rye and barley that can cause digestive upset in some people. When cooked, amaranth is pleasantly sticky and mild tasting.

To cook: Boil one cup of amaranth grains in two-and-a-half cups of water or broth for 20 minutes or until tender. If desired, season with herbs, pepper and a bit of olive oil. Or use milk as part of the cooking liquid and add sweet spices, such as cinnamon and cardamom. Also try amaranth flakes as a breakfast cereal...amaranth crackers...and amaranth flour, swapping it for one-third of a recipe's white flour.

Buckwheat, a gluten-free grain, offers plenty of protein...the heart-healthy flavonoid rutin...plus bone-building magnesium and other minerals. It is strongly flavored, so serve it as a side dish paired with robust entrées, such as those made with red wine or balsamic vinegar. Cook the hulled, crushed kernels by simmering one cup of buckwheat in two cups of water for about 10 to 15 minutes (avoid overcooking so it doesn't become mushy)...then flavor with onions, mushrooms and whatever else you like.

Kamut, the brand name for an ancient relative of wheat, provides protein, fiber, vitamin A, iron and zinc (it does contain gluten). With their nutty, buttery taste, kamut kernels make a great substitute for rice in recipes. Note that the cooking time is around 90 minutes…or you can soak the kernels overnight to reduce cooking time to about 30 minutes. Kamut flour can be used to bake bread, tortillas, cookies and more.

Recipes: Kamut.com.

Quinoa is a tiny gluten-free grain rich in essential amino acids (protein building blocks that our bodies must get from dietary sources) as well as iron, magnesium, phosphorus, potassium and protein.

To cook: Simmer one cup of quinoa and two cups of water or broth for 15 minutes or until water is absorbed. Add cooked quinoa to omelets or soups…or combine with vegetables, nuts and spices for a tasty side dish.

White whole wheat is an unrefined variety of wheat with a light-colored kernel. It has a lower gluten content than the red wheat used to make regular whole-wheat flour, so it produces foods with a softer texture and sweeter flavor. It provides nutrient and fiber content similar to that of regular whole wheat, though it is lower in some antioxidants (which accounts for its lighter color).

In recipes: Substitute white whole-wheat flour for half of the refined flour or for all of the regular whole-wheat flour.

You Can Break the Sugar Habit

Jacob Teitelbaum, MD, director of the Practitioners Alliance Network, an organization for health providers dedicated to improving patient care. He is coauthor of *The Complete Guide to Beating Sugar Addiction*…the website Vitality101.com…and the free smartphone app Cures A-Z.

People may joke about having a "sweet tooth," but it's really no laughing matter.

The craving for sweets can be just as intense as cravings for drugs or alcohol. The comparison is apt because sweets trigger some of the same brain changes that occur in people who use cocaine or other highly addictive substances—and can be even harder to give up. So what's the harm in having a daily sugar fix?

What the research now says: While we've long known that overindulging in sugar can lead to cavities and weight gain (and related risks such as diabetes), a growing body of research now shows a far broader range of potential harms. These include increased risks for high blood pressure and heart disease…certain types of cancer (such as malignancies of the breast and pancreas)…kidney disease…liver failure…migraines…osteoporosis…and cognitive decline. Too much sugar has also been linked to fatigue, anxiety and depression.

Wondering if you are a sugar addict? As with most addictions, if you feel the need to ask the question, you likely are! (See the box on the next page for a self-test.)

Sugar Overload

A little sugar won't hurt, but most people get much more than the daily maximum amount of added sugar recommended by the American Heart Association (AHA)—100 calories for women and 150 calories for men, which is roughly equal to six to nine teaspoons of sugar (or 25 g to 37 g).

And it adds up fast. Most sodas and many fruit drinks have up to three-quarters of a teaspoon of sugar per ounce. It's also hidden in places you might not expect. Many flavored six-ounce yogurts have seven teaspoons of sugar…a half-cup serving of coleslaw has 2.5 teaspoons…and one-half cup of spaghetti sauce has almost two teaspoons.

Cut the Cravings

With sugar's addictive qualities, cutting back is no easy feat. Some people try to go cold turkey for a few days (forgoing even foods that contain natural sugar) to prime themselves for a longer-term low-sugar diet. For many people, however, this approach is too drastic.

A gentle way to rein in your sugar intake: Start by cutting back on the highest-sugar foods in your diet—sweet beverages, candy and other sugary desserts. You'll still be getting some added sugar in foods you may not expect (such as condiments, including salad dressing, sauces and ketchup...granola...and even many types of bread). But if sugar is listed as one of the top three ingredients on a food or drink label (meaning the sugar content is high), don't have it.

Important: When you're checking labels, be aware that added sugar may appear under such terms as sucrose, maltose, glucose or dextrose...and, of course, high-fructose corn syrup, molasses, honey, etc. A lot of restaurant food is also notoriously high in sugar—including ethnic foods, such as Chinese and Thai.

Keep it simple: Your goal is to significantly cut back on added sugar—that is, sugars and syrups added to food or beverages during preparation and processing. Aim for the AHA's guideline (six teaspoons a day for women... and nine for men). To calculate teaspoons, divide the number of grams by four. Also avoid foods with white flour, found in many breads and pastas—the body rapidly converts it to sugar. But if it's a whole food without a label—such as a fruit or veggie—then you can safely assume that it's OK to eat.

If you've been getting too much sugar, you'll probably experience irritability, loss

---

What Type of Sugar Addict Are You?

Here are the four main types of sugar addiction...

TYPE 1: **Low energy.** Do you repeatedly crave sweets or caffeine to give you the energy you need to get through the day?

What helps: Take a multinutrient powder. Nutrient deficiencies can cause fatigue while increasing both appetite and sugar cravings.

Good product: Energy Revitalization System multinutrient powder.*

Take one-half to one scoop daily. You can blend it with milk, water or yogurt. For extra energy, add a scoop of ribose (see main article).

TYPE 2: **Overtaxed adrenal glands.** Do you constantly feel stressed out? Are you irritable when you're hungry? These are both red flags for another common cause of sugar addiction—adrenal insufficiency, a stress-related reduction in adrenal hormones.

What helps: Drink one cup of licorice root tea each morning. This helps the adrenal hormones that are made by your body last longer.

Caution: If you have high blood pressure or take any type of medication, ask your doctor before trying licorice root tea. Adrenal function is also supported by vitamins C and B-5 (the Energy Revitalization System multinutrient powder mentioned above provides healthful levels).

TYPE 3: **Candida overgrowth.** Do you have chronic nasal congestion, sinusitis or irritable bowel syndrome? These conditions may indicate hidden Candida (yeast) overgrowth. Yeasts thrive on sugar and release a chemical that causes sugar cravings.

What helps: A good enteric-coated probiotic (such as Optima) will fight Candida overgrowth. It is also worth seeing a holistic physician (check the website of the American Board of Integrative Holistic Medicine, *ABIHM.org*, for a referral) to help you get rid of Candida.

TYPE 4: **Imbalanced hormones.** In premenopausal and menopausal women, changes in estrogen and progesterone can lead to mood changes that improve when sugar is eaten. Men can be affected by midlife drops in testosterone, which also can trigger sugar cravings.

What helps: Eating a handful of edamame daily may help balance hormone levels in women with premenstrual syndrome (PMS) and ease menopausal symptoms, such as hot flashes. Women and men who suffer from hormonally driven sugar cravings may also want to ask their doctors about natural hormone replacement.

*Dr. Teitelbaum formulated this product and donates 100% of royalties from sales to charity.

When to Have Your First Cup of Coffee

Wait to have your first cup of coffee until between 9:30 and 11:30 am.

Reason: For most people, the body naturally produces cortisol—a hormone that makes us feel alert, between 8:00 and 9:00 am, so you don't need caffeine that early to help you wake up.

And: Drinking caffeine too early can lead to too much cortisol, and that can disturb your body's circadian rhythms.

Psychology Today. PsychologyToday.com

of energy and other withdrawal symptoms when you first cut back, but they usually fade within 10 days.

Helpful while you're cutting back...*

• **Replace added sugar with stevia.** This plant-based sweetener has no calories, and it doesn't cause the insulin spikes that occur with sugar ...or increase risk for diabetes.

Stevia is 200 to 300 times sweeter than sugar, so you can use just a small amount in your coffee or tea...and use it for baking (follow label instructions for the correct amount). Some brands of stevia have a bitter aftertaste due to poor filtering.

Good products: Body Ecology's Liquid Stevia Concentrate, Stevita, Truvia, and Pure Via.

• **Take ribose.** It's a special type of sugar that is made by the body to create energy. You can use ribose in supplement form to replace the sugar energy "high" you may miss when you phase out sweets. Research has shown that it increases healthy energy by an average of 60% within three weeks.

My advice: Add a 5,000-mg scoop of ribose powder twice daily to any food or drink. Ribose powder looks and tastes like sugar but doesn't raise blood sugar (it can lower blood sugar in people with diabetes). Use less if you feel too energized.

*If you have diabetes or take any type of medication, consult your doctor before changing your diet and/or taking supplements.

• **Eat low-glycemic foods.** The glycemic index (GI) rates foods by how quickly they raise blood sugar. High-glycemic foods, such as white bread and white rice, raise blood sugar nearly as quickly as pure sugar—and increase sugar cravings.

Foods rated 70 or above cause rapid rises in blood sugar...those with a GI below 55 have little effect (those in between have an intermediate effect). Choose foods at the lower end of the scale.

Examples: Whole grains, legumes, nonstarchy vegetables, nuts and eggs.

To find the GI of specific foods, go to *GlycemicIndex.com* and use the search function.

Soy May Counter Effects of BPA in Women Undergoing Fertility Treatments

Journal of Clinical Endocrinology & Metabolism, news release.

A soy-rich diet may protect women undergoing infertility treatments from the harmful effects of a chemical widely used in food containers, a new study suggests.

Bisphenol A (BPA)—which is found in such items as polycarbonate plastic water bottles and can linings—can mimic estrogen, one of the two main sex hormones found in women, and the chemical has been linked to reproductive disorders.

More than 96% of Americans have BPA in their bodies, according to the U.S. Centers for Disease Control and Prevention.

This study included 239 women, aged 18 to 45, who underwent at least one in-vitro fertilization (IVF) cycle between 2007 and 2012. They completed questionnaires about their eating habits (176 consumed soy foods) and their urine was analyzed to measure BPA levels.

Among women who did not eat soy foods, those with higher BPA levels had lower rates of embryo implantation, fewer pregnancies that advanced to the point where the fetus could be seen on an ultrasound, and fewer live births than those with a soy-rich diet, the researchers found.

Among women who regularly consumed soy, BPA levels had no impact on IVF outcomes, according to the study.

"Our study is the first to show a possible interaction between soy and BPA in humans," first author Dr. Jorge Chavarro, from Harvard School of Public Health and Brigham and Women's Hospital and Harvard Medical School, all in Boston, said in a journal news release.

"Although it is recommended that women trying to get pregnant reduce their exposure to BPA, our findings suggest that diet may modify some of the risks of exposure to BPA, a chemical that is nearly impossible to completely avoid due to its widespread use," study senior author Dr. Russ Hauser, from Harvard School of Public Health, Massachusetts General Hospital and Harvard Medical School, said in the news release.

"Additional research could help identify other diet and lifestyle changes that may modify the effects of not only BPA exposure, but also exposure to other chemicals," Chavarro said.

The U.S. National Institute of Environmental Health Sciences has more about BPA at *niehs.nih.gov/health/topics/agents/sya-bpa/*.

Why Sardines Are So Healthy

Karen Collins, MS, RDN, registered dietitian nutritionist, syndicated columnist and nutrition adviser to the American Institute for Cancer Research. She was an expert reviewer for the Institute's international report, *Food, Nutrition, Physical Activity and the Prevention of Cancer: A Global Perspective.* KarenCollinsNutrition.com

What makes sardines the sea's superfood? Canned sardines have more omega-3 fatty acids than most fish. And because they're a small fish that's low on the food chain, they contain less mercury than many other fish. They're also inexpensive and are a sustainable source of protein. So why do Americans eat only minnow-size amounts?

Sardines are an oily fish, and oily fish can taste a little...well, fishy. You might prefer sardines that are lightly smoked or sardines nestled in mustard or tomato sauce.

Here, more on the health benefits of sardines...

Great for omega-3s: A recent report from the USDA concluded that 80% to 90% of Americans eat less than eight ounces of fish a week, the minimum recommended amount. This means that you're probably not getting enough omega-3s, beneficial fats that have been shown to reduce the risk for heart disease and that may protect against cancer, depression, rheumatoid arthritis and other serious conditions.

All cold-water fish provide omega-3s, but sardines are among the best. A four-ounce serving of sardines has about 1.1 to 1.6 grams. That's right up there with salmon (1.2 to 2.4 g depending on the salmon) and much higher than cod (0.2 g) or the most common types of tuna (0.3 g).

Your body needs these important types of fats. A study published in *Neurology* found that people who ate fish three or more times a week were about 26% less likely to have silent *infarcts*, damaged brain areas that can lead to dementia and stroke. Omega-3s have been found to reduce heart irregularities (arrhythmias) that can be deadly and even may provide some blood pressure control help. Some experts speculate that the anti-inflammatory effects of omega-3s could help prevent some cancers...and eating more fish can help people eat less red meat or processed meat, important for decreasing the risk for colorectal cancer.

Other health benefits: Sardines are high in protein, vitamin D and selenium—and sardines with bones give an extra shot of calcium. A three-ounce serving of bones-in sardines has as much calcium as a glass of milk.

Less mercury: Some people avoid seafood altogether because they're worried about mercury, a contaminant found in virtually all fish, including farmed fish.

Good news: Sardines are among the lowest-mercury fish in the sea. They do contain trace amounts, but that might be offset by their high selenium content. The research isn't conclusive, but it's possible that a high-selenium diet could reduce the risks of mercury, either by "binding up" the mineral or by reducing its oxidative effects.

The health benefits of sardines and other fish more than outweigh the potential downsides of mercury—so much so that the EPA's and FDA's recently revised guidelines encourage pregnant women and young children (who are particularly susceptible to mercury) to eat eight to 12 ounces of low-mercury fish a week.

The Healthiest Olive Oil

Study titled "New Drugs from Ancient Natural Foods. Oleocanthal, the Natural Occurring Spicy Compound of Olive Oil: A Brief History" by researchers at University of Santiago de Compostela, Spain, et al., published in *Drug Discovery Today*.

Study titled "Oleocanthal Rapidly and Selectively Induces Cancer Cell Death via Lysosomal Membrane Permeabilization" by researchers at Hunter College of the City University of New York, et al., published in *Molecular & Cellular Oncology*.

Pizzicante. That's the Italian word for the pungent, back-of-the-throat, peppery, almost burning, bite found in some olive oils.

• **Oleocanthal.** That's the scientific term for the compound that gives these oils their bite.

It's an amazing compound, one that may be responsible for some of the extraordinary health powers of the Mediterranean diet.

A Dietary Painkiller...and Much More

Oleocanthal is one of the many antioxidant compounds found in extra-virgin olive oil. Almost a decade ago, it was first identified as a natural nonsteroidal anti-inflammatory (NSAID)—much like *ibuprofen* (Advil, Motrin). A synthetic version is patent-pending as a possible new painkiller.

Recent research has uncovered even more tantalizing health properties...

• **Killing cancer cells.** Our bodies kill cells all the time—it's one of our protections against cancer. Oleocanthal may enhance this. Researchers at Hunter College in New York City recently reported that, in the lab, a purified version of oleocanthal killed cancer cells—without damaging healthy cells. It does so by disrupting the membrane of a cellular organelle known as the lysosome, which is enlarged and more fragile in cancer cells.

• **Detoxing the brain.** Alzheimer's disease is marked by tangled neurons and the buildup of the toxic compound beta-amyloid. Researchers at the University of Louisiana at Monroe have found that oleocanthal interferes with this process. In mice given oleocanthal, two proteins key to transporting beta-amyloid out of the brain worked significantly better.

It's early work, but it may shed light on the anticancer and dementia-protective properties of the traditional Mediterranean diet. In one Spanish study, women who followed the diet over five years were 68% less likely to develop breast cancer, while in an American study, men and women who ate Mediterranean over 14 years were 32% less likely to develop Alzheimer's. There are many nutrients and compounds that may play a role in these protective benefits, of course, but a group of scientists believe that oleocanthal is an important part of the story.

How to Eat More Oleocanthal

It's not available as a supplement—at least not yet—so the best approach is to seek out olive oil that is likely to be high in this bracing compound. Start with extra-virgin olive oil (EVOO), since the harsh methods of extraction used for "pure" oils destroys antioxidants, including this one.

Then go rustic: The highest levels are typically found in green, early harvest EVOO, since levels decline as the olive fruit ripens, according to a study of Greek and California olive oils. If you have a good specialty shop, ask the vendor for a good green olive oil with a pungent flavor.

The best way to tell? Taste. Swallow a spoonful of EVOO, and wait for a peppery sensation in your throat. If you "feel the burn" after a few seconds, you have the real thing. No burn, not much oleocanthal.

Pizzicante EVOO isn't for every dish—or every palate. If you don't like it, you can rest assured that it's but one of the hundreds of health-protective compounds in the traditional Mediterranean diet, with its emphasis on vegetables, fruit, beans, nuts, whole grains, seafood, fermented dairy products and wine. But if you do like an assertive EVOO, there's a good argument that you're enjoying the healthiest olive oil money can buy.

The Truth About Those Anti-Kale Rumors

Katherine Zeratsky, RD, LD, registered dietitian, Mayo Clinic, Rochester, Minnesota.

Oh, how Superfood Kale seems to have fallen. Here are some headlines collected recently by the media watchdog group *Health News Review*…

"Find Out Why This Superfood Is Actually Super-Poisoning"

"Is Kale Making People Sick?: The Dark Side of Everyone's Favorite Superfood"

You know that kale is packed with a stunning amount of nutrients. But could you be poisoned by America's favorite superfood?

Kale Fail

Headlines like those above have their origins in an article in *Craftsmanship* magazine, later amplified in a *Mother Jones* magazine article entitled "Sorry, Foodies: We're About to Ruin Kale."

The story: A molecular biologist who works at an integrative health clinic in Cali-

fornia theorized that high levels of the heavy metal thallium from soil were seeping into kale—and may be causing a variety of ailments including chronic fatigue, hair and skin problems, cardiac arrhythmias, neurological problems and "foggy thinking."

The "kale-is-making-us-sick" hypothesis, however, is based on shaky information—anecdotal statements from people with various symptoms who said they liked to eat kale, and the results from a single lab that said it found high levels of thallium in kale samples. (That lab has been the subject of controversy and lawsuits over faulty testing, so at a minimum one would want to see its results replicated at other labs.) Nor has there been any evidence published in a peer-reviewed scientific journal that links kale intake with any disease or symptoms.

Here's what's known: Thallium is poisonous, and kale can accumulate thallium from soil. So can many other cruciferous vegetables such as broccoli, Brussels sprouts, cauliflower and cabbage…as well as canola, the plant used to make cooking oil. But most thallium is found very deep in the earth's crust, far below the soil level, so it's not likely to get anywhere near the kale plant's roots. As one molecular biologist interviewed by a reporter for *VOX* magazine put it, "It is close to impossible for humans to be poisoned by eating kale from normal soil." The exception is soil that is very near coal-burning power plants, since coal ash can contain high levels of thallium, or soil that is contaminated with industrial wastes. (Thallium is used in manufacturing electronic devices and semiconductors.)

So…unless your kale is grown on property that has been contaminated by nearby industrial activity, you're probably just fine. The real issue is contaminated soil, and that affects all of agriculture, not just one food. If any real evidence about kale or cabbage or any other food does show up to the contrary, we'll be sure to let you know.

In the meantime, though, there actually are some evidence-based reasons that some people may want to steer clear of kale.

Kale Precautions

Please enjoy this nutritious vegetable in the safest, healthiest way. *A few tips…*

• **Rinse it.** Although it's not easily absorbed by plants, lead-containing dust formed by the soil lands on the leafy greens and settles in the crevices. The solution—a good rinse under running water. Don't use soap or detergent.

• **If you have a thyroid condition,** such as hypothyroidism (low thyroid hormone levels), don't overdo raw kale (or other cruciferous vegetables)…as in juicing. It contains compounds that may affect the thyroid in people with this condition. That's not a concern for people with normal thyroid function, and even if you have hypothyroidism, cooked kale a few times a week is fine. Cooking destroys most of these compounds.

• **If you're on a blood thinner,** talk to your doctor about foods such as kale that are rich in vitamin K, which helps blood clot. For the medications to work right, you need a consistent amount of vitamin K in your diet, so you may be told to limit or avoid foods such as kale.

• **Eat a variety of foods,** including a variety of green vegetables, and you'll get a wider array of nutrients…and if there are contaminants in a particular food, you won't be exposed to large amounts.

Is Bacon the New Smoking?

Study titled "Carcinogenicity of Consumption of Red and Processed Meat" by scientists at the International Agency for Research on Cancer (IARC), Lyon, France, for the World Health Organization, published in *The Lancet Oncology*.

The WHO recently declared that processed meats such as ham, bacon and hot dogs were "human carcinogens." That's the same category as tobacco or asbestos. WHO also classified unprocessed red meat (such as steak and burgers) as a "probable carcinogen."

You might wonder if the new report means it's time to say bye-bye to burgers and sayonara to sausage…and to start wondering, Is eating bacon as bad for me as smoking?

Far from it. Here's why: The WHO classification system has nothing to do with actual risk. It's about the strength of the evidence. They're saying that the evidence is as strong about processed meats as about smoking. *But the risk is pretty darn different…*

• **If you eat a daily average of 50 grams of processed meat**—about two slices of ham—your risk of developing colorectal cancer goes up 18%.

• **If you eat a daily average of 100 grams of red meat**—about 3½ ounces—your risk for colorectal cancer goes up by 17%.

Compare that to tobacco…

• **If you smoke,** your lifetime risk of developing lung cancer, compared to people who never smoke, goes up 24 times—that is, by 2,400%!

A Place for Bacon and Burgers

The recent report is no reason to panic. While the new WHO classification is big news, it's not really surprising to health researchers that processed meats and, to a lesser degree, red meats can modestly increase your risk for colon cancer. That research is part of the reason why the Dietary Guidelines 2015 recommends that a healthy dietary pattern is "lower in red and processed meats." Of course, the American meat industry isn't too happy about either the WHO report or the Dietary Guidelines.

Nevertheless, it's a good idea to take a look at how much meat, especially processed meat, you're eating. While the WHO report didn't specify a safe limit, Dariush Mozaffarian, MD, DrPH, dean of the School of Nutrition and Science Policy at Tufts University, told NPR that he recommends eating no more than one or two servings of processed meats a month, and no more than one or two servings of red meat a week.

Easy Ways to Fix 4 Nutrient Deficiencies...

Dennis Goodman, MD, cardiologist and clinical associate professor of medicine in the Leon H. Charney Division of Cardiology and director of Integrative Medicine, both at NYU Langone Medical Center in New York City. He is the author of *Magnificent Magnesium, The Thrill of Krill and Vitamin K2*. Dennis GoodmanMD.com

If you eat a balanced diet, you may assume that you're getting all the nutrition you need. To play it safe, you might even take a multivitamin-mineral supplement. But is that enough? Probably not.

Four missing nutrients: Increasing evidence shows that there are four little-known nutritional deficiencies—each of which can threaten your health. The problem is, these deficiencies are not remedied by a typical multivitamin-mineral supplement and are extremely difficult to reverse through diet alone—even if you eat organic foods, which provide higher levels of some nutrients. *Here's what you're likely missing—and the nutrient fix you need...* *

Vitamin K-2

Vitamin K isn't even on most people's radar. But there are more than a dozen subtypes of this vitamin, including an important one known as menaquinone (vitamin K-2).

K-2 is crucial for your bones and heart. Without enough K-2, osteocalcin, a protein that binds calcium to bone, cannot be activated. When calcium doesn't stay in bones, it can end up clogging your arteries, causing a heart attack or stroke.

*If you take medication, check with your doctor before trying any of these supplements to avoid potential interactions.

Important finding: People with the lowest blood levels of vitamin K-2 had a 57% greater risk of dying from heart disease than those with the highest levels, according to research published in *The Journal of Nutrition*. People with low K-2 levels also are at increased risk for osteoporosis and bone fractures.

K-2 is found mainly in meat, eggs and dairy. But to get a bone- and heart-protecting level of K-2 from animal sources, you'd have to include in your daily diet at least eight pounds of beef, a gallon of milk, eight egg yolks and a gallon of yogurt. The only good nonanimal sources of K-2—fermented soybeans, found in foods such as tamari, miso and natto—aren't eaten regularly by most Americans.

My advice: Take a K-2 supplement—at least 45 micrograms (mcg) daily. Look for MenaQ7 (MK-7), a long-acting and better-absorbed variety.

Good products: MenaQ7 from NattoPharma, MenaQ7.com...and MK-7 from NOW Foods, NowFoods.com.

Caution: If you take *warfarin* (Coumadin), ask your doctor before trying vitamin K-2—it can alter the drug's effectiveness.

Coenzyme Q10

Coenzyme Q10 (CoQ10) helps the body make adenosine triphosphate (ATP), the main energy source for cellular activity. But modern life steals CoQ10. You are probably deficient in this nutrient if you take a cholesterol-lowering statin...if you're exposed to high levels of air pollutants...or if you have a chronic disease. Research links low levels of CoQ10 to heart disease, Parkinson's disease, type 2 diabetes, male infertility and fibromyalgia.

CoQ10 is found in such foods as broccoli, nuts, beef and fatty fish—but only in small amounts.

My advice: Take a 100-mg CoQ10 supplement daily. If you have side effects from taking a statin—such as muscle pain and weakness—consider taking 200 mg of CoQ10 daily. In my cardiology practice, I recommend SmartQ10, from Enzymatic Therapy, *EnzymaticTherapy.com*.

Omega-3s

Chronic, low-grade inflammation underlies many chronic health problems, including heart disease, type 2 diabetes, arthritis, cancer and Alzheimer's disease.

Omega-3 essential fatty acids—found in fatty fish, such as salmon, mackerel and tuna, and in oil-rich plant foods, such as walnuts and flaxseeds—are anti-inflammatory. In contrast, omega-6 essential fatty acids—found in baked goods (such as chips, crackers and cookies), cooking oils (such as corn oil, cottonseed oil and sunflower oil) and meat (especially processed meats and non-lean red meat)—are pro-inflammatory. Because the typical American diet has far too much omega-6 and not nearly enough omega-3, the majority of us have an omega-3 deficiency.

My advice: Take 500 mg of krill oil daily. I choose krill oil for myself and my patients rather than fish oil. Krill—small, shrimplike crustaceans—are at the bottom of the oceanic food chain and mostly harvested in the pristine waters around Antarctica, so their oil is less likely to be contaminated with mercury.

Krill oil also contains phospholipids, fatty substances that optimize the absorption of omega-3s. And because of that superior absorption, you need less—500 mg of krill oil is the therapeutic equivalent of 1 g to 2 g of fish oil.

If you are allergic to shellfish: Do not take krill oil.

Magnesium

Eight out of 10 Americans unknowingly suffer from a chronic deficiency of this crucial nutrient. That deficiency causes or contributes to health problems, including heart attacks and other forms of cardiovascular disease (such as arrhythmias, heart failure and stroke), some forms of cancer, type 2 diabetes, obesity, osteoporosis, fatigue, depression and anxiety, migraines, muscle cramps and insomnia.

My advice: Magnesium is the most important supplement anyone can take. I recommend that women take 400 mg to 500 mg daily…and men take 500 mg to 600 mg daily. You can take it all at once or in divided doses—just take it! (If you have insomnia, consider taking your daily dose before bedtime to help you sleep.) I recommend Jigsaw Magnesium, from Jigsaw Health, *JigsawHealth.com*. A well-absorbed form of magnesium malate, its sustained-release formula helps prevent diarrhea, a possible side effect of magnesium.

Vitamin D for Muscle Strength

A vitamin for weight loss?

Vitamin D supplements will not cause you to lose weight, but people who are vitamin D–deficient may experience muscle weakness, fatigue and joint pain, which could result in weight gain. Adults should take 1,500 IU to 2,000 IU of vitamin D day. If you're obese, you may need more.

Michael F. Holick, PhD, MD, professor of medicine, physiology and biophysics at Boston University School of Medicine.

Strong Muscles Postmenopause

Vitamin D supplements may help women build muscle after menopause. In a Brazilian study, postmenopausal women in their 50s and early 60s who took 1,000 international units (IU) of vitamin D-3 daily for nine months had 25% more muscle mass than women who took placebos. Many of the women had low vitamin D levels at the start.

Study titled "Effect of Vitamin D Supplementation Alone on Muscle Function in Postmenopausal Women: A Randomized, Double-Blind, Placebo-Controlled Clinical Trial" published in *Osteoporosis International*.

L.M. Cangussu, PhD, Botucatu Medical School, Sao Paulo State University, Brazil.

Whatever brand you use, look for magnesium malate, magnesium citrate or magnesium glycinate—the most absorbable forms. Avoid magnesium oxide—unless you want its stool-loosening effect to help ease constipation. You can also get magnesium in spray or cream forms online (check *Ancient-Minerals. com* or *Amazon.com*)—and by using Epsom salts (which is hydrated magnesium sulfate) in your bath!

7 Common Mistakes People Make When Taking Vitamins

Jacob Teitelbaum, MD, holistic physician and nationally known expert in the fields of chronic fatigue syndrome, fibromyalgia, sleep and pain. He is author of numerous books, including *The Fatigue and Fibromyalgia Solution* and *Pain-Free 1-2-3*. Vitality101. com

Many of us take vitamins and other nutritional supplements. In fact, researchers from Harvard analyzed data from nearly 125,000 middle-aged and older people and found that an astounding 88% of women and 81% of men took supplements.

Unfortunately, a lot of us take nutritional supplements wrong.

We don't take high-enough doses…or we take them at the wrong time of day…or we combine them with other supplements, foods or drugs that can block absorption.

Good news: I've counseled thousands of patients on the best ways to take vitamins, and I can assure you that taking them correctly can be simple and straightforward.

What you might be doing wrong—and how to quickly fix the problem…

VITAMIN MISTAKE #1: **You take a dose that's too low.** There are many nutrient-nutrient interactions that can reduce the absorption of individual nutrients by 5% to 10%.

Example: Iron cuts the absorption of zinc—the more iron in a supplement, the less zinc you're likely to absorb.

My advice: Don't take a multivitamin that supplies 100% of the "Daily Value" of nutrients, a level intended only to prevent deficiency diseases. Instead, take a multivitamin that supplies an optimal amount of nutrients—an amount that will easily overcome every absorption issue caused by nutrient-nutrient interactions.

For simplicity, use the B-vitamins as your reference point. Look for a product that supplies about 40 milligrams (mg) each of thiamin, riboflavin, niacin and vitamin B-6 (pyridoxine), and 200 micrograms (mcg) of vitamin B-12. These levels are safe and therapeutic, improving energy and mental clarity. When a product contains the above levels of these nutrients, it usually will have optimal levels of other nutrients as well.

VITAMIN MISTAKE #2: **You take a dose that's too high.** It can be detrimental to your health to take high doses of vitamin A and vitamin E.

Reasons: Taking more than 3,000 international units (IU) of vitamin A (retinol) daily can increase your risk for osteoporosis, the bone-eroding disease. Vitamin E actually is a family of eight compounds called tocopherols and tocotrienols. Alpha-tocopherol—the compound commonly found in multivitamins—can be toxic in doses higher than 100 IU daily.

My advice: Take a multivitamin that contains no more than 3,000 IU of vitamin A total, with approximately one-half from retinol and one-half from beta-carotene (which turns into vitamin A in the body and does not cause osteoporosis).

Choose a multivitamin with no more than 100 IU of vitamin E. If you take the nutrient as a separate supplement for a specific condition, such as for breast tenderness, take it in the form of mixed tocopherols and tocotrienols.

VITAMIN MISTAKE #3: **You try to take vitamins two or three times a day.** Taking vitamins in divided doses—two or even three times a day—is ideal because the body sustains higher blood levels of the nutrients. But very few people can stick with this type of regimen.

My advice: Take vitamins first thing in the morning, with breakfast. (The fat in the meal will help you absorb vitamins A, D and E, which are fat-soluble.) Yes, there's a tiny trade-off of effectiveness for convenience, but it's worth it.

Exception: If you take magnesium as a separate supplement, you might want to take it at bedtime for deeper sleep. Avoid magnesium oxide and magnesium hydroxide, both of which are poorly absorbed. Magnesium glycinate or magnesium malate is preferred.

VITAMIN MISTAKE #4: **You take a second-rate formulation.** Vitamins come in a range of forms—tablets, caplets, capsules, chewables, softgels, liquids, powders—and some are better than others.

Vitamin tablets, for example, are a poor choice. They may not dissolve completely—and you can't absorb any nutrients from a pill that doesn't dissolve. Tablets (and some of the other forms listed above) also may contain binders, fillers and other additives. These supposedly "inert" compounds may have all kinds of unknown effects on the body.

My advice: I recommend powders, which are highly absorbable. Just add water and stir. My favorite is the Energy Revitalization System, from Enzymatic Therapy, which I formulated. (So that I can't be accused of profiting from my recommendation, I donate 100% of my royalties from sales to charity.) I recommend one scoop each morning combined with 5 grams of ribose (a naturally occurring sugar) to optimize energy.

Don't like drinks? Try a combination of My Favorite Multiple Take One by Natrol plus two tablets of Jigsaw Sustained Release Magnesium plus two chewable ribose tablets (2 grams to 3 grams each).

VITAMIN MISTAKE #5: **You take calcium.** One-third of people who take supplements take calcium—and I think just about

every one of those people is making a mistake. The scientific evidence shows that taking a calcium supplement provides little or no protection against bone fractures, and research now links calcium supplements to increased risk for heart attacks and strokes.

My advice: I strongly recommend that you get your calcium from food, eating one or two servings of dairy a day. Almonds, broccoli and green leafy vegetables such as kale also are good calcium sources. Unlike supplemental calcium, calcium from food is safe. If you decide to take a calcium supplement for stronger bones, take no more than 100 mg to 200 mg daily, and always combine it with other bone-supporting nutrients, such as vitamin D, magnesium and vitamin K. Take these at night to help sleep.

VITAMIN MISTAKE #6: **You don't realize that your medication can cause a nutrient deficiency.** Some medications block the absorption of specific nutrients. *In my clinical experience, the two worst offenders are…*

•**The diabetes drug metformin,** which can cause a B-12 deficiency.

What to do: Metformin is an excellent medication, but be sure to take a multivitamin containing at least 200 mcg of B-12 daily.

•**Proton pump inhibitors** such as Nexium *(esomeprazole),* which block the production of stomach acid and are prescribed for heartburn, ulcers and other gastrointestinal problems. Long-term use can cause deficiencies of magnesium and B-12.

What to do: Take a multivitamin with 200 mcg of B-12 and additional magnesium (200 mg daily)—and talk to your doctor about getting off the drug. (A gradual decrease in dosage is safest.) Proton pump inhibitors are toxic when used long term and addictive, causing rebound acid hyper-secretion when stopped. The solution? Improve digestion using plant-based digestive enzymes, deglycyrrhizinated licorice (DGL), marshmallow root and other stomach-healing supplements. Follow directions on the labels.

Matcha Tea Can Be Super-Healthy—If You Heed This Warning

Health Insider research.

You know green tea is really good for you. Its antioxidant compounds show up in studies as protective against heart disease, diabetes, cancer, dementia, obesity and more. But you're probably not going to start drinking four or more cups every day—even 10 cups a day in some studies—like many Chinese and Japanese people do. How to get the bennies without all the cuppas?

The models at Fashion Week in New York City had a solution. Backstage, for energy and Zen balance, they sipped little shots of matcha green tea, a specific kind that contains unusually high levels of antioxidants. There's also matcha tea powder that has become today's "it" ingredient in everything from smoothies to latte to fruit pops to very, very green muffins. Matcha, it seems, is suddenly and literally on everyone's lips.

Does it deserve the hype? There's no question that it can be a very healthy beverage or even recipe ingredient. But now that it's a fad, and everyone's getting into the act, be careful about matcha products that are unhealthy—or even unsafe...because they are contaminated with heavy metals. So it pays to be matcha savvy. Here's what you need to know to safely benefit from this unique form of green tea.

Good Stuff in a Small Package

For matcha, concentration is the name of the game. It's made from green tea, so it contains the powerful antioxidant epigallocatechin gallate (EGCG), responsible for many of green tea's health benefits, as well as the amino acid L-theanine, which has antianxiety properties (more about that in a moment).

It has about three times as much EGCG as standard brewed green tea, according to some estimates. It also has about as much caffeine as a cup of coffee.

How does matcha deliver this bioactive bounty? It's a combination of how it's grown and how it's prepared. Unlike with other varieties, a few weeks before harvest, the plant is covered from the sun, which causes it to produce more EGCG and L-theanine.

Another unusual step: After harvest, the leaves are ground into a fine powder. And matcha is also prepared differently. When you drink matcha, you're actually drinking a "suspension" of ground leaves infused in water, rather than a typical brew where leaves are steeped and then removed from the cup or pot. Hence, you are actually consuming the leaves and, along with them, more green tea compounds.

The L-theanine may be responsible for one of matcha's coveted benefits—a pleasant sense that users say it brings that may be described as "alert calmness." Credit caffeine for the alertness, of course. L-theanine, on the other hand, has been shown in studies to reduce anxiety.

Matcha Dos—and One Big Don't

Matcha has long been appreciated in the East. In Japan it forms part of the traditional tea ceremony and is the most revered form of tea. Because matcha involves consuming the entire tea leaf, however, the origin of any matcha powder you consume is extremely important for your safety. *Here's what you need to know...*

• **Tea plants grown in soil that is contaminated with lead will absorb it into the leaves,** and, because you are consuming the entire leaf, more lead may wind up in your cup. In one study from the research organization ConsumerLab, tea grown in China had high lead concentrations.

• **Your best bet—**Stick to matcha teas grown in Japan, and look for brands that report consistent testing for the presence of heavy metals. In the ConsumerLab's study, for example, the one tea tested that came from Japan, Teavana, had no detectable lead.

• **The highest-quality matcha comes from the southern regions of Japan**—Kyushu, Nishio, Shizuoka and Uji.

• **Good-quality matcha is bright, vivid green and will have a fine powdery consistency**—anything yellowish or coarse is not likely to taste very good.

• **Expect to pay about $26 to $32 for a standard 30-gram tin (about an ounce).** Anything cheaper is not likely to have good flavor.

• **One cup of matcha calls for about one gram of dry powder,** so a 30-gram tin should give you a cup of matcha tea every day for a month. (You can get a special measuring spoon from a matcha supplier, along with a whisk to prepare the tea in a bowl.)

• **Now that matcha has become popular in the US,** some prepared versions may have plenty of added sugar. Skip them, and make the real thing yourself.

• **Ready to try it?** Kenko Tea, an Australian brand that gets its matcha from the Nishio region of Japan, is a good choice and ships worldwide. Other reputable brands include DoMatcha and MidoriSpring.

So go ahead, enjoy your own tea ceremony. Matcha has a grassy, slightly bitter flavor…some people compare it to that of kale or spinach. You can try it the traditional way or experiment with adding the powder to recipes. Just remember that tossing matcha into your 1,000-calorie ice cream milkshake doesn't suddenly turn it into a health drink!

To Burn Fat, Pair Green Tea With Your Exercise

Study titled "Green Tea, Intermittent Sprinting Exercise, and Fat Oxidation" by researchers at Charles Darwin University and University of New South Wales, both in Australia, published in *Nutrients*.

You may already know that short bursts of high-intensity exercise make your body more efficient at burning fat even when you aren't exercising. Now a new study from Australia shows that adding green tea extract to your exercise routine gives that fat burn an extra boost.

In the study, fat oxidation was calculated in a group of women who exercised intensely for 20 minutes on exercise bikes. The day before each exercise day, half the women took capsules containing green tea extract—the other half got a placebo (cellulose). As you'd expect, both groups showed more fat burned after exercising compared to before…but the women who took green tea extract burned significantly more.

So if you're struggling to lose your belly, see if green tea extract will help. Like tea better? The amount of active ingredients in the green tea extract was equivalent to about two or three cups of green tea.

For Lifelong Weight Control, Walking Beats the Gym

Study titled "Do All Activities 'Weigh' Equally? How Different Physical Activities Differ as Predictors of Weight" by researchers at London School of Economics, School of Economics, University of Queensland, Australia, and Indian Institute of Technology Kanpur, India, published in *Risk Analysis*.

When it comes to keeping your body weight in check, brisk walking almost every day is proving to be the best exercise.

In an analysis of a large British multiyear survey, women who engaged in brisk walking for 30 minutes or more a day about five days a week weighed about 11 pounds less—and men about 6 pounds less—than their sedentary counterparts.

By contrast, those who went to the gym or played sports just as frequently as the walkers didn't fare as well. Compared to the sedentary types, women weighed about six pounds less (and men just 1.8 pounds less). Other activities done for the same time/frequency—heavy housework (moving furniture, walking with heavy shopping bags, scrubbing floors) or manual activities (digging, chopping wood, moving heavy loads)—were only weakly linked to a lower body weight.

It's just an association, not proof, but the research does suggest that the one exercise we can do almost anywhere, almost any time, for free, is a good lifelong defense against weight gain.

Get Off That Couch Together

Mona Xu, PhD, an assistant professor of experimental psychology at Idaho State University (ISU) and director of the ISU Social, Health and Neuroscience Lab, which studies the interplay between close interpersonal relationships and behavioral health.

For better or worse, your significant other's health habits strongly influence your own. Got a spouse who thinks that walking to the kitchen is exercise, and you're less likely to stay fit yourself. And there's research to back this up.

Important new finding: In a study of 3,722 adults, nearly 70% of men took up physical activity if their wives did, while only one-quarter of men became active without their spouses as inspiration. Women are similarly affected by their husbands but to a lesser extent.

If you're single: Having a supportive friend who exercises may give you the incentive to get moving yourself.

Motivation and More

Why does it help to have an active partner? For starters, it is a great form of motivation.

Seeing your partner exercise reminds you to work out. An active partner also lends social support, acting as your cheerleader and sharing strategies for coping with setbacks such as sore muscles or trepidation when trying a new activity. Your partner can provide accountability, too—you are less likely to skip a workout if someone is planning on joining you.

An added perk: Because exercise has been repeatedly linked with better heart health and lower rates of cancer, diabetes and depression, this means that the two of you will increase your odds of having more higher-quality years together.

Working out as a team (for example, going on long walks or jogs together) allows you to talk and reconnect.

Bonus: These opportunities contribute to a satisfying and committed relationship, which will help ensure that your partnership will stay strong.

Attempting shared goals, such as completing a 5K walk or run, gives you the chance to grow and celebrate as a duo. If the exercise is something novel—this could be snowshoeing, tandem bicycling or hiking a beautiful new route—you may get an extra benefit. Couples report feeling happier with their relationships and more in love with their partners after completing an exciting physical activity together…perhaps because you associate your partner with fun and adventure.

How to Be the Catalyst

If you're the more active one in your marriage—or simply the one taking the lead in making exercise a priority—your first step is to light a fire under your more sedentary partner.

Caution: Nagging him to join you can backfire—especially if your partner's weight is a touchy subject or if he finds exercise to be intimidating or stressful.

Helpful: Think of some activities your partner might enjoy. Then start with a low-key conversation, explaining that you're planning to try some new activities that are fun and healthy. Explain that you'd be happy for your partner to join you but that you understand if he isn't interested or wants to exercise alone. You might also offer support by, say, taking over some household chores to give your partner time to exercise.

What works well: Suggest enjoyable activities that don't seem like exercise but will improve fitness—for example, ballroom dancing, kayaking, a walk in the woods, golf or tai chi. You might also find local clubs focused on these activities.

Note: You need not exercise together in order to experience the benefits above—such as supporting one another and sharing advice on workout challenges. In fact, exercising independently is helpful when one partner prefers the meditative aspects of yoga, for example, while the other enjoys the competitiveness of basketball.

Ask your partner how you can help—maybe he would like some suggestions on finding a class or sport to try...perhaps she's anxious about shopping for the right workout gear or embarrassed about being in a gym setting.

Offer reassurance, then step back and see what happens. Resist the urge to pressure your partner...stay active yourself...and be supportive. Instead of saying, "You should work out more," try, "My hike is getting kind of stale—would you come with me and keep me company?"

Making It Work

Exercise within a marriage is not a competition. Just because your partner has been running for years, it doesn't mean that you need to attempt an hour-long run on your first day—or even that you need to run at all. If one of you is much stronger than the other and you have decided to try exercising as a team, pick activities that allow you to tailor your workout according to your own fitness level.

Good choices: Spin class, where you control the resistance on your bike...hiking (one person could wear a weighted vest)...a beginner-to-intermediate yoga class...or an indoor rock-climbing wall.

Also helpful: Use exercise as an opportunity for a date night—research shows this can strengthen a relationship. To ensure follow-through, put it on your calendar and go out for a healthy bite afterward.

Try, Try Again...

If you and your partner are fighting as a result of your repeated efforts to motivate him to exercise, back off for a few months and re-strategize. But don't give up—suggest a new activity, offer encouragement and keep up your own exercise habit. When it comes down to it, you want your partner—and your marriage—to be healthy.

7 Ways to Plank for Strength, Flexibility and Balance

Lee Jordan, certified American Council on Exercise (ACE) health coach and personal trainer based in Jacksonville, Florida.

Jim White, registered dietitian, certified fitness instructor, and owner, Jim White Fitness & Nutrition Studios, Norfolk, Virginia. He is spokesperson for the Academy of Nutrition and Dietetics, Chicago.

he Plank. We're not talking about carpentry or what pirates make prisoners walk off, but an amazing exercise that simultaneously strengthens many of your body's most critical muscles—your core.

It tightens your belly...provides better support for your lower back...increases flexibility in your shoulders and the arches of your feet and your toes...improves your posture...and helps you keep your balance when you're out and about during your busy day.

How can one single exercise that you do for only 30 seconds to a minute do all this? We'll tell you. And we'll show you seven ways to do it, from easy to challenging, with variations to strengthen different muscle groups...

Plank 101

The main focus for any plank pose is on the area between your hips and your shoulders—your core.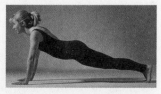
All of the plank positions below work your core, and all but the last one work your glu-

Do This Together...

Try this fun "full-body" move with your partner. It gives your shoulders, arms, back and legs a nice stretch, which improves flexibility before or after exercise...

What to do: Warm up with a few minutes of easy walking, then begin by sitting on the floor. Face your partner and place the bottoms of your feet against his/her feet. Each of you should grab one end of a towel or resistance band. Slowly lean backward, gently pulling the towel or band so that your partner must lean forward until he feels a stretch in his hamstrings. Hold for 10 to 30 seconds, then return to the starting position and have your partner lean back. Repeat the entire sequence three to five times.

Caution: If you've had hip or back surgery, check with your doctor before trying this stretch.

—Dr. Mona Xu

teals—your butt muscles. The variations target specific muscle groups—to strengthen the muscles in your chest, shoulders, arms, legs and back.

The first one, the High Plank, is the basic form. It's the best one to get started with—and also the easiest one to customize. If you want a little more challenging core workout, try the Front Plank.

With each position, start by holding it for 10 to 15 seconds. As you get stronger, increase the time—aiming for a goal of one minute. Start with the stationary poses first. Once you can hold a stationary pose for one minute, challenge yourself with one or more of the mobile poses. It's fine to increase your planking time if you want even more challenge!

STATIONARY PLANKS
High Plank

Tones your core and gluteals (butt muscles).

Lying on your stomach, lift your body so that you're supported on your hands (flat on the floor) and your toes, arms straight.

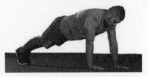

It looks like a push-up. Pay attention to keeping your abdominals taut and maintaining your body in a straight line from your head to your ankles.

Front Plank

Tones your core and gluteals and also your chest, shoulders, arms and legs.

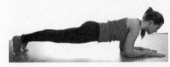

Lying on your stomach, lift your body so that you are supported by your forearms and your toes. Your elbows should align under your shoulders. Maintain your body in a straight line from your head to your ankles, making sure not to lift your head or arch or curve your lower back. Squeeze your gluteal and abdominal muscles while pressing your elbows into the floor.

Side Plank

Tones your core and gluteals and also your obliques (muscles on the side of the torso that help you turn from side to side) and hips.

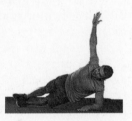

Lying on your right side, prop yourself up on your right elbow and forearm, with your elbow aligned directly under your shoulder and your feet stacked. Now tighten your abdominals and lift your hips off the floor. Your head, shoulder, hips and feet should line up straight. As you lift your hips, push your elbow into the floor for stability.

Switch sides and repeat.

MOVING PLANKS
High Plank with Alternating Shoulder Touch

Tones your core and gluteals and also your upper chest, back and legs.

Start with the High Plank. In a smooth, alternating movement, balance on your left hand only and touch your right hand to your left shoulder...then bring your right hand down, and touch your left hand to your right shoulder. Repeat for one minute (or however long you can).

Plank Jacks

Tones your core and gluteals and also your legs.

While holding a Front Plank position, continuously move your legs together and then apart—as if you were doing jumping jacks. Keep your upper body stable, maintaining a straight line...avoid raising your hips out of alignment.

Mountain Climber Plank

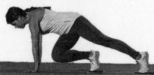

Tones your core and gluteals and also your upper arms and legs.

While holding a High Plank position, bring your left knee in toward your chest, pointing your toe, and then extend it back to its starting position. Bring your right knee in toward your chest and extend back to start. Continue alternating legs in a smooth movement while maintaining your upper body in a stable position.

Twisting Plank

Tones your core and also your obliques, shoulders and arms.

Begin in a Front Plank position. Then turn your body so that you're supported on just your right forearm and lift your left arm straight up toward the sky. Bring your arm back down into the Front Plank...then turn and do the same on your left side, lifting your right arm toward the sky. Alternate side to side, aiming for a goal of holding for 30 seconds on each side.

Here's to happy planking—and a stronger, more supple, flexible and injury-resistant body!

Note: The images in this story that demonstrate High Plank, Side Plank, and Mountain Climber Plank are used with permission, courtesy of the American Council on Exercise. You can see more in their Exercise Library.

---

5 Exercises That Make Everyday Life Better...and Keep Your Body Younger

Beth and Lee Jordan, both certified American Council on Exercise (ACE) health coaches and personal trainers based in Jacksonville Beach, Florida.

Jim White, registered dietitian, certified health fitness instructor, and owner, Jim White Fitness & Nutrition Studios, Norfolk, Virginia. He is spokesperson for the Academy of Nutrition and Dietetics, Chicago.

What are your fitness goals? Amazing endurance? Extraordinary strength? Lightning speed? If so, more power to you—literally. But many of us just want to stay healthy so we can keep doing the activities we need to do...and activities we love to do...for a good long time.

Try this test: Can you put your socks on standing up? Can you stand up from a chair without using your arms, sit back down, and repeat another 11 times within 30 seconds? Can you stand on one foot for 30 seconds? These are tests of functional fitness, sometimes called neuromotor or neuromuscular fitness.

The good news is that you can improve your functional fitness level with simple exercises. The goal is to increase your ability to do the activities that you need to do every day at home, at work and during recreational fun... such as lifting work files or children or grandchildren...carrying the laundry down to the basement and back...bending down to garden...keeping your balance getting in and out of the tub and when you're out for a nice hike. It's a combination of balance and power.

"Functional fitness exercises combine upper- and lower-body movements into what are known as compound exercises, while emphasizing core stability," explain Lee and Beth Jordan, a husband-and-wife team of personal trainers with the American Council on Exercise (ACE). "They often mimic real everyday movements."

These exercises are especially important as you age, when your muscles weaken and simple activities can feel more difficult. All the things you used to barely give a thought to can become challenging if you don't give those muscles some extra attention.

Get started with these five functional exercises designed to help you keep living the active life you enjoy…for a long, long time.

Bent-Over Dumbbell Row

What it helps you do: Bend over to reach things…and pick up an object such as a laundry basket, package of mulch or bag of groceries.

How to do it: Use a dumbbell with a weight that challenges you but that you can lift repeatedly. Stand next to a bench or chair and, holding the dumbbell in 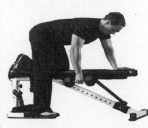 your right hand, bend at a 90-degree angle so that your back is parallel to the floor. Brace your left hand and left knee on the bench or chair. You weight will be on your right foot, and your right hand should hang down directly under your shoulder, holding the weight. Keeping your back straight, head in line with your spine and abdominal muscles taut, pull the dumbbell up toward your shoulder as far as you can. Your elbow should remain higher than the dumbbell. Then lower the weight by straightening your arm toward the floor. Repeat several reps and then switch sides.

Single-Leg Squat

What it helps you do: Control and balance your own weight when walking on unstable ground, going up and down stairs, getting out of bed and getting up out of a chair.

How to do it: Start by standing with your feet hip-width apart, one foot several inches in front of the other, with feet parallel. Slowly squat down as far as you're able to, without losing balance and keeping your bent knee of the leg in front behind your toes. Your hands can be on your hips 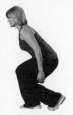 or your arms can be extended straight out in front of you. Rise to your starting position. Perform several reps and then switch legs.

Forward Lunge

What it helps you do: Move with ease during activities such as yard work, vacuuming and putting groceries in your cupboard.

How to do it: Start in a standing position. Keeping one leg in place, step your other foot out in front of you and bend your knees—your ultimate goal is for them to both reach 90-degree angles. (Once you get good at this, your front thigh and back shin should be parallel to the floor.) Push off with your front leg to return to your starting position. Maintain a straight spine and taut abdominals throughout the movement, keeping your arms at your sides or your hands on your hips. Perform several reps, alternating legs with each lunge. (Once you're comfortable with the forward lunge, try side lunges and walking lunges with twists.)

Superman

What it helps you do: Maintain a healthy posture while sitting, standing and walking.

How to do it: Lie on your stomach, facing straight down, with your head in line with your spine, legs extended straight, toes pointing, and your arms extended straight out in front of you, palms facing each other. Simultaneously, lift both your arms and your legs a few inches off the floor. Make sure your head stays aligned with your spine during the entire movement, and avoid arching

your back or
lifting your
head. Hold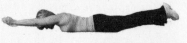
the lift for a few seconds, and then gently
return your arms and legs to the starting position. Perform several reps.

Farmer's Walk

What it helps you do: Increase your grip
strength and improve coordination when
walking and carrying items at the same time.

How to do it: You'll need to walk during
this exercise. Don't worry if you don't have
much space—this is fun if you have a lawn,
driveway or walkway to use, but you can also
just go in circles inside. Start in a
standing position with a dumbbell
beside each foot. (Choose a weight
that's challenging for you but not
so heavy that you can't lift it.)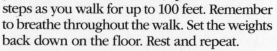
Keeping your back straight, squat
down and grip the handles of the
weights, lifting them as you stand
back up, keeping your weight on
your heels. Then take short, quick
steps as you walk for up to 100 feet. Remember
to breathe throughout the walk. Set the weights
back down on the floor. Rest and repeat.

Getting Started With a Functional Fitness Routine

How often should you do these exercises? The
American College of Sports Medicine recommends about two or three 20-to-30-minute
sessions each week. You'll still want to keep
up a regular routine of aerobics, strength
training and flexibility exercises, too.

As with any new exercise routine, it's always a good idea to check with your doctor
before getting started...and that's especially
true if you have any joint problems or other
physical challenges. And as with any physical activity, if it starts to hurt, stop.

Are these five exercises the only way to improve functional fitness? Of course not. Yoga
and tai chi are also great, and they "count" toward the recommendations. You can even do
functional exercises with a paper towel tube.

But if you're looking for a streamlined routine, the five exercises above all work together to improve your ability to do the things
that matter every day.

Note: The images in this story that demonstrate each exercise are used with permission, courtesy of the American Council on
Exercise. You can see more in their Exercise
Library.

Appendix 2
GET THE BEST MEDICAL CARE

Don't Fall for These Medical Care Myths

H. Gilbert Welch, MD, MPH, an internist at White
River Junction VA Medical Center, Vermont, and a
professor of medicine at The Dartmouth Institute for
Health Policy & Clinical Practice, where he specializes in the effects of medical testing. He is author
of *Less Medicine, More Health: 7 Assumptions That
Drive Too Much Medical Care.*

I t's natural to assume that more health care
is better than less—that checkups, tests
and treatments make people healthier.
But that isn't always the case.

Obviously, people who are sick need to see
doctors and get the necessary tests. Those
who are healthy may benefit from preventive
medicine. But many of the assumed benefits
of medicine don't always pan out.

Here are four common but false assumptions about medical care...

***FALSE*: It's always better to find it
sooner.**

The argument for cancer screening seems
obvious. If you had cancer, wouldn't you
want to know as soon as possible? Screening (looking for disease in large populations)
does turn up a lot of cancers. Does this save
lives? Less often than you might think.

Take mammography. It's been used for widespread screening for 30 years, yet the number of women who are diagnosed with metastatic breast cancer is about the same now as it was before. For every 1,000 women who get the screenings, at most three (likely closer to less than one) will avoid dying from breast cancer as a result. The numbers are roughly the same for men who are screened for prostate cancer.

The benefits are huge if you happen to be in one of these small groups, but what about the rest? They're faced with the cost and inconvenience of the initial test. Many will be advised to get biopsies or other follow-up tests. Some will have surgery or radiation for cancers that probably would have done nothing.

I'm not saying that screening tests are all bad—just that they aren't all good.

My advice: Ask your doctor if he/she is confident that you, as an individual, will benefit from screening tests.

FALSE: It never hurts to get more information.

It would seem that getting as much medical information as possible would be a good thing. Not necessarily.

More data can produce more problems, which require more tests, which can create problems of their own. And all this can cost you real money—yet not improve your health.

More data also can distract your doctor. Minor laboratory abnormalities identified during a routine visit—such as slightly elevated cholesterol or slightly depressed thyroid function—often draw physicians away from the problems you want to talk about.

My advice: Expect more and more opportunities to get tested for a variety of conditions. Know that while all these tests may serve the financial interests of their manufacturers, they may not serve your interests. Before agreeing to any test, ask your doctor what he/she is looking for. Is there a specific problem you are likely to have? Or is it a fishing expedition? Avoid the latter—it's too easy to catch trash fish (meaningless abnormali-

> ## Exercise and Varicose Veins
> Can exercise cause varicose veins?
> No. Exercise can actually help prevent or slow the progression of this common condition. These bulging, twisted veins (which often appear on the legs) form when blood flow backs up and pools in veins. Walking, swimming, cycling, cross-country skiing and other low-impact exercise improve blood flow through veins. Wear compression stockings for extra support when doing high-impact exercise, such as jumping rope or running.
> Erez Salik, MD, a vascular and interventional radiologist, The Greenwich Vein Center, Greenwich, Connecticut. GreenVein.com

ties). Also, ask your doctor whether more information will change what you should do. If not, don't seek more information.

FALSE: It's always better to fix the problem.

All medical treatments are a bit of a gamble. You might improve when a problem is "fixed." Or things could go wrong and you could get worse. It's often better to manage a problem than to bring out the big guns.

Consider coronary artery disease. It's potentially life-threatening, so it needs to be treated. Many doctors recommend balloon angioplasty, a procedure to expand the arterial opening and restore normal blood flow. It can eliminate symptoms almost immediately, but it also carries significant risks to the patient.

With medical management, on the other hand, your doctor will treat the problem with medications and advice for a healthier lifestyle. You'll still have the underlying problem, but you'll learn to live with it.

How do the approaches compare? One large study found that patients with stable angina who had balloon angioplasty were no less likely to die or have a heart attack than those who depended on lower-risk medical management.

My advice: When you're faced with a medical decision—scheduling a test, having surgery, starting medications—tell your doctor that you want to take a stepwise approach. Start with the easiest, safest treatments first. You can always add more aggressive treatments later.

Think about upper-respiratory infections. Sure, you could get pneumonia, and you might eventually need antibiotics. But most people can just wait it out. Don't get tests or treatments unless your doctor convinces you, with good evidence, that you need them.

FALSE: Newer treatments are always better.

There's a saying in medicine, "When you have a new hammer, everything looks like a nail." When doctors discover a new treatment, such as a drug or a particular surgery, they tend to want to use it again and again.

Some new drugs really are superior to old ones—but not that often. Vioxx is a good example. It's an aspirin-like arthritis drug that got a lot of attention because it was somewhat less likely than similar drugs to cause stomach bleeding. But a few years after it was approved by the FDA, it was removed from the market because it was found to increase the risk for heart attack and stroke.

New drugs are tested in relatively small numbers of people. It can take many years before their benefits and risks become fully apparent.

My advice: Unless you have to take a new, breakthrough drug, tell your doctor that you would prefer something tried and true—preferably a drug that's been on the market for seven years or more.

Is Your Doctor Choosing the Right Care for You?

Harold Sox, MD, an internist, clinical epidemiologist and the director of research portfolio development at the Patient-Centered Outcomes Research Institute (PCORI) in Washington, DC. PCORI.org

I f you've got symptoms that might indicate a serious medical problem, your doctor will first choose the tests that he/she be-

lieves will lead to an accurate diagnosis. Then he will choose the treatments that he thinks are most likely to work for your condition.

But how does your doctor make these important decisions? Often, there is no clear evidence and it comes down to an educated guess—but guesses aren't what you want when you're facing a life-changing decision...

Better Medical Research

Traditional medical research has inherent limitations. Industry-sponsored studies, for example, often compare new drugs to placebos. To make real-life decisions, however, doctors and patients need to look to comparative effectiveness research (CER). This type of study makes head-to-head comparisons among existing treatments...and attempts to tailor them to individuals rather than the "average patient."

The Patient-Centered Outcomes Research Institute (PCORI), authorized by Congress in 2010, funds this type of comparative research (more than 280 studies so far) on medical conditions ranging from depression to stroke and cancer. Among recent CER findings from studies funded by PCORI or the federal government–sponsored Agency for Healthcare Research and Quality...*

Kidney Stones

Every year, about half a million Americans go to ERs with the fearsome pain of kidney stones. Doctors usually order an abdominal computed tomography (CT) scan to make the diagnosis. CT scans are the most sensitive test, but they're expensive...often reveal incidental (and usually harmless) abnormalities that lead to unnecessary tests...and expose patients to high doses of radiation that may increase cancer risks. Ultrasound, which is also used to diagnose kidney stones, is cheaper and safer. But until recently, experts didn't know if it was equally effective.

*For recent studies funded by PCORI, go to *PCORI.org* and click on "Research & Results."

The study: 2,759 patients suspected of having kidney stones were randomly assigned to have CT scans or ultrasounds.

Results: Ultrasounds and CT scans were found to be equally accurate. Patients given these tests had similar rates of adverse reactions (such as subsequent complications from kidney disease). But the ultrasound patients were exposed to far less radiation than those given CT scans.

Conclusion: Ultrasound should usually be the first choice when diagnosing kidney stones.

Diabetes

More than a decade ago, the landmark Diabetes Prevention Program study found that lifestyle changes (exercise, healthful eating, etc.) reduced the risk for diabetes by 58%. The study also found that the diabetes drug metformin reduced diabetes risk by 31%.

However, few at-risk patients take advantage of either of these approaches, most likely because lifestyle improvement programs can be expensive and time-consuming. PCORI researchers wondered if it might be possible to identify those patients who would strongly benefit from these approaches.

The study: In a re-analysis of data from the original study, complex statistical models were used to correlate diabetes risk factors—age, body mass index, waist circumference, physical activity, etc.—with treatment outcomes.

Conclusion: Metformin was clearly effective, but only in the 25% of patients with the highest risk of developing diabetes (based on highest glucose levels, waist circumference and other factors). Those in lower-risk groups showed little benefit from metformin. Lifestyle changes were found to offer good protection to virtually all patients.

Spinal Stenosis

Spinal stenosis, an often-painful narrowing of the spinal canal that may require surgery, is typically treated with injections that combine a glucocorticoid (a type of steroid) with an anesthetic such as lidocaine. It's estimated that more than 2.2 million of these epidural injections are given every year. But the benefits have never been proved in rigorous, randomized, controlled clinical trials. Nor has it been shown that this drug combination is more effective than a single-drug injection.

The study: 400 patients with spinal stenosis were given one or two injections of either the two-drug shot or the lidocaine alone. They were then evaluated by doctors three and six weeks later.

Results: Patients given glucocorticoids plus lidocaine reported less leg pain and better physical function than those given lidocaine alone—but only at the three-week examination. At six weeks, patients in both groups had the same improvement in pain scores.

Conclusion: The steroid adds very little benefit. This is an important finding because even the short-term use of glucocorticoids can suppress calcium absorption and cause a reduction in bone density, which increases the risk for bone fracture. PCORI has funded a longer-term follow-up to this study.

Stroke

Previous studies have shown that the blood-thinning drug *warfarin* (Coumadin) can lower stroke risk for stroke survivors with atrial fibrillation (AFib), a dangerous heartbeat irregularity. But these past studies have tended to exclude the elderly and patients with more than one health problem and not taken into account the impact of warfarin on the quality of life after stroke.

The study: Researchers looked at 12,552 patients in all age groups who had AFib after a stroke to determine if warfarin decreased the number of days spent in the hospital after treatment and discharge.

Results: Patients who were treated with warfarin at discharge from the hospital had 47 more days at home during the two-year follow-up. They also had improvements in standard cardiac outcomes, such as the number of heart attacks, etc.

Conclusion: Warfarin provided these benefits to all patients studied, but the benefit was slightly stronger in women, patients older than age 80 and those who had more severe strokes (groups less likely to be treated with warfarin in the past).

Note: Warfarin can raise risk for bleeding, so risks and benefits should be carefully considered.

Better Medical Care... Even If You're on Medicare

Robert Wergin, MD, family physician, Milford, Nebraska, board chair of the American Academy of Family Physicians, and medical director, Crest View Healthcare Center, Milford, Nebraska.

Imagine calling your doctor on the day you need to see him/her, heading over and spending a half hour or more discussing the full range of your health concerns. He knows you well and even reminds you about some issues to discuss. Your doctor tells you that he wants look into one of your health issues more carefully, do some research and talk with a specialist, and he promises to call you back with a treatment plan—and he encourages you to e-mail or call him any time you have questions.

You notice that not only do you feel better about your doctor, but, compared with your last one, he seems less stressed and appears to enjoy providing such unrushed, attentive and personal care.

Is this all a dream? In a way, it is—an alternative to insurance-based fee-for-service health care dreamt up by primary care doctors including internists and family physicians who are fed up with the current high-pressure system that serves neither doctors nor patients well.

It's called direct primary care (DPC). It's a tiny movement, but it's growing. It shares some features of concierge medicine, but it's much less expensive and caters to the middle class rather than the affluent.

Can you believe its promises? And if so, would it work for you and your family? Here's what you need to know.

How DPC Works

Most direct primary care practices don't accept insurance, and they do charge a retainer, usually between $40 and $100 a month per person. Some charge on the lower end of that range for kids and on the higher end for older patients, who tend to have chronic conditions. In addition, some charge a small payment per visit, usually $5 to $20.

While DPC physicians don't take insurance, if you use one, you'll still want to carry some insurance. However, you can buy a less expensive, high-deductible plan...just enough to cover specialty care, emergencies and hospitalizations, such as a "bronze" plan under the health exchanges. If DPC gains popularity, more insurers will likely begin offering plans specifically tailored to work with the DPC model.

If you have Medicare, DPC can work, too, but it depends on the individual practice you sign up with. Since Medicare is insurance, many DPC physicians will not accept Medicare patients. But if you find a practice that does, you can work with them to have Medicare cover the services that the DPC doesn't cover—you'll also need to make sure that Medicare isn't billed for services that the DPC covers, which would be illegal.

If you have a health savings account, you can still see a DPC physician, but you will not be allowed to pay the retainer with the HSA money. Bipartisan federal legislation is pending to remove this restriction.

The DPC Promise

Why pay an extra fee each month? DPC advocates argue that the benefits are worth it, such as...

•**Easier appointments—and more time with your doctor.** DPC physicians tend to have a total of 600 to 800 patients rather than the typical 2,000 to 2,500. That makes it easier for your doctor to accommodate same-day visits and longer office visits. Most DPC doctors see 10 to 15 patients a day rather than the standard 20 to 30.

•**More help from your doctor when you're not there.** With fewer patients, DPC doctors can build time into their schedules to communicate with patients via e-mail, Skype and phone consultations. Some offer this kind of access to your own doctor 24/7.

•**Less paperwork.** That means not only no insurance claims for usual care, but also that your doctor isn't required to be typing documentation into a tablet or computer while he or she is supposed to be examining and advising you. "I didn't go into medicine to be a computer programmer—I did it to work with patients," says Robert Wergin, MD, board chair of the American Academy of Family Physicians, who still practices within the traditional insurance-based model but sees value in the DPC model.

The range of services that are included with the DPC retainer varies among physicians and is typically spelled out in a contract. But most provide everything you'd need for regular preventive care and sick care.

If you need a specialist, the physician will guide you and also negotiate fees for you. (Your insurance may pay as well, if you've met your deductible and copay requirement.) If you need a CAT scan, MRI or other imaging test, most DPCs negotiate with imaging centers to keep the costs down—and again, your insurance might well cover it. Some DPC physicians are also purchasing medications from pharmaceutical companies and distributing them to patients at cost.

Is DPC Right for You?

DPC sounds great, but it's important to note that it's so new that it hasn't been studied extensively by objective researchers. One recent report found that the overall patient costs are lower because the extra retainer costs are less than the money saved by buying cheaper insurance—but that study was done by a firm that consults for DPC physicians. Nor is there objective research that documents that the promises of DPC, such as more time with patients and greater patient satisfaction, regularly occur. There is also concern within the medical establishment that the DPC trend might leave out people who can't afford the retainer, widening the already existing class system in medicine. And it's so new that many states are still working out the regulatory requirements to set up practices.

Whether DPC is right for you depends on how comfortable you are with your current primary care provider—and what insurance policy you carry. If you don't want to switch doctors, for example, it's clearly not a good fit.

If you want to explore this new approach to medical care, the best action to take is to contact a local DPC practice and ask a lot of questions—what the fee is, what kinds of services are covered, what kind of insurance they recommend and, if you're on Medicare, whether the practice is set up to accommodate you. Currently there are 141 practices with 273 locations spanning 39 states, with more on the way. Some are listed with the Direct Primary Care Coalition on its website (*DPCare.org*). Or you can also search online for "direct primary care" in your area.

If DPC does turn out to be a good fit, you may be able to benefit from one of the most encouraging new trends in primary care medicine—a medical practice designed to meet the needs of patients...rather than insurance companies.

When a Doctor Is Not Enough

Charles B. Inlander, a consumer advocate and health-care consultant based in Fogelsville, Pennsylvania. He is the author or coauthor of more than 20 consumer-health books.

Several years ago, a friend of mine was diagnosed with fibromyalgia after suffering from severe fatigue and aches and pain all over her body. Her doctor, a highly trained neuromuscular specialist, provided her with written information about the condition and explained the various treatment options that he suggested she try.

But according to my friend, the doctor's best recommendation was to join a patient-assistance group sponsored by a local hospital—a type of free program that is enormously helpful for people who are newly diagnosed and long-term patients with conditions ranging from cancer to arthritis. My friend's group met regularly (most groups meet monthly), but her fellow fibromyalgia patients were also available around the clock and provided her with guidance on how to handle the side effects of her medications… recommended nearby stress-reduction classes that were a big help…and even suggested some local primary care doctors who had a good understanding of her condition.

Studies show that patients often find fellow patients more helpful than medical professionals when dealing with the day-to-day challenges related to a specific medical condition. In patient-assistance groups sponsored by hospitals, self-help groups or advocacy organizations dedicated to specific conditions, such as the American Cancer Society, American Heart Association or the Arthritis Foundation, the volunteers can be especially helpful because they are usually well trained to address common issues. How to benefit from a patient-assistance group…

•**Realize that there's probably a group for you.** No matter what your condition, there is likely a patient-assistance program ready to help you. Among the most common are those for people with breast and other forms of cancer (and survivors undergoing follow-up treatment and/or monitoring)…coronary bypass and other heart conditions…Parkinson's disease…arthritis…lung disorders…and post-stroke issues. If you have a rare disorder or live in a rural area, national organizations have programs that can match you up one-to-one with fellow patients for phone calls, Skype visits or one-on-one meetings.

Important: Patient-assistance groups should not be used as a substitute for a doctor but rather as an adjunct to your overall care.

•**Get a good referral.** Start with your doctor. Ask if he/she can recommend a patient-assistance group in your area. You can also check with your local hospitals—speak to the hospital's social work department or volunteer coordinator. To find out what is available in your area, you can also go online or call national disease-specific advocacy groups, such as the American Cancer Society. For less common conditions, contact the National Organization for Rare Disorders (*RareDiseases. org,* 203-744-0100).

•**Know what help is available.** In addition to the benefits listed above, patient-assistance groups can give you firsthand feedback, based on other patients' experiences, on what to realistically expect from treatments…advice on what questions to ask your health-care providers as issues arise…and, in many cases, even the opportunity to have another person, with a similar situation, accompany you to your medical appointments. You won't get this kind of personalized attention from your doctor!

Don't Let Your Doctor Get It Wrong

Helen Haskell, MA, president of Mothers Against Medical Error, a nonprofit patient-safety organization, MAMEmomsonline.org. In 2015, she was named one of the top 50 patient-safety experts in the country by Becker's Hospital Review.

Fifteen years ago, my teenage son Lewis went to the hospital for an elective surgical procedure. After the operation, his doctors failed to notice that he was suffering from an undetected infection and blood loss from an ulcer caused by pain medication. They believed his symptoms were an indication of constipation from other pain medications he was taking. This mistake cost my son his life—he died four days after entering the hospital.

Now: I teach patients skills that can help them avoid a similar tragedy.

A "Blind Spot" in Medicine

A groundbreaking new report from the prestigious Institute of Medicine (IOM) concluded that most Americans will experience at least one diagnostic error—that is, an inaccurate, missed or delayed diagnosis, as determined by later definitive testing—at some point in their lives.

The IOM report called diagnostic errors a "blind spot" in the delivery of quality health care. Each year, about one in 20 patients who seek outpatient care will suffer from a wrong or delayed diagnosis. According to autopsy studies, diagnostic mistakes contribute to about 10% of patient deaths. Unfortunately, diagnostic errors haven't gotten as much attention as treatment and surgical errors—for example, operating on the wrong body part—partially because the latter are easier and quicker to identify. Now patient-safety experts are taking steps to better understand why diagnostic errors occur. *Key reasons…*

•**Tests help—and hurt.** Patients may be given a staggering number of tests—X-rays, blood tests, biopsies and more. The process of ordering, conducting and conveying the results of a test, however, can be complex and poorly organized.

•**Poor communication.** Can you count on the internist to talk to the nurse? Will the radiologist convey all of the pertinent information to the surgeon? Don't count on it. Patients also play a role. They should tell their doctors about all the symptoms they're having and whether they're getting better or worse after starting a new treatment.

•**Snap judgments.** Doctors often develop a working diagnosis within the first few minutes of hearing the patient's reported symptoms. The danger is that doctors can develop a so-called anchoring bias that leads them to cling to their initial diagnosis and prevents them from fully considering new information or looking for other possibilities.

How to Make Sure Your Doctor Gets It Right

Major medical groups, including the Society to Improve Diagnosis in Medicine, have identified a number of institutional factors—such as stronger teamwork—to reduce errors. But no one has more at stake in these situations than the patients themselves. Four steps you can take to avoid a misdiagnosis…

STEP 1: **Organize your thoughts.** Most of the time, doctors have only 15 minutes with each patient, so you need to make the most of your time together.

Plan ahead: Your medical history—including a description of symptoms and when the problem started—is the most important part of an exam. Describe the nature and context of your symptoms in as much detail as you can. When do you feel them? What makes them worse or better? Why are you worried? Keep it concise and on topic, but include your own thoughts so the doctor can address the issues that concern you.

My advice: If possible, before you see the doctor, use the Internet to investigate your symptoms and the likely causes. Your findings should not be used to challenge your doctor, but rather as a way to have a more informed conversation. If you don't have confidence in your own abilities to do research, take advantage of a service like Expert HealthSearch (*ImproveDiagnosis.org/ ?page=ExpertHealthSearch*), a free service that puts you in touch with a medical librarian who can search the literature for you.

STEP 2: **Don't be afraid to question test results.** They are more prone to error than most people imagine. In one study, experts who reviewed biopsies of more than 6,000 cancer patients concluded that 86 had been given a wrong diagnosis. Samples can be too small or even contaminated…technicians can make mistakes…and there can be false-negatives or false-positives. Results can be misinterpreted, or even more often, they can go unreported to the patient.

My advice: If a test result seems to fly in the face of the symptoms you are experiencing, consider asking to repeat the test or have a second doctor review it. And never assume that no news is good news. Follow up to be sure that your test results have been received and reviewed and that you know what they are.

STEP 3: Ask about alternatives. Many common symptoms—such as fatigue, muscle aches and abdominal pain—are known as nonspecific symptoms. They can be caused by dozens of conditions.

My advice: To help understand your doctor's thinking, ask him/her this question: Could you please explain your differential diagnoses? This is a list of possible diagnoses ranked in order of likelihood. It's a thought process that helps a diagnostician avoid overlooking any likely possibilities. The most serious conditions on the list should be ruled out before settling on a less serious diagnosis, and the doctor should be looking for causes and not just treating symptoms.

What to ask: If there is any question about a diagnosis, patients can help assess the "fit" by asking three important questions: Does this diagnosis match all my symptoms? What else could it be? Could there be more than one thing going on?

STEP 4: Don't skip the second opinion. I cannot stress this enough. In the study of cancer patients cited earlier, Johns Hopkins University researchers found that one to two of every 100 who got a second opinion with definitive testing after a tumor biopsy had gotten a wrong diagnosis the first time.

My advice: It's not always possible to get a second opinion—sometimes in medicine you have to move fast. But if you can, a second (or even a third) opinion is smart when symptoms seem severe…if your doctor is recommending surgery…or if you are told that you have a rare or fatal condition. Check first, but usually insurance will pay for a second opinion. Outside of emergencies, most of the time a brief delay in treatment while you get a second opinion will not affect your outcome.

How to Get an Appointment with Your Busy Doctor

Charles B. Inlander, a consumer advocate and health-care consultant based in Fogelsville, Pennsylvania. He was founding president of the nonprofit People's Medical Society, a consumer advocacy organization, and is author or coauthor of more than 20 consumer-health books.

Over the past few years, more and more patients have been complaining about how long it takes to get appointments with their doctors—even doctors they have been seeing for years. While the problem tends to occur more often with specialists, who are harder to come by than primary care doctors in some locales, the declining number of primary care doctors is creating a backlog for some practices, too. But with the help of the following secrets, you'll greatly increase your chances of getting a medical appointment sooner. *What works best…*

• **Talk to the right person.** The receptionist answering the phone at a medical practice usually has little discretion over scheduling. Ask to speak to the nurse who works with your doctor. Even if you have never been to the practice before, this usually works.

Insider secret: Don't cry wolf. When you talk to the nurse, give a legitimate medical reason (such as a recurrence of a previously treated condition) for the expedited appointment.

• **Do not ask about a "waiting list."** If you can't get through to the nurse, you'll probably assume that you should ask to be put on a waiting list (so you'll be called if there's a cancellation). Don't do that!

Insider secret: Instead of mentioning a waiting list, ask the receptionist if you can be put on the "quick call" list. This is the term that most medical practices use when referring to the list for people who get priority appointments when a cancellation or opening occurs. Asking for the quick call list tells the receptionist that you are something of an insider, which will help you get priority status.

•**Consider an urgent-care center.** If you are having a nonemergency problem (such as flulike symptoms or pain due to a minor injury) but cannot get a timely appointment with your primary care doctor or a specialist, head to your nearest hospital-affiliated or freestanding urgent-care center or even one at your local drugstore or supermarket.

Important: For serious problems, such as chest pains, high fever, breathing difficulties or burns, go to an emergency room!

•**Get a new doctor.** If one of your current doctors regularly makes you wait several weeks or longer for an appointment, don't hesitate to find a new doctor. While he/she may be busy, your time is valuable too, and it's reasonable to expect to be seen within a month for a routine appointment or within a few days for a special need.

Is Genetic Testing Right for You?

Robert Nussbaum, MD, chief medical officer at Invitae, a genetic information company based in San Francisco. He is also the coauthor of more than 200 scientific publications in human genetics and coauthor of the textbook *Genetics in Medicine.*

G enetic testing can save lives by alerting individuals to risk factors for diseases that may be hiding in their genes. But most patients are missing out on these benefits because the tests aren't well understood. Traditionally, genetic testing has been used to screen newborn babies for treatable conditions and by prospective parents concerned about passing on genetic diseases to their children.

What few people realize: There are now many tests that are useful for adults who may wonder about conditions, such as certain types of heart disease, cancer, Alzheimer's disease or Parkinson's disease, that tend to develop later in life. In fact, there are more than 1,000 genetic tests to detect the "variants" in genes (DNA) that can cause or complicate such health problems—before symptoms develop.

Predictive Testing

This type of genetic testing (typically based on an analysis of blood or saliva) predicts your risk for a specific disease long before symptoms appear. A marked family history of the disease (in a first-degree relative such as a parent or sibling, for example) usually prompts a doctor to recommend the test. Predictive testing can be helpful for…

•**Breast and ovarian cancer.** If there is a history of breast or ovarian cancer in your family, with two or more relatives affected at a relatively young age (before age 50), ask your doctor if you should have a test for BRCA1 and BRCA2 genetic mutations.

An unexpected risk: These genetic mutations are also found in about 5% of patients with prostate and pancreatic cancer. Therefore, both women and men may want to consider the BRCA1 and BRCA2 test if these cancers have occurred in two or more of their family members before the age of 60.

•**Colon cancer.** If you have a first-degree relative who had colon cancer before age 50, you may have the APC mutation, which causes familial adenomatous polyposis, a precursor to colon cancer. Or you may test positive for Lynch syndrome, a hereditary predisposition to colon cancer that carries a lifetime risk for the disease of 10% to 74%, depending on the specific gene and mutation. Lifetime colon cancer risk for the general population is about 5%.

Depending on the results of your test, you and your doctor may decide that you should…

•Have a colonoscopy every year, not every 10 years, if you test positive for the APC mutation or Lynch syndrome…or have a total colectomy (removal of the colon) as a preventive measure.

• Get more frequent screening for ovarian and uterine cancer—risk for both cancers is also significantly increased in women with Lynch syndrome. You may also consider prophylactic surgery to remove the ovaries and/or uterus.

• Receive a customized chemotherapeutic regimen proven to have greater efficacy in people with Lynch syndrome if you do develop colon cancer.

• **Heart disease.** People whose first-degree relatives have had (at any age) certain cardiac conditions (see below) may be predisposed to sudden cardiac death or heart disease. *Genetic testing is recommended for disorders including…*

Hypertrophic cardiomyopathy, an inherited disease that causes thickening of the left ventricle, one of the four chambers of the heart…ventricular tachycardia, a faster-than-normal heartbeat that starts in the heart's lower chambers…or atrial fibrillation, an irregular heartbeat caused by a misfiring of the heart's electrical system. If testing reveals one of these conditions, your doctor will be able to treat you sooner.

Getting Tested

Among the issues for you and your doctor to deal with in the process of deciding to get a genetic test…

• **Usefulness of the results.** Deciding before the genetic test how you will use the results is an important part of the test process. For example, if Alzheimer's disease runs in your family, you may decide to be tested for a genetic variant in the APOE gene that indicates an increased risk for the illness.

The dilemma: If the test results reveal you have the APOE variant, there is no medicine or surgery that can address your genetic risk. However, you may be more motivated to make lifestyle changes, such as eating a Mediterranean diet or walking regularly, since studies show these can lower the risk for Alzheimer's. You might also change your long-term planning—such as moving closer to your family.

• **Health insurance.** In the APOE example above, it is likely that your insurer would not pay for this genetic test because the result would not affect your medical treatment.

Similarly, if you are concerned about breast cancer and want a test for BRCA1 and BRCA2, the insurance company may deny the request because the insurer may believe that your family history doesn't warrant the testing.

Helpful: If the test is not covered, you may try to get authorization for it by asking your doctor to write a letter indicating that the testing is a medical necessity and providing the relevant supporting data.

Good news: The Genetic Information Nondiscrimination Act (GINA) of 2008 prohibits most group health insurers from denying insurance coverage or adjusting group premiums based on the genetic information of members of the group.

• **Psychological repercussions.** Before receiving a genetic test from your doctor, talk to a genetic counselor. The counselor can help determine if you need the test, provide psychological support when you receive results and also help determine whether or not family members should be informed about the results of your test, which could be meaningful for their own health. A genetic counselor can also help you through the maze of health insurance.

To find a genetic counselor: Ask your doctor for a referral or consult the National Society of Genetic Counselors (*NSGC.org*).

4 Mistakes to Avoid During an Emergency

Leslie D. Michelson, founder and CEO of Los Angeles–based Private Health Management. He is the author of *The Patient's Playbook: How to Save Your Life and the Lives of Those You Love.*

There are no two ways about it—medical emergencies fill us with fright, confusion and sometimes panic. While you may think that you can't prepare for an unexpected health crisis, the truth is that you can—and should.

Whether you're dealing with a stroke, heart attack or even a relatively minor injury such as a broken ankle, the consequences of not being prepared can be quite serious. In the most extreme cases, it can result in a preventable medical error, which studies show is a leading cause of death in the US.

Below are four common mistakes that patients make during the first 24 hours—and simple steps you can take to avoid them...

MISTAKE #1: **Not calling 911.** In the first moments of a health crisis, it's hard to know what to do. Simply render aid? Call 911? Or load the patient in the car and take him/her to the hospital yourself?

What to consider...

•**What's the nature of the problem?** If it's a minor injury to a limb (arm or leg) or an extremity (hand or foot), it's generally less urgent than an injury to the head or torso, where vital organs are located. (Note: If bleeding from a limb or extremity won't stop even when pressure is applied or there is a very long or deep cut, the situation may be serious and warrants a 911 call.)

If there's no visible injury but the person is experiencing troubling symptoms, be sure to pay close attention. Does he have unexplained shortness of breath? Is he clammy and cold or faint and dizzy? (All are potential heart attack signs.) Is the pain getting worse? Does he appear to be having an acute allergic reaction or asthma attack? Any of these scenarios could become life-threatening and should prompt an immediate call to 911.

If the patient is stable, talking coherently and none of the above symptoms are present, it's helpful to call the patient's primary care physician and ask if the situation can be handled in an office visit. If you can't reach the doctor or you have any doubts, call 911.

•**What's the age and health status of the patient?** If you're dealing with someone who's in his 70s or older and/or has a chronic condition such as diabetes, heart disease or cancer, it's best to err on the side of caution

and call 911 if there is any question whether the person requires emergency treatment.

MISTAKE #2: **Heading to the wrong hospital.** When a patient realizes that he is at a hospital that simply doesn't have the expertise and resources to properly render care, it can require dozens of phone calls over days and pushback from the insurance company to get a transfer to another hospital. Instead, get to the right hospital the first time. *Here's how...*

•**Before there's ever an emergency, check to see if you have a designated "trauma center" in your area.** An emergency room is considered a trauma center when it has the manpower and technology to handle the worst physical injuries—such as those from car crashes, high falls, etc. There are five different levels of trauma centers—a Level I center has the most resources while a Level V center would provide basic trauma care. To find out if you have a trauma center near you, go to *FACS.org/search/trauma-centers*.

If your condition is not life-threatening, you can ask the ambulance driver to take you to your preferred hospital. If he resists, request that the driver contact his supervisor for permission. However, if it's a true emergency, such as a heart attack, you should be taken to the closest ER available.

Important: When you reach an emergency department (or even while in transit, if possible), call your doctor. This will enable the medical staff to more accurately place your diagnosis in the context of your medical history.

Note: If you have the choice of going to a trauma center (not all locations will have one) or the hospital where your doctor has privileges (meaning he has been cleared to use the hospital's facilities), you need to consider the specific situation. For example, if it's a chronic problem that might require a lengthy stay, having your primary care physician present becomes more important. If you've been in a car accident, a trauma center is likely better.

MISTAKE #3: Not communicating clearly. Once you're at the emergency room, you (or your loved one) will need to convey a lot of information fast. And that might not be so easy. *What helps…*

• **Don't assume that electronic medical records will be in place.** In this age of electronic medical records, that advice to carry an up-to-date medical information card in your wallet is no longer valid, right? Oh yes, it is! The electronic medical record systems of many hospitals and doctors' offices are not compatible at this point, so it's still wise to have that card with you at all times. Be sure to include any allergies, chronic conditions such as asthma or diabetes, medications (and dosages) and phone numbers for emergency contacts.

• **Make sure you are heard.** Studies show that the average ER patient gets interrupted after 12 seconds of explaining his symptoms. For the best care, it's crucial to give the medical staff your full range of symptoms and medical history, so be clear and detailed. Also, be assertive if you are interrupted and let your needs be known.

MISTAKE #4: Giving up your power. When illness strikes you or a family member, it's easy to believe that if you simply obey the doctors and nurses, all will be well. Not so. The patient is ultimately in charge of his own health destiny. *What helps…*

• **Find out who is treating you.** If you're at a teaching hospital, it can be difficult to tell whether it's an attending physician, a resident or an intern who might be working in the emergency room. It's perfectly reasonable to ask, "Could you tell me what your title is?" If your health issue is complex, politely request to be examined by the attending physician. This way, you'll be sure to have a doctor who has completed his training (and is actually supervising the others) caring for you.

• **Don't forget your records.** By federal law, all your medical records belong to you. Before you're discharged after an ER visit, ask for copies of all of your medical records in case you encounter complications down the road and the doctors treating you need to know your medical history. The cost for these copies varies by state.

Don't Skip Your Follow-Up After an ER Visit

If you go to the ER for chest pain, treatment guidelines urge you to see a physician for further evaluation within 72 hours of being released. But a new study of nearly 57,000 such patients showed that 25% of them did not get this follow-up—increasing their risk for future problems such as heart attack.

Dennis Ko, MD, senior scientist, Sunnybrook Research Institute, University of Toronto, Canada.

Going to the Hospital for Surgery? Vitamin D May Protect Your Mind

Study titled "Association Between Pre-hospital Vitamin D Status and Hospital-Acquired New-Onset Delirium" by researchers in the department of medicine, Harvard Medical School, and Brigham and Women's Hospital, both in Boston, published in *British Journal of Nutrition*.

Delirium in the hospital is more common—and more dangerous—than you may think. It's a severe condition that mostly affects older patients (although not only older patients) and is often missed by hospital staff, especially in emergency rooms. If it's not treated promptly, it can lead to longer hospital stays and poor health outcomes, including permanent cognitive problems and even a higher risk for mortality. It's more common if there's already some cognitive impairment, but research shows that between 3% and 29% of "low-risk" patients without any existing cognitive problems succumb to delirium after a hospital stay. A combination of surgery, infection, social isolation, dehydration, poor nutrition and mind-affecting pharmaceuticals such as painkillers, sedatives and sleeping pills can bring it on...quickly.

You can't control all of these factors, especially in the heat of the moment during emergency treatment. But researchers have discovered a nutritional factor that may protect against hospital-induced delirium...vitamin D.

D Is for...No Delirium

Compared with patients who had blood levels 30 ng/mL and over, patients with levels from 10 ng/mL to 20 ng/mL were 50% more likely to develop delirium—and those with levels under 10 ng/mL faced double the risk. And that wasn't just a handful—about one in six (16%) of all the patients studied had levels under 10 ng/mL. Adjusting for other possible factors, including history of depression, calcium level and season of vitamin D testing, didn't change the results.

A No-Brainer Approach to Protecting the Brain

It was an observational study, which means it can't prove (or disprove) that a lack of vitamin D caused delirium, so it's possible that whatever caused delirium in these patients also made their vitamin D levels plummet. Nor does this study show that bringing vitamin D levels up to speed proactively prevents delirium. More studies will be needed to explore that hypothesis.

But it's a reasonable hypothesis, and there is good reason to believe that vitamin D may play a specific role in protecting the brain and the mind. The brain has vitamin D receptors throughout, and there is evidence that the active form of vitamin D may remove plaque, a hallmark of Alzheimer's, from brain cells, scientists have recently discovered. Research has shown that low blood levels of vitamin D are linked with dementia, Alzheimer's disease and depression.

In a way, though, the exact question is beside the point. Medicine is about balancing benefit and harm, and in this case, if you're vitamin D–deficient, there's no harm, and potentially much benefit, in bringing your body's vitamin D level up to normal! According to the National Institutes of Health, 77% of Americans are deficient in vitamin D, with blood levels under 30 ng/mL, and 6% have levels under 10 ng/mL. Even if you don't know your level, taking a daily supplement that contains up to 2,000 IU or 3,000 IU is considered safe.

An even better idea: Get a blood test. It's simple, quick, and inexpensive. If your level is low, your health-care provider may prescribe a higher dosage for a while or even recommend vitamin D injections to get your level up to normal quickly.

If you are going into the hospital or know someone who is, the idea of getting tested for vitamin D beforehand...and reaching a normal level with a supplement if need be... is a no brainer. It may prevent a scary form of delirium that can take hold in the hospital and lead to a downward health spiral. Even if it doesn't, it's a healthy thing to do.

More Ways to Prevent Hospital Delirium

Ensuring you get enough vitamin D is something you can do before hospitalization. Once there, there are additional steps you can take to avoid delirium...or arrest it before it gets too bad. Whether it's you or a loved one, make sure that items such as eyeglasses or hearing aids are readily available, books and other familiar objects are nearby, and that the patient walks around if possible, stays hydrated, and gets as much sleep as possible in the sleep-depriving hospital environment. Regular visits from friends and family are key, since being (and feeling) isolated can lead to loneliness and fear that in turn can be a factor in delirium. Monitor medications carefully, especially pain and sleep drugs, which can contribute to confusion and push a patient toward delirium. If you're caring for a loved one who does become agitated, confused or disoriented while in the hospital—even if it comes and goes, a common feature of hospital-induced delirium—alert the staff and ask specifically for a delirium evaluation from a mental health care provider. Basic treatment, including making sure the patient is well hydrated and nourished...stops taking dangerous medications if possible...gets daily exercise...is surrounded by familiar objects...and stays connected to family and friends, can often turn incipient delirium around before it gets too bad.

FDA Tightens Rules for Using Mesh Implants in Women's Surgery

U.S. Food and Drug Administration, news release.

The U.S. Food and Drug Administration has strengthened rules regarding the use of vaginal mesh implants to treat pelvic organ prolapse in women.

The devices have been reclassified from a "moderate" to "high" risk category. Manufacturers must now submit pre-market approval applications to the FDA to help the agency better assess the implants' safety and effectiveness.

Pelvic organ prolapse involves a weakening or stretching of internal structures that support organs such as the bladder, bowel and uterus. It can happen in women after childbirth, a hysterectomy or menopause. It can cause pelvic pain, constipation and urinary leakage, and often affects sexual activity.

Surgeons have long used the mesh implants to reinforce weakened pelvic floor muscles and repair pelvic organ prolapse. But, problems afterwards such as pain, infection, bleeding, urinary problems and pain during intercourse are common, the agency said.

"These stronger clinical requirements will help to address the significant risks associated with surgical mesh for repair of pelvic organ prolapse," Dr. William Maisel, deputy director of science and chief scientist at the FDA Center for Devices and Radiological Health, said in an agency news release.

"We intend to continue monitoring how women with this device are faring months and years after surgery through continued post-market surveillance measures," he added.

The updated requirements apply to surgical placement of the mesh implants through the vagina (transvaginal) to treat pelvic organ prolapse. The new rules do not apply to other uses of surgical mesh.

Makers of transvaginal mesh implants already on the market now have 30 months to submit pre-market approval applications, while makers of new devices must submit an application before they can be approved for sale in the United States, the FDA said.

New Discovery Helps You Stay Calm During Surgery

Pornpattana Vichitvejpaisal, MD, researcher, Chiang Mai University, Thailand.

Being awake during an operation in which you're given local—not general—anesthesia can be nerve-wracking.

But did you know that you have the ability to reduce your anxiety without (hardly) lifting a finger or spending lots of money?

You've probably heard that listening to music mixed with nature sounds may help keep you calm, but new research finds that listening to something else in addition to that may help even more...

Soothing Sounds

A few years ago, researchers evaluated the effects of something called binaural beat audio therapy. It's when you listen to one sustained tone in your right earphone and a different sustained tone in your left earphone simultaneously—and each tone is at a slightly different frequency than the other. (If you listen to the tones without earphones, such as through a stereo, each tone would come from a different speaker.) To both ears, the combined beats tend to sound like a single, vibrating tone. Prior research has indicated that this sound triggers alpha-frequency brainwaves, which can reduce fear and pain perception and induce feelings of relaxation.

Researchers wanted to see whether binaural beats mixed with music (such as melodies and rhythms) and nature sounds (such as the sounds of waterfalls, birds, oceans, rivers and forests) would relax patients undergoing surgery more than the same audio mix of music and nature sounds without the binaural beats...or more than no audio at all. They referred to their three groups of test subjects as "the binaural/music group," "the music group" and "the control group." Researchers decided to work with patients having cataract surgery because it's one of the most common operations done worldwide and because it requires local (not general) anesthesia, so a patient remains awake throughout the procedure.

Patients' anxiety levels were measured in three ways—through a blood pressure measurement...a heart-rate measurement...and self-reported feelings of anxiety.

Results...

Blood pressure: The control group's blood pressure went up during surgery, indicating rising anxiety. In contrast, blood pressure actually fell (in a healthy way) during surgery for both the binaural/music group and the music group—with the music group's pressure falling the most. So in this category, the music group (with no binaural beats) did best.

Heart rate: The control group's heart rates rose during surgery, indicating anxiety. Again, in contrast, heart rates fell in both the binaural/music group and the music group—but in this case, the binaural beats group did much better.

Self-reported anxiety: Right after the surgery, patients were asked to report how anxious they had felt during the surgery. The binaural/music group did best by far.

In other words, listening to music combined with nature sounds may help you relax during surgery, but hearing those sounds with binaural beats may help you relax during surgery even more.

Low-Cost Ticket to Lower Anxiety

According to lead study author Pornpattana Vichitvejpaisal, MD, almost anyone having surgery with local anesthesia could benefit from the soothing effects of binaural beat audio, and the fact that it's low cost and non-invasive makes it easy to try. The only types of people he excluded from his study were those with epilepsy, those with blood pressure over 160/100 and those with hearing problems or ear infections—anyone in those groups should consult a doctor before trying binaural therapy to make sure that it's safe and likely to be effective.

The cheapest and easiest way to listen to binaural beats mixed with music and nature sounds is to go online and grab the sounds off of YouTube (on the site, search for "binaural beats, music, nature"). If you aren't allowed to do that during surgery (or if you don't want to have to rely on an Internet connection), you can download and save a file on your smartphone or MP3 player ahead of time. If you'd prefer to do the latter, buy a digital audio track or CD of binaural beats mixed with music and nature sounds. Many companies sell them—for example, there are hour-long files on *Amazon.com* for about $1 apiece.

Getting Cataract Surgery? Don't Pay for These Unnecessary Tests

Catherine L. Chen, MD, MPH, department of anesthesia and perioperative care, Center for Healthcare Value, University of California, San Francisco. Her study was published in *The New England Journal of Medicine*.

Some doctors take surprising precautions with a simple, safe and quick outpatient surgery. We're talking about cataract surgery, which takes about 20 minutes and is performed 1.7 million times a year in the US. The only anesthesia is eye-numbing drops. Complications are exceedingly rare.

So why are more than half of people scheduled for cataract surgery made to undergo pre-op tests such as a complete blood count, urinalysis, cardiogram, chest x-ray, stress tests, pulmonary function tests…sometimes five or more tests?

If you are scheduled for cataract surgery, it turns out, it's not your medical condition that's the primary driver in the decision to get these expensive and usually unnecessary tests.

It's who your ophthalmologist is.

A Cavalcade of Unnecessary Tests

The research is equally clear—routine preoperative testing (i.e., getting extra tests because you're scheduled for surgery) doesn't make a bit of difference in how well you'll do during cataract surgery. *Here's why…*

• **Serious adverse complications such as a heart attack are just as rare** (less than 1%) in people who didn't have preoperative testing as in those who did.

• **The effectiveness of the operation for patients is just as good whether or not testing is performed.**

• **A group of professional medical societies issued guidelines stating that routine preoperative testing before standard cataract surgery is not needed…**and that was back in 2002! Yet 13 years later, doctors still aren't heeding this message.

In fact, according to a new study, the guidelines may not be making a difference at all in how doctors behave. Researchers analyzed 440,857 Medicare patients from around the country who had cataract surgery in 2011. The records told the story—each patient's health status…whether he or she went for a presurgical evaluation by a doctor other than an ophthalmologist (such as a cardiologist, internist, general practitioner, anesthesiologist or geriatric special-

ist)…and whether the patient had any of the common preoperative tests.

Result: More than half (53%) had at least one preoperative test and about the same number had a preoperative office visit with a doctor other than the ophthalmologist. About 13% of beneficiaries had five or more tests.

A Minority of Doctors Order Most of the Tests

In this latest study, sicker patients were just a tad more likely to get pre-op testing. People who had their cataract surgery in a hospital outpatient department rather than an ambulatory surgery center were also slightly more likely to get pre-op tests. But the health of the patient and the type of institution where the surgery was performed were not the most important predictors of who got tested.

In fact, the biggest predictor by far of being sent for these tests, or being referred to another doctor for an additional visit, was… the identity of the eye doctor that patients happened to go to. Although it was hard to tell whether the ophthalmologists were the ones who were actually ordering the extra tests, the data showed that the patients of some eye doctors had more pre-op tests than patients of other eye docs. In fact, approximately one-third of doctors ordered tests on more than three-quarters of their patients. And about 8% ordered pre-op tests on every single patient. In the end, just 36% of the ophthalmologists, who operated on 26% of the patients, accounted for 84% of all testing. The nearly 800,000 tests ordered cost more than $16 million, and the extra office visits added another $28.3 million. Even if your out-of-pocket expenses aren't very high, eventually these costs come back to bite all of us in the form of higher health insurance premiums.

The most disturbing finding is that the clear, evidence-based medical guidelines that conclude that routine pre-op testing is unneeded has still not been incorporated into everyday practice. Indeed, the rate of pre-op testing before cataract surgery is virtually the same as it was 20 years ago—before the guidelines were developed.

What to Do Before You Get Cataract Surgery

If you need cataract surgery and your doctor hands you a stack of referrals for presurgical medical clearance or testing, ask questions. Is this referral really necessary? Do I need to take all these tests? If so, why—specifically? Your surgeon may be routinely recommending testing for reasons other than to evaluate your health—to protect himself/herself from a lawsuit...or because the surgery center where the operation is taking place requires it...or maybe it's just an innocent habit from a long time ago.

However, if you or your ophthalmologist have genuine concerns about your ability to safely undergo cataract surgery, don't hesitate to get checked out by your primary care doctor, cardiologist or other relevant specialist, who may or may not choose to send you for testing. Guidelines aren't hard-and-fast rules. They're suggestions based on evidence, and the final discretion lies with your health-care provider and you.

Common Meds That Slow Surgery Recovery

Patients sometimes take antianxiety drugs to calm themselves before surgery. But people who took *lorazepam* (Ativan) before a surgical procedure requiring general anesthesia needed ventilation tubes longer, had poorer-quality postsurgical sleep, had more postsurgery amnesia and took longer to recover cognitive abilities than people who took a placebo or nothing.

Study led by researchers at Timone Hospital, Marseille, France, of 1,062 patients admitted to French hospitals, published in *JAMA*.

Medications That Hurt Your Eyes

Jeffrey R. Anshel, OD, optometrist and founder of Corporate Vision Consulting, which addresses visual demands in the workplace. He is author of *The Ocular Nutrition Handbook*. He maintains a private practice in Carlsbad, California.

Are your eyes dry or sensitive to light? Do you have blurred vision or "floaters"? These and other eye problems could be side effects of common medications.

Few people make the connection between changes in their eyes and medications they take—yet the truth is that many prescription and over-the-counter drugs cause ocular side effects. *Here are common symptoms and the drugs that could be causing them...*

Important: Contact your physician (eye doctor or primary care) if you have any of these symptoms. Most are not dangerous, and minor eye problems may be a reasonable trade-off for a potentially lifesaving drug. Always bring with you to the doctor a complete list of the medications you take—prescription and over-the-counter—and the doses. Stopping the medications can reverse the symptoms in many cases.

•**Abnormalities in pupil size.** Discrepancies in how your pupils react to light (called aniscoria) can be caused by a variety of medications, including Catapres (for hypertension), Donnatal (irritable bowel syndrome/ulcers), Humulin (diabetes) and Tavist (allergies).

If your pupils aren't always the same size—especially if only one pupil is abnormally enlarged—it's important to go to the emergency room immediately. The brain controls pupil size, so a disturbance there can cause pupils to be different sizes.

•**Cataracts.** If you live long enough, you eventually will develop cataracts (lenses that have clouded over, making it more difficult to see). Certain drugs may speed the process, including Coumadin (for heart disease), Plaquenil (malaria, rheumatoid arthritis and lupus) and most steroids.

•**Difficulty focusing.** The medical term for this condition is "accommodative insufficiency." It grows more common with age and also is a side effect of some medications. These include Adipex (for obesity), Enduron (hypertension), Norpramin (depression) and Xanax (anxiety).

•**Double or blurred vision.** There are many potential causes for seeing double or for vision that suddenly blurs. Medications that can cause this include Adipex (for obesity), Celebrex (inflammation), Lamictal (seizures), Mevacor (elevated cholesterol), Tylenol (pain relief) and Zantac (ulcers).

If your blurred or double vision is sudden, severe and unrelenting, go to the emergency room immediately. This visual impairment is not only unsafe (for instance, when you are driving), but it could be a sign of a serious medical problem such as a stroke or brain lesion.

•**Dry eyes.** Many factors (including computer use, wearing contact lenses and allergies) can reduce tear production and cause dry eyes—and so can certain medications, such as Actifed (for allergies), Catapres (hypertension), Detrol (bladder control) and Paxil (depression).

Until you see your doctor, self-treatment options for dry eyes include blinking as often as possible…use of artificial tear solutions (available in drugstores and chain stores)…avoiding irritants, including eye makeup and air pollution…and wearing sunglasses. Or try an oral gamma-linolenic acid (GLA) product such as BioTears.

•**Eye irritation.** Redness in the whites of your eyes or irritations on your eyelids can be caused by medications such as Aricept (taken to improve cognitive loss), Cardizem (heart disease), Enduron (heart disease) and Voltaren (rheumatoid arthritis, osteoporosis).

•**Floaters and other visual disturbances.** Flashes of light or color, floaters and other visual disturbances can occur for a host of reasons, including as a side effect of a drug. Medications linked to visual disturbances include Benadryl (for allergies), Cardizem (heart disease), Elavil (depression) and Xanax (anxiety).

The causes of visual disturbances can range from inconsequential to potentially serious, so they should be checked out by your eye doctor as quickly as possible. This is especially true if you suddenly see flashes of light or if numerous new floaters appear—that could be a sign of a retinal detachment.

•**Light sensitivity.** Though there are other possible causes, light sensitivity may be a side effect of drugs (including recreational drugs such as cocaine and amphetamines). Drugs linked with light sensitivity include Diabinese (for diabetes), Dilantin (epilepsy), Lipitor (high cholesterol/heart disease), Pepcid (gastric ulcers) and Viagra (erectile dysfunction). If light sensitivity is severe and your pupils are enlarged—especially if only one pupil is enlarged—go to the ER. It could be a sign of stroke or a brain tumor.

•**Yellowed eyes.** Several conditions can cause the white parts of the eye to turn yellow, including illness, sun exposure and drugs such as Diabinese (for diabetes), Elavil (depression) and Librium (anxiety). Yellowing may be a sign of cirrhosis or hepatitis. It is important to see your doctor quickly to have this checked out.

These Everyday Drugs Can Mess with Your Mind

Jack E. Fincham, PhD, RPh, a professor of pharmacy administration at Presbyterian College School of Pharmacy in Clinton, South Carolina.

You wouldn't be surprised if a narcotic painkiller made you feel a little sleepy or you developed an upset stomach after taking an aspirin-like painkiller for a few days.

What most people don't know—and their doctors don't talk about—is that popular prescription and over-the-counter (OTC) drugs can affect your body and your mind.

Common offenders you need to know about—psychiatric side effects can occur with any dose, but the greater the drug amount, the greater the risk...

Painkillers

Naproxen (Aleve, Naprosyn and others). It's one of the most popular pain relievers because it's less likely to cause stomach upset than other nonsteroidal anti-inflammatory drugs (NSAIDs), such as aspirin or *ibuprofen* (Motrin). But it's more likely than other OTC painkillers to cause depression.

How it hurts: The exact mechanism isn't clear, but naproxen affects the central nervous system in ways that other NSAIDs do not. Some people who take naproxen every day—for chronic arthritis, for example—have reported drowsiness, reduced concentration and/or depression.

My advice: Be aware of your mood when using naproxen. Even though this drug is less likely to cause stomach upset than other NSAIDs, you should watch for signs of depression while taking naproxen. If depression develops, ask your doctor for advice.

Blood Pressure Drugs

Beta-blockers, such as *propranolol* (Inderal) and *sotalol* (Betapace), work by blocking the effects of *epinephrine* (also known as adrenaline), thus slowing the heart rate.

How they hurt: Damping down the heart's action can cause fatigue and depression. Because these drugs affect many different body systems, including the brain, they've also been linked to mania and other mood problems in some people.

My advice: Beta-blockers are typically used to treat serious conditions such as high blood pressure and cardiac arrhythmias, so never stop taking this medication without consulting your physician. You may be able to switch to a different drug (such as a calcium channel blocker) for high blood pressure.

If you must take a beta-blocker, use non-drug approaches to improve your energy levels and mood. Be sure to exercise regularly, rely on positive thinking and get enough sunlight, which the body uses to produce vitamin D (low levels have been linked to depression).

Cold Remedies

•*Guaifenesin.* This is one of the most common ingredients in OTC decongestants and cold remedies, such as Robitussin and Mucinex. As an expectorant, guaifenesin thins mucus, making it easier to cough it up.

How it hurts: Guaifenesin has wide-ranging effects on the central nervous system. In some people, these changes can lead to fatigue and/or depression. When guaifenesin is combined with other ingredients such as pseudoephedrine (a common decongestant), side effects can also include anxiety.

My advice: For most people, drinking water helps to thin mucus about as well as a pharmaceutical expectorant does. When you're stuffed up, drink a few more glasses of water—or tea or juice—than you usually consume during an average day.

Allergy Drugs

•**Nonsedating antihistamines.** Don't believe the labels—so-called "nonsedating" allergy drugs may have less noticeable side effects than older antihistamines (such as Benadryl), but they are sedating.

Some people with seasonal or year-round allergies who use drugs such as *loratadine* (Claritin) or *cetirizine* (Zyrtec) complain about drowsiness—and depression.

How they hurt: All antihistamines have anticholinergic effects (caused by blocking a neurotransmitter in the central nervous system). While some people have no side effects, others notice that they're agitated and/or confused. For some people, these antihistamines also may lead to depression or concentration problems.

My advice: Since unwanted sedation is the most common side effect, take antihistamines at bedtime. Pollen counts and allergy symptoms tend to be worse in the morning, so taking an antihistamine at night will also help you feel better when you wake up.

Worth a try: Break the tablets in half (assuming that the medication isn't timed-release). Many people get the same allergy relief with fewer side effects from a lower dose.

Heartburn Medications

•**H2 blockers.** Some patients who take these heartburn drugs, including *cimetidine* (Tagamet) and *ranitidine* (Zantac), have reported suffering from depression, confusion and even hallucinations. These and other side effects usually occur in older adults, who tend to accumulate higher drug levels in the body.

How they hurt: Ironically, the psychiatric side effects of H2 blockers are probably related to lower stomach acidity—the effect that these drugs provide to fight heartburn. Too much stomach acid (or a weak esophageal muscle that allows acid reflux) is obviously a problem, but reduced acid may have its own risks. For example, people who take

these drugs every day tend to absorb smaller amounts of folate and other nutrients—an effect that can lead to mood problems.

My advice: Most people can reduce—or even eliminate—heartburn without the daily use of potent drugs. Simple approaches that work include not eating within a few hours of bedtime…and avoiding "trigger" foods such as chocolate or alcohol. If you need more relief, you may be able to get by with the occasional OTC antacid, such as Mylanta or Maalox.

The Overdose Danger

Jack E. Fincham, PhD, RPh, a professor of pharmacy administration at Presbyterian College School of Pharmacy in Clinton, South Carolina.

When you get a new prescription, the first thing your doctor does (after choosing the drug) is decide on the dose.

What most people don't think about: Your doctor's dosing decision is crucial—getting even slightly more of a medication than you need can greatly increase your risk for side effects. Correct dosing, however, can lessen (or even eliminate) side effects.

Each year in the US, drug side effects are estimated to cause more than one million hospitalizations and more than 100,000 deaths. Yet many doctors reflexively prescribe "average" doses without checking recommendations for optimal dosing based on such factors as age, sex and body weight.

For example, a 100-pound woman might be given the same dose as a 200-pound man… and a 75-year-old may be given the same dose as a healthy college student. It's not hard to guess who is more likely to have preventable side effects. While many people know that taking a blood thinner in a dose that's too high can have devastating consequences, recent research is focusing on other drugs that can also have dangerous side effects.

Important new finding: With blood pressure drugs and diabetes medication, in particular, excessive doses can increase risk for dizzy spells, confusion, falls and even death—especially among adults age 70 and older, according to recent research in *JAMA Internal Medicine*.

Dosing Dangers

Common drugs to watch out for…*

•**Sedatives.** Valium and related drugs, known as benzodiazepines, are commonly prescribed sedatives in the US, but the standard doses can be much too high for women as well as older adults.

Medications such as *diazepam* (Valium), *triazolam* (Halcion) and *zolpidem* (Ambien) accumulate in fatty tissue. Since women have a higher percentage of body fat than men, the drug effects can linger, causing next-day drowsiness or a decline in alertness and concentration. In older adults, the drugs are metabolized (broken down) more slowly, causing unacceptably high levels to accumulate in the body.

My advice: Women who are given a prescription for one of these drugs should always ask if the dose is sex-specific. They can ask something like, "Do I need a lower dose because I'm a woman?"

Also, in my opinion, people age 65 or older should avoid these drugs altogether unless they have to take them for a serious problem, such as a seizure disorder. If your doctor says that you need a sedative, ask if you can use a shorter-acting drug such as *lorazepam* (Ativan)…if you can take it for a short period of time (less than a month)…or if you can get by with a lower dose.

Important: These drugs should never be combined with alcohol. The combination increases the sedative effects.

•**Blood pressure drugs.** About 25% of patients who take one or more of these medications stop using them within six months because of side effects, and up to half quit taking them within a year. The majority of people who take blood pressure drugs will

*Never change a medication dose without consulting your doctor.

initially suffer from dizziness, unsteadiness, falls or other side effects. Alert your physician if you experience any of these side effects. Even though the discomfort typically wanes over time, it can often be prevented altogether by starting with a lower dose of medication.

Beta-blockers, such as *metoprolol* (Lopressor) and *propranolol* (Inderal), are particularly dose-sensitive. So are alpha-blockers, such as *prazosin* (Minipress). Women who take these drugs tend to have a greater drop in blood pressure/heart rate than men, so they typically need a lower dose. The same may be true of patients who have both high blood pressure and lung disease, who often suffer shortness of breath when they take excessive doses. People who take multiple blood pressure medications are also more likely to have side effects.

My advice: Tell your doctor that you would like to start with one drug. Emphasize that you'd like to take the lowest possible dose—and that you're willing to be retested (or check your own blood pressure at home with an automated blood pressure monitor) to make sure that the treatment is working.

•**Diabetes medications.** The risks for diabetes complications—such as nerve damage, blindness, stroke and heart attack—are so great that doctors tend to treat it aggressively. But oral diabetes drugs given in high doses can easily cause blood sugar to fall too low.

Example: Patients who take *glyburide* (Micronase) or *repaglinide* (Prandin) often develop hypoglycemia, excessively low blood sugar that can cause dizziness, confusion and other symptoms. Even if the initial dose was correct, physiological changes as you age and/or changes in your lifestyle could make that starting dose too potent. For example, suppose that you start exercising more and eating a healthier diet. You'll probably need a lower drug dose than you did before, but your doctor might not think (or know) to change the prescription.

My advice: Tell your doctor right away about any lifestyle changes that could affect your blood sugar levels, such as exercise frequency (or intensity), changes in meal timing, etc. Keep careful tabs on your blood sugar with home tests. If your blood sugar is consistently testing at the lower end of the recommended range (or below it), call your doctor and ask whether you should switch to a lower drug dose.

• **Painkillers.** Aspirin, *ibuprofen* (Motrin) and other nonsteroidal anti-inflammatory drugs (NSAIDs) are widely available and effective. But they're also dangerous at high doses. One study found that more than 70% of people who take these drugs daily on a regular basis suffer at least some damage to the small intestine. Like the blood thinner *warfarin* (Coumadin), they're a common cause of excessive bleeding.

My advice: Take the lowest possible dose…use painkillers as rarely as possible… and always take them with food. People assume that over-the-counter drugs are safe, but none of these medications are meant to be used long term (more than four weeks).

If you can, switch to one of the many brands of *acetaminophen* (such as Tylenol). It has about the same pain-relieving effects, but even with its increased risk for liver damage, acetaminophen (taken at the recommended dosage) is less likely than an NSAID to cause side effects.

To Read more about a drug you're taking: Go to *Drugs.com.*

Are You Taking the Wrong Drug?

Dietrich Stephan, PhD, chairman of the department of human genetics at the University of Pittsburgh Graduate School of Public Health. He leads research in public health genetics at the Institute for Personalized Medicine at the University of Pittsburgh and the University of Pittsburgh Medical Center.

When your doctor writes you a prescription, you may assume that it's just a matter of matching the med-

ication to the condition that's being treated. Not so.

In reality, doctors are trained to narrow down the medication options—sometimes several of them—by taking into account such factors as your age, sex and weight. Until recently, that's all doctors have had to go on.

Now: The medication-choosing process has become far more sophisticated. With pharmacogenomics, also known as drug-gene testing, your doctor can use your genetic profile (genotype) to determine in advance if a drug is likely to be effective…the best dose…and how likely you are to have side effects. This breakthrough is now available for many commonly used medications, including heartburn drugs, painkillers, antidepressants, statins and certain cancer drugs.

Here's how to put drug-gene testing to work for you—or a loved one…

Personalized Prescriptions

The genes that you inherited from your parents largely determined what you look like—and even, to an extent, how you act and feel. Are you tall or short? What's your blood type? Are your eyes blue or brown?

Genes, the chemical sets of instructions that the body uses to build proteins, play an important role in making you you—and that includes how you respond to medications. In the future, it's likely that every drug—including over-the-counter standbys such as aspirin—will take genetics into account.

Less Guesswork

Suppose that you have colon cancer and will need chemotherapy. Your oncologist will pick the drugs with the best record of success. For example, two of the most effective drugs for this cancer are *cetuximab* (Erbitux) and *panitumumab* (Vectibix). Yet research has shown that they're not the best choice for about 40% of patients with a particular genetic profile.

Another example: Patients with cardiovascular disease are often given *warfarin* (Coumadin), a blood thinner. It's very effective at preventing clots, but it has a high risk for side effects, such as excessive bleeding—particularly when the dose isn't exactly right. For those with a particular genetic profile, the drug is up to three times more potent than in those with different genes. These patients should be given a much lower dose.

What to Expect

For now, genetic tests are available for more than 150 FDA-approved drugs. (For a complete list of FDA-approved drugs with pharmacogenomic information on the label, go to the FDA website at *snip.ly/P4XQ*.)

If your doctor plans to start you on one of these medications, ask him/her about going to a laboratory to give a blood/saliva sample. This can be used to create your unique genetic profile.

Important: A single test can't predict how you'll respond to all medications. You might need additional tests if you're taking more than one drug—although some test "panels" will include information on multiple medications.

The cost of a drug-gene test can be as little as about $100. More specialized tests—for the drugs used to treat some cancers, for example—can be as high as $7,000. Check with your health insurer to make sure the cost of the test is covered.

Can You Benefit?

Genetic variations could account for anywhere from 20% to 95% of the difference in individual responses to various medications, according to a recent review of studies that appeared in *The New England Journal of Medicine*.

Because there's such a high probability that drug-gene testing may yield helpful information, it's wise to discuss with your doctor whether genetic testing is available for any medication he may prescribe for you. The results could affect the prescribed dose…the likelihood of side effects…or even cause your doctor to choose a different drug. *Examples…*

• **Statins.** Depending on the drug, this class of medications can lower LDL "bad" cholesterol by up to 55%—in some people. In others, the results can be quite different. For example, one large study found that more than 13% of participants who took the statin *pravastatin* (Pravachol) failed to lower their LDL by even 10%.

Reason: Some genetic variations make people "poor responders" to statins. They might require a higher-than-normal dose…or a different drug altogether, such as a fibrate like *gemfibrozil* (Lopid). Other genetic variations cause people to metabolize statins too quickly, which increases the risk for muscle pain or other side effects.

• **Proton pump inhibitors (PPIs).** Drugs in this class, such as *omeprazole* (Prilosec) and *lansoprazole* (Prevacid), inhibit the production of stomach acid and are widely used to treat heartburn and stomach and duodenal ulcers. Researchers have identified a number of genetic variations that affect how well these medications work.

Patients who are "extensive metabolizers," for example, will require a higher dose than those who have genetic factors that cause them to metabolize the drugs more slowly.

• **Selective serotonin reuptake inhibitor (SSRI) antidepressants.** SSRIs require a lot of trial and error. About half of patients with depression don't improve on their first drug. Their success on second and third drugs is even lower.

With genetic tests, psychiatrists can make more than an educated guess about which drug and doses to try. An analysis of studies presented at a meeting of the International College of Neuropsychopharmacology found that genetics-based prescribing for SSRIs doubled response rates as well as the rate of remission.

• **Painkillers.** Codeine is among the most effective (and least expensive) analgesics, but some individuals have a genetic variation that inhibits their ability to convert it into morphine (the mechanism that provides its pain-relieving effect). They usually require a higher dose—or sometimes a different medication, such as fentanyl or hydromorphone.

Another genetic variation causes codeine to be metabolized much more rapidly than normal. These patients are more likely to suffer serious side effects, including impaired breathing, when they're given a standard dose.

This Dangerous Moment Leads to Painkiller Addiction

Survey titled "Changes in Substance Abuse Treatment Use Among Individuals With Opioid Use Disorders in the United States, 2004-2013," Johns Hopkins Bloomberg School of Public Health, Baltimore.

Study titled "Opioid Prescribing at Hospital Discharge Contributes to Chronic Opioid Use," University of Colorado Denver School of Medicine, et al., published in *Journal of General Internal Medicine*.

Other sources include the Centers for Disease Control & Prevention, the Centers for Medicare & Medicaid Services and *The New York Times*.

There's a painkiller addiction epidemic—and almost anyone is vulnerable. You are vulnerable.

Don't believe it? Prescription painkillers—which don't work very well in the first place when used long-term—kill 46 Americans daily.

And you can get addicted from a hospital stay.

The primary drivers of this plague? Doctors, according to a *New York Times* piece by Richard A. Friedman, MD, director of the psychopharmacology clinic at Weill Cornell Medical College in New York. Twenty years ago, opioids were primarily used to treat acute pain such as cancer pain or post-surgery recovery, but now they are widely prescribed for chronic conditions such as low-back pain and sciatica. Opioid addiction is driving the new heroin plague, too. Many people who find it hard to get, or afford, prescription narcotics are turning to heroin, which is illegal but often cheaper.

For many Americans, the issue hits close to home—39% of us know someone personally who has been addicted to painkillers, according to the latest Kaiser Family Foundation poll.

The Riskest Addiction Moment—Hospital Discharge

Here's the scenario: You're not currently taking opioid medications at all. You need to have a procedure at a hospital. When you get discharged, you are given a prescription for an opioid painkiller for the pain. It might be *hydrocodone* (Vicodin, Zohydro), *oxycodone* (Oxycontin, Percocet) or *hydromorphine* (Dilaudid).

Here's why it's risky: Compared with someone given a different kind of painkiller prescription or no prescription at all, you are five times more likely to be a chronic opioid user over the following year. So report researchers at the University of Colorado Anschutz Medical Campus in the *Journal of General Internal Medicine*. One reason, the researchers speculate—the drugs work for pain but also provide euphoria, and it's easy to get addicted even after original post-surgical pain is gone.

Better Solutions for Chronic Pain

Chronic pain affects about 100 million Americans, but relying on opioid prescriptions, especially for long-term relief (more than 90 days), greatly increases the risk for adverse side effects—constipation, drowsiness, concentration problems, driving accidents, vision impairment, reduced immunity and, for men, reduced testosterone levels.

Taking opioid medications for chronic pain is a dangerous, and sometimes deadly, slippery slope. To take a different path, work with a knowledgeable practitioner to start by exploring drug-free ways to handle pain.

Do Doctors in Your State Overprescribe Opioids?

Where you live can be a risk factor, too. The states with the highest prescription opioid addiction rates, according to the Centers for Disease Control and Prevention, are Alabama, Arkansas, Indiana, Kentucky, Louisiana, Michigan, Mississippi, North Carolina, Ohio, Oklahoma, South Carolina, Tennessee and West Virginia. Similar geographical differences also show up in Medicare claims. A map from the Centers for Medicare & Medicaid Services lets you see how your state stacks up against the national average in prescription opioid Medicare claims. Go to *cms.gov* and search "Opioid Drug Mapping Tool."

There are many reasons why some states have more opioid prescriptions (and addiction) than others, but one factor may be the prescription patterns of area doctors. So if you live in a high-use state, you may need to be extra-vigilant to avoid falling into a prescription addiction for chronic pain. Ask your doctor if there are better solutions for you.

The Truth About Blood Thinners

Stephen Kimmel, MD, MSCE, professor of medicine and epidemiology at University of Pennsylvania School of Medicine in Philadelphia.

For people at risk of developing dangerous blood clots—a main cause of stroke and other serious conditions—*warfarin* (Coumadin) has long been the granddaddy of anticoagulant medication. This pill is taken by about 3 million Americans.

Recent development: The FDA has approved four newer oral anticoagulants. (Other anticoagulants such as *enoxaparin* and *heparin* are available only as injections.) While the newer oral anticoagulants may offer certain benefits over warfarin, they are not the best choice for everyone.

Why this matters: Using the wrong anticoagulant drug (or dose) can have dire consequences, such as life-threatening bleeding in the brain or gastrointestinal tract.

Why an Anticoagulant?

Anticoagulants are used by people who are at increased risk for ischemic (caused by a blood clot) stroke and transient ischemic attacks, or "ministrokes"...or deep vein thrombosis (a blood clot in a deep vein), which can lead to a deadly pulmonary embolism (a blood clot in the lung). Anticoagulants also help prevent clots from forming in people who have an abnormal heartbeat (atrial fibrillation)...or have received a heart-valve replacement.

The Warfarin Standard

Warfarin has been used in the US for decades and is very effective at protecting high-risk people from blood clots. It's the only anticoagulant approved for use in people with mechanical heart valves.

Here's the catch: The amount of warfarin in the body must be regularly measured via a blood test called the International Normalized Ratio (INR). This allows doctors to monitor and customize the dosage for each individual patient, but it also means that you'll need frequent blood tests—weekly or monthly—to make sure that the drug is working properly. This testing is crucial, but not all patients do it as often as they should.

In addition, when you take warfarin, you must closely monitor your diet. Foods that contain vitamin K, such as leafy greens, broccoli and spinach, help your body make normal clotting proteins, which means they will work against the drug's action. For this reason, you should be consistent in the amounts of vitamin K–rich foods that you eat. Otherwise, the drug's effectiveness will be affected.

Also, warfarin interacts with more than 700 prescription and over-the-counter drugs as well as many supplements, including ginkgo biloba, St. John's wort, coenzyme

Q10 and others. You need to keep your doctor informed about everything you take. The newer drugs have far fewer interactions.

Better Than Warfarin?

Four alternatives to warfarin are now available in the US—*dabigatran* (Pradaxa), *rivaroxaban* (Xarelto), *apixaban* (Eliquis) and *edoxaban* (Savaysa). Clinical trials show a lower risk for hemorrhagic (bleeding) stroke with the newer drugs compared with warfarin. There is also a reduction in overall strokes with some of the newer drugs.

Other differences include…

•**No regular blood work.** There is no good way to monitor levels of these new drugs in the body, but they have proved effective without monitoring levels, so you won't have to endure weekly or monthly blood tests, as needed when using warfarin. However, the complete safety profile of new drugs is also unknown, and doctors cannot customize dosing for each individual.

•**There are no foods that work against the newer drugs, as there are with warfarin.** The newer drugs are as effective as warfarin no matter what you eat.

•**No antidote.** If a patient's blood becomes too thin and bleeding becomes uncontrollable, there is nothing to reverse it when using one of the newer anticoagulants. Warfarin does have an antidote.

Editor's note: More than 100 lawsuits have been filed on behalf of patients who were injured or died due to a major bleeding event after taking Xarelto. The manufacturer of Pradaxa agreed to pay $650 million in 2014 to settle about 4,000 similar claims.

•**A link to kidney function.** The newer drugs can be affected by your kidney function, so your doctor will need to consider this when choosing a medication and its dose.

How to Choose?

If you're taking warfarin and doing well, you don't need to think about trying one of the newer drugs—unless there are strong, compelling reasons to do so (such as an inability to get necessary blood work). Remember, newer drugs don't have as long a track record as older ones. That's why it's important to thoroughly discuss your medication options with your doctor.

What to consider…

•**If you have difficulty remembering to take pills throughout the day,** once-a-day Xarelto or Savaysa may be best for you.

•**If you play sports or have a hobby that may cause a bleeding accident,** warfarin might be best, since it is the only anticoagulant with an antidote that allows doctors to stop uncontrolled bleeding.

•**If you have a history of stomach problems or gastrointestinal bleeding,** you may want to avoid Pradaxa and Xarelto—both medications have the highest risk for these complications.

•**If cost is an issue, you may want to consider warfarin.** The newer anticoagulants are marketed only in brand-name versions that are much more expensive (even with insurance coverage) than warfarin, which is available in generic form. With warfarin, you also have the cost of the necessary routine blood work, but this expense may be covered by your insurance.

Caution: Do not stop using an anticoagulant without consulting your physician—this drug helps control your increased risk for stroke and other blood clot complications. Because of the bleeding risk associated with anticoagulants, people who use these drugs should wear a medical identification bracelet.

OTC Painkillers That Can Be Deadly

The Food and Drug Administration recently strengthened an existing label warning that non-aspirin nonsteroidal anti-inflammatory drugs (NSAIDs) increase the risk for heart attack and stroke. Popular over-the-counter medications including *ibuprofen* (Advil and Motrin) and *naproxen*

(Aleve) are among the products affected. Taking these regularly for as little as a few weeks can put people's lives at risk…as could exceeding recommended dosages.

What to do: If you take an NSAID, keep your dose as low as possible and your duration of use as short as possible. People who have a history of heart disease, kidney disease or stroke should be especially careful to limit NSAID use.

Hidden danger: When you take a cold medication or sore throat medication, check the ingredients on the label for NSAIDs. If you see these, avoid extended use and do not take these medications if you also are taking a painkiller that contains any NSAID—the combined dose could put you in danger.

Lynn R. Webster, MD, vice president of scientific affairs with PRA Health Sciences, and author of *The Painful Truth: What Chronic Pain Is Really Like and Why It Matters to Each of Us.* ThePainfulTruthBook.com

APPENDIX 3
OPTIMUM AGING

Stress Adds Years to Your Face: How to Erase It

Sanam Hafeez, PsyD, founder and clinical director of Comprehensive Consultation Psychological Services, with offices in New York City, Forest Hills and Uniondale, New York. Her research/clinical interests include neuropsychology, behavior modification and psychopathology. ComprehendTheMind.com

Compare the faces of two people in your life. Person One is happy, relaxed and pleased with life. Person Two is overworked, stressed and harried. Guess which face appears younger and more attractive?

Stress can add years to your looks. When you're stressed, your body churns out cortisol, the hormone that primes you for action. Some cortisol is helpful (and motivating), but too much triggers inflammation, which affects every organ in your body, including the skin.

Experts have coined a term for the link between emotions and the skin—psycho-dermatology. This new field is based on research that shows that chronic stress and other psychological issues can trigger or exacerbate skin changes. But you can reverse those changes using emotional strategies and other lifestyle changes.

Example: Critically ill children who were given relaxing massages showed improvements in itching, redness and other skin conditions, according to researchers at the Touch Research Institute at University of Miami.

You can spend a fortune on anti-aging products and cosmetic procedures, but unless you manage stress at the same time, you'll still look older than you should.

What Stress Does to Skin

Stress can cause blotches, itching, redness and acne. The cortisol-driven rise in inflammation damages tissues and capillaries that are readily apparent in the mirror. *Stress also causes…*

• **Dryness.** The constant bombardment of cortisol in women with chronic stress can mean a drop in estrogen that's been called mini-menopause. Estrogen is largely responsible for the differences in appearance between young women and older ones. Women who are frequently stressed tend to develop dryness and a loss of skin elasticity.

While women need estrogen more than men and are more impacted on a monthly basis by its regulation, hormonal imbalance also happens in men with the excess secretion of the stress hormone androgen, as well as glucocorticoids. This can cause a loss of estrogen, leading to dryness in both men and women and an overproduction of sebum (an oily secretion of the sebaceous glands), which can trigger acne and razor bumps.

• **Wrinkles.** There's a reason that forehead furrows, between-the-eye creases and other wrinkles are known as "frown lines," "worry lines" or even "battle lines." Repeated expressions can etch themselves permanently in your face.

• **Circles under the eyes.** They make you look tired and can age your appearance even more than wrinkles. Some people are genetically prone to under-eye circles. They also can be caused by sun exposure, a lack of sleep or allergic skin conditions, along with stress.

What happens: Stress increases blood flow, and the tiny capillaries under the eyes become engorged. Those dark circles really are blood vessels that are visible through the skin.

• **Under-eye bags.** Like circles under the eyes, these puffy areas are partly due to genetics. But they're also common in people whose stress keeps them up at night. A lack of sleep causes fluids to accumulate under the eyes and makes your face appear puffy and tired.

What to Do

Take "mini-vacations." Almost everyone can benefit from frequent "mini-vacations" that provide a break from stress. These can be as simple as a lunchtime walk…admiring a piece of art…or listening to a favorite song.

• **Eat an estrogen-enhancing diet including fresh fruits and vegetables, salmon and whole grains.** These antioxidant-rich foods fight inflammation. Fruits and vegetables also are naturally rich in phytoestrogens, plant compounds that mimic the effects of estrogen in the body. Estrogen "plumps" the skin and gives women and men a healthy glow.

• **Avoid excess sugar in all forms,** including refined carbohydrates, alcohol and highly processed foods, such as cake and cookies. These cause the body to produce advanced glycation end-products, toxins that trigger inflammation in the skin. The sugars in carbohydrates attach to certain proteins and can break down skin collagen, causing a loss of elasticity and the plumpness we associate with young skin.

• **Drink more water.** People who stay hydrated tend to have plumper, younger-looking skin. Also, water can flush excess salt from the body, which reduces under-eye puffiness. If you don't care for regular water, try coconut water. It is a natural source of electrolytes that help to keep you hydrated.

• **Relax your face.** You're probably not aware of your facial expressions, but you can learn to relax your face. When you're feeling stressed, remind yourself not to squint or frown. Be mindful of your expressions. Eventually, not frowning will become a habit. If you find yourself frowning, make it a habit to smooth your hand over your forehead and think happy, tranquil thoughts until your face naturally relaxes to a resting state.

• **Get a good night's sleep.** Even if you find that you can't log a full eight hours, at least make sure that the sleep you get is quality sleep. If you can't fall asleep in 15 or 20 minutes, get up and do something relaxing, such as gazing out the window or holding a yoga pose. You want to stay within yourself instead of engaging with electronics or the outside world until you're tired enough to try again. If you find yourself becoming anxious about all the things you have to do, make a list of what needs to be done.

Sleep with your head slightly elevated—a thick pillow will do it. The increased pull of gravity will help fluids drain away from your eyes.

• **Exercise.** Exercise relieves stress. You'll almost instantly see a difference when you attend a yoga class or go for a power walk. Your face will look smoother and younger.

Can Home Ultrasound Give You Better-Looking Skin?

Jennifer Peterson, MD, dermatologist and dermatologic cosmetic surgeon, private practice, Houston.

Dermatologists and plastic surgeons use ultrasound all the time. A well-placed ultrasound device can, for example, help tighten skin to reduce the appearance of lines, wrinkles and loose skin. The machines are big, powerful—and expensive.

But now less expensive and less powerful ones are available to use at home, for a few hundred dollars or even less. The claim is that home ultrasound machines make regular skin-care products more effective. But do they? Are they safe?

We took a close look at the website claims of one of the most popular products—the JeNu Ultrasonic Infuser System. It's a cordless rechargeable device about the size and shape of an electric razor. The instructions are simple—apply your regular skin-care product as you do normally, then put a small amount of conducting gel (a 60-day supply comes with the machine) on the head of the ultrasound wand and gently massage the area with the wand for a minute. The device is marketed as a cosmetic device, with no claims to cure or treat any skin condition.

To learn more, we spoke with Jennifer Peterson, MD, a dermatologist who is also board-certified in dermatologic cosmetic surgery. Dr. Peterson uses a commercial-grade ultrasound device in her office to provide cosmetic treatments for her patients, but she's also very familiar with JeNu, as many of her patients use it.

How Home Ultrasound Works: Tiny Hammers to Let Products In

The outer layers of your skin act as a barrier against the outside world, protecting the more delicate layers and everything else underneath. The top layer of skin is mostly dead skin cells...called keratinocytes...waiting to be shed. Living, healthy keratinocytes, which regenerate skin, sit a few layers lower, so skin-care products you put on your skin don't always penetrate well and reach them.

Ultrasound opens the way for better absorption. That conducting gel you apply to the wand, Dr. Peterson explains, has tiny "microspheres" that bounce around in response to the ultrasound energy. "The spheres are like tiny hammers that gently open up spaces between the cells and push the skin-care product inside, thus allowing the skin-care product to reach the healthy keratinocytes below."

Now let's take a look at JeNu's website statement—JeNu triples the absorption of skin-care products, based on an "independent lab test."

Here's the real story: The research wasn't published in a peer-reviewed scientific journal, so it did not have to meet the most rigorous standards. It was done at an independent lab, however, using objective and validated measurement techniques.

Result: While JeNu may have tripled absorption in certain parts of the test, the average increase was a more modest 45%, according to the lab report.

So this home ultrasound machine does improve absorption of products you put on your skin. But is that a good thing?

The Sound—and Risky— Use of Ultrasound

For the most part, Dr. Peterson thinks that at-home ultrasound devices are perfectly fine and can be a great help, especially for hydrating dry skin. When used as instructed on healthy, intact skin, they won't irritate or burn your skin. (If you have a skin rash or other condition, on the other hand, ultrasound could be irritating.) And those "little hammers" are so tiny that you won't feel them.

Now for the big "but." Not all skin-care products are meant to be absorbed at higher than the normal rate. For example, Dr. Peterson said, skin-care products containing salicylic acid, glycolic acid or lactic acid, which chemically exfoliate the skin, or retinols, which increase skin-cell turnover and slow the breakdown of collagen, can cause skin irritation when the "dose" your skin gets is higher than what the manufacturer intended. You don't need to avoid these products when using ultrasound, but be very cautious at first. Use every other day for a week, suggests Dr. Peterson. If there's no irritation, try increasing to daily use.

For regular over-the-counter moisturizers and other products without potentially irritating ingredients, it's fine to try them with ultrasound once a day and see how your skin reacts to the increased absorption. If you're OK after a few days, you can go up to twice a day. (If your products contain sunscreen, that's fine and unlikely to be irritating—but you won't get additional benefit, since sunscreen is supposed to be on top of your skin—it's a barrier.)

JeNu's website has similar precautions, including not using it if you have a skin condition or open sores and starting with just one minute per area each day to see how you react at first. Don't overdo it, says Dr. Peterson: "Most antiaging and antiacne skin-care products aren't meant to be applied three or more times a day."

Prescription skin-care products, on the other hand, are another thing entirely. You definitely don't want to be absorbing more of these until you find out from a health professional whether that's actually a good idea. Says Dr. Peterson, "Always check with your doctor before using JeNu, or any other ultrasound device, with any prescription medication."

Help for Old-Looking Hands

Prominent veins and tendons, thinning skin and brown spots (also known as "liver spots" or "sun spots") are very common as we age. Topical skin lighteners, such as over-the-counter Lumixyl, can be used at home. There are also many in-office treatments for brown spots and crepey skin, including chemical peels, microneedling and laser therapy.

Until recently, little could be done for the veiny hands that often betray our age. But the FDA has now approved Radiesse, a calcium-based volumizing filler that recontours hands and camouflages veins and tendons. Hyaluronic acid fillers have also been successfully used off-label for hand rejuvenation. The cost of these treatments is not covered by insurance.

Nelson Lee Novick, MD, clinical professor of dermatology, Icahn School of Medicine at Mount Sinai, New York City. YoungerLookingWithoutSurgery.com

No More Hot Flashes!

JoAnn V. Pinkerton, MD, executive director of The North American Menopause Society, Menopause.org. She is professor of obstetrics and gynecology and division director of Midlife Health at the University of Virginia Health System in Charlottesville.

Imagine trying to function in the world when, at any moment, you can be randomly dropped into a self-generating sauna. That's what it's like for women who have hot flashes.

While hormone therapy, hands down, works the best for most women, it's not a universal answer. Some women don't want to take hormones because the treatment has been linked to increased risk for breast cancer and heart disease. And hormone therapy is inappropriate for women who have had an estrogen-sensitive cancer or a history of blood clots.

Scientists have begun solving some of the mystery of what causes hot flashes. And research has recently revealed which non-hormonal treatments really help against hot flashes.

Solving the Mystery

New research has changed what we know about hot flashes. *Key findings…*

Before: Experts believed that symptoms of menopause lasted only about six months to two years.

Now: Research published in the April 2015 edition of *JAMA Internal Medicine* revealed that hot flashes go on for much longer than anyone thought—7.4 years, on average…and the earlier the symptoms started in perimenopause, the longer they were likely to continue after menopause.

Before: Hot flashes were believed to be an unfortunate but benign "side effect" of menopause.

Now: Recent research from the University of Pittsburgh School of Medicine published in *Obstetrics & Gynecology* suggests that hot flashes may be a marker for more serious disease processes. For example, studies have shown that women who have hot flashes are more likely to have higher levels of triglycerides and LDL "bad" cholesterol, putting them at greater risk for cardiovascular problems. This was true for all women who experienced hot flashes, but the risk was greater for women who had them frequently—on at least three days a week.

Another important study found that women with physiologically measurable hot flashes at night have more white matter hyperintensities—changes in the cerebral white matter (nerve fibers that connect brain cells) that could indicate a loss of blood flow in the brain.

Best Drug-Free Therapies

In November 2015, The North American Menopause Society (NAMS) published the results of its review of hundreds of scientific studies focusing on nonhormonal treatments for hot flashes. The goal was to determine which treatments really worked. In the NAMS review, two therapies stood out as providing significant relief from hot flash symptoms without hormones or other medication...

• **Cognitive behavioral therapy (CBT).** CBT is designed to help people change their underlying emotions, thinking and behavior patterns. The first step in CBT for hot flashes is relaxation—a clinical psychologist trains women in paced, slow breathing and stress-reduction techniques. Then women talk about their experience with hot flashes and learn how to manage their reactions. For example, instead of thinking, Hot flashes are ruining my life or I hope I don't get a hot flash in the middle of the meeting, women might learn to change their thoughts to, Hot flashes are temporary…They only last a few seconds…I know how to handle this. Over time, negative beliefs recede and the experience is less upsetting.

CBT can take a number of forms—individual or group therapy, or even take-home books or recordings. This is short-term therapy, usually requiring no more than eight hours spread over four to eight weeks.

Studies showed that after CBT, though the number of hot flashes didn't change, about 75% of participating women perceived the hot flashes differently and seemed psychologically better able to handle them. This improvement remained steady even six months later.

CBT is covered by some health insurance, but check with your provider. To find a therapist familiar with CBT, talk with your primary care physician or gynecologist. Or you can search for a therapist in your area by visiting the website for the Association for Behavioral and Cognitive Therapies at *ABCT.org*.

• **Clinical hypnosis.** This is a newer therapy for hot flashes that may provide even greater relief than CBT. You start by getting into a deeply relaxed state. Then the therapist uses individualized mental imagery (such as coolness, relaxation or a safe place) and suggestions to change the body state—in this case, from one that is susceptible to hot flashes to one that is not.

Two studies from Baylor University showed remarkable results from clinical hypnosis. Participants had about a 55% drop in hot flash frequency and a 65% drop in hot flash intensity. Hypnosis has also been shown to improve sleep.

The downside of clinical hypnosis is the effort required. In the study, participants attended weekly training sessions for five weeks and had to practice with an audio recording at home every day. Plus, not everyone can enter the state of deep relaxation necessary for hypnosis. The first step is to find a qualified practitioner through the National Board for Certified Clinical Hypnotherapists (*NatBoard.com*). Before your first visit, ask if the hypnotherapist has experience treating menopause symptoms.

For More Help

If you need more help for bothersome hot flashes, see a menopause expert (find one in your area at *Menopause.org* under the "For Women" tab). The physician can do an evaluation of the severity of your symptoms and work with you to find the best solution, whether or not that includes hormone therapy.

Women who have more than seven hot flashes per day or 50 per week, which disrupt their ability to function or sleep, or who experience heavy sweating are often good candidates for therapy. Don't suffer in silence. Ask for help!

Hormone-Free Help for Hot Flashes

Julia Schlam Edelman, MD, board-certified gynecologist and certified menopause clinician in private practice in Massachusetts. She is author of Menopause Matters: Your Guide to a Long and Healthy Life. JuliaEdelmanMD.com

---

About 75% of menopausal women experience these sudden rushes of heat that can leave them dripping with perspiration (so if you are approaching midlife and it hasn't happened to you yet, chances are that it will someday). Yet many are understandably reluctant to resort to the conventional treatment, hormone therapy, because it can increase the risk for heart disease, stroke, blood clots and breast cancer.

So here are some alternative therapies that have credible scientific evidence for being safe and effective at reducing hot flashes. For certain women whose menopausal symptoms are debilitating and whose risk for cardiovascular problems and breast cancer is low, the benefits of hormone therapy may outweigh the risks—but even so, it just makes sense to try safer alternatives first. *Here's what really works…*

Body-Cooling Breathing Technique

It sounds almost too good to be true, but paced respiration—a form of very slow, deep breathing—has been found to decrease the frequency and severity of hot flashes by up to 80%. To teach yourself paced respiration, sit comfortably in a quiet place where you won't be interrupted. Slowly inhale for five seconds

(counting to yourself, "one, one thousand… two, one thousand" etc.). Don't hold your breath after inhaling—instead, exhale in the same slow manner for five seconds (silently counting backward, "five, one thousand… four, one thousand" etc.). The goal is to take five to seven breaths per minute rather than the typical 12 breaths.

Practice twice a day until you can comfortably perform the technique continuously for 15 minutes—this trains your body to breathe slowly on command. Then, to reduce hot flash frequency, do paced respiration for five to 15 minutes each morning and evening. Also do the technique whenever you experience a hot flash or awaken from a night sweat—this makes symptoms subside more quickly.

Bonus: Paced respiration also reduces blood pressure.

Nutritional Heat Soothers

Various studies indicate that certain dietary approaches can help reduce hot flashes. *What works best…*

•**Flaxseed.** In a small study from Mayo Clinic, women who had at least 14 hot flashes weekly added four tablespoons of crushed flaxseed per day to their diets. After six weeks, they reported that their hot flashes had decreased in frequency by half and in severity by 57%, on average.

Theory: Flaxseed contains lignans, antioxidants that may have estrogenic effects. More research is needed, but in the meantime, flaxseed looks promising—plus it contains heart-healthy omega-3 fatty acids.

Try it: Add crushed flaxseed to cereal, juice, yogurt or fruit dishes. To avoid constipation (or even intestinal blockage), be sure to drink plenty of water at the same time.

Caution: Do not consume flaxseed within two hours of taking oral medication—flaxseed may interfere with medication absorption.

•**Fiber.** Research suggests that women whose daily diet includes at least 30 grams of fiber have fewer hot flashes than women who consume less fiber. The research is on fiber from foods rather than supplements, so to boost your fiber intake, eat more fruits, vegetables, brown rice and whole grains.

•**Vitamin E.** Though studies have had mixed results, some research indicates that vitamin E does help ease hot flashes. Taking up to 400 international units (IU) daily is safe for most women, though as with any nutritional supplement, check with your doctor before beginning.

Caution: To avoid bleeding problems, do not take vitamin E if you take blood-thinning medication, such as aspirin or *warfarin* (Coumadin), or an anti-inflammatory drug, such as *ibuprofen* (Motrin) or *naproxen* (Aleve)…if you supplement with evening primrose oil, ginkgo biloba, garlic or ginger…or if you have ulcers or heavy periods.

•**Cutting back on caffeine.** While any hot liquid can trigger hot flashes, caffeinated coffee is a particular problem because it disrupts sleep and promotes night sweats. Simply avoiding caffeine in the evening isn't enough—because six hours after you ingest caffeine, half of it still remains in your system. "This means that if you drink a medium cup of coffee containing 200 mg of caffeine at 4 pm, 100 mg of caffeine will still be left in your body at 10 pm," Dr. Edelman said. Tea has less caffeine than coffee but still may cause problems if you are sensitive to caffeine.

Abruptly eliminating caffeine can bring on severe headaches, so instead, cut back on your caffeinated beverage intake by two ounces for seven days…then cut back by another two ounces for seven more days. If your hot flashes disappear, you can continue drinking that amount…otherwise, keep reducing by two ounces per week. Does it really work? "I've had patients who completely got rid of their hot flashes this way."

A Juice That Relieves Menopause Symptoms

Women who drank about seven ounces of unsalted tomato juice twice a day for eight weeks reported a 16% improvement in hot flashes, fatigue and irritability.

Reason for the improvement: Tomatoes contain lycopene and gamma-aminobutyric acid (GABA). Lycopene reduces stress, and GABA helps ease hot flashes.

Study of 93 women by researchers at Tokyo Medical and Dental University, Japan, published in *Nutrition Journal*.

Coffee Drinkers Live Longer

Neal D. Freedman, PhD, MPH, cancer prevention fellow, division of cancer epidemiology and genetics, National Cancer Institute, Rockville, Maryland.

Coffee has already been shown by numerous studies to do plenty of wonderful things for your body.

For example, it's well known that coffee boosts concentration and reduces the risk for heart disease, type 2 diabetes, liver disease, Parkinson's disease, depression and Alzheimer's disease.

Recent research takes this good news a step further, showing that coffee lowers the risk for death from a wide variety of major diseases. In fact, it's the largest study to ever look at the link between coffee and health.

But how many cups do you really have to drink to potentially tack on years to your life? Is it a practical amount…or one of those absurd laboratory amounts that you often see in studies?

Brewing Health Benefits

At the start of the study, researchers at the National Cancer Institute in Rockville, Maryland, gave questionnaires to more than 400,000 men and women ages 50 to 71 and asked them to report their coffee intake. They noted whether they drank mostly caffeinated or decaf coffee, what type (regular ground, instant, espresso, etc.) and whether they added products such as cream or sugar.

Results: Regardless of the drink's caffeine content, the way the coffee was made or how much milk and/or sugar was used, the more coffee that people drank—up to about five cups a day—the lower their risk for death at the end of the 13-year study from health problems including heart disease, respiratory conditions, diabetes, stroke and infection. *Check out this chart...*

Coffee per day	Reduced risk of dying
8 ounces	5% to 6%
16 to 24 ounces	10% to 13%
32 to 40 ounces	12% to 16%
48 ounces or more	10% to 15%

Alas—no association was seen between coffee and death from cancer.

Results differed a little bit between men and women, with the association being slightly stronger for women than men.

Mo' Joe, Anyone?

Coffee's association with a lower death risk doesn't mean that a cause-and-effect relationship between the two was established.

And it's impossible, at this point, to know exactly what properties of coffee may be helpful in preventing death. Coffee's most famous constituent is caffeine, of course, but in reality coffee contains more than 1,000 compounds, including antioxidants and many others. Any of these could play a role.

Back in the mid-1990s, when the study began, a typical cup of coffee out on the street was actually a cup—about eight ounces. But with the rise of specialty coffee shops, today's "cup" is more like two or three cups. (Starbucks' "venti" large size for a hot beverage, for example, is 20 ounces or two and one-half cups—and for a cold beverage, it's 24 ounces or three cups.) So if you're downing a few of today's "mega-cups" of coffee each day, you're getting more ounces than you might realize. But that seems fine. In some people, lots of coffee can lead to side effects, such as the jitters and insomnia—but this study suggests that there's perhaps also a fantastic benefit to America's big coffee habit.

How to Get the Nap You Need

Sara Mednick, PhD, assistant professor, department of psychology, University of California, Riverside. Dr. Mednick is author of *Take A Nap!*

What if there were a safe, nontoxic, simple, free way to increase your alertness...boost your creativity... improve your memory...reduce your stress... and even reduce your risk for heart disease, all in just 20 minutes a day? There is. It's called a nap.

Napping Without Guilt

In our work-driven, activity-driven society, the hardest part of taking a nap is getting past that little voice in your head telling you that napping is a sign of laziness.

Reality: People who nap tend to be more productive, not less.

When you allow yourself that brief period of rest and refreshment, you wake up alert and energized, ready to be active for the rest of the day. The time you spend sleeping is more than made up for by the improved work or activity time a nap can give you.

Instead of a nap, you could just have coffee or another form of caffeine to perk yourself up, but a nap is a better idea. Caffeine

How Long Hot Flashes Can Last

Hot flashes may continue for 14 years. And the sooner they begin, the longer a woman is likely to have them. Women who started having hot flashes before they stopped menstruating were likely to continue having hot flashes for years after menopause. The median duration of hot flashes is almost seven-and-a-half years.

Study of 1,449 women led by researchers at Wake Forest School of Medicine, Winston-Salem, North Carolina, published in JAMA Internal Medicine.

makes you more alert, but it doesn't give you any of the other benefits of napping.

Example: Napping enhances performance on a wide range of memory tests. Studies show that a 90-minute nap is as good as a full night's sleep for improving memory.

The Sleep Cycle

To understand why napping can be so valuable, it helps to understand the basic concept of the sleep cycle and how it applies to both nighttime sleeping and daytime napping.

Through the night, your sleep moves through a consistent pattern of four distinct phases…

• **Stage 1.** This occurs when you're just falling asleep and generally lasts for only a few minutes. Your structured thinking gradually gives way to dreamlike imagery.

• **Stage 2.** After you've fallen asleep, stage 2 sleep takes over. During this time, many parts of your brain are less active, but stage 2 sleep is the sleep that restores alertness and helps consolidate motor learning—anything that involves muscle movements such as dancing or driving.

• **Stage 3.** When you move into stage 3 sleep, your brain waves slow down, so much so that this stage is also called slow-wave sleep (SWS). In SWS, your body repairs itself because growth hormone is secreted during this phase, which helps with muscle fiber growth and repair as well as bone growth—basically, the antidote to cortisol, a stress hormone—and consolidates memory, such as new information you've just learned (a phone number, for example) so that you'll remember it.

• **Stage 4.** During stage 4, you move into rapid eye movement (REM) sleep, or dreaming. REM sleep is when you consolidate more complex information and learning, such as a vocabulary list in a foreign language.

In the course of the night, you generally go through stage 1 sleep only once, just as you fall asleep. After that, you cycle through stage 2, stage 3 (SWS) and stage 4 (REM) sleep several times through the night. Each cycle takes about 90 minutes. Of that, about 60% is spent in stage 2 sleep. The amount of time spent in SWS and REM sleep varies through the cycles.

Your Optimum Nap

Most people feel a natural lull in their energy levels sometime during the afternoon. That's the natural time for napping—and in many countries, the traditional siesta happens then. Ideally, because one sleep cycle takes about 90 minutes, you would nap for that long and awaken feeling refreshed and alert.

Not too many of us can manage a full 90 minutes in the middle of the day, however, and not everyone feels the need to nap that long. *To choose the best nap length for you, decide what you want to get from your nap…*

• **Stage 2 nap.** Reduces sleepiness, heightens alertness, increases concentration, enhances motor performance and elevates mood.

Sleep for: 15 to 20 minutes.

• **Stage 3 (SWS) nap.** Clears away useless information, improves conscious memory recall and restores and repairs tissues.

Sleep for: 60 minutes.

• **Stage 4 (REM sleep) nap.** Increases creativity, improves perceptual and sensory processing, and improves memory for complex information.

Sleep for: 90 minutes.

The best time for your nap depends on several factors, including when you woke up and what type of sleep you want to get from your nap. Nap Wheel, explained on the next page, will help you determine when the ideal time for your nap is.

Napping and Your Health

We know that lack of sleep is definitely bad for your health, but is napping good for it? That has actually been a hotly debated question. Over the years, some studies seemed to show that people who often napped had a greater risk for death, especially from heart disease.

A Harvard University study, however, strongly suggests the opposite. In the study, more than 23,000 people in Greece were followed for an average of 6.3 years. None of the individuals had a history of heart disease, stroke or cancer at the start of the study, and they ranged in age from 20 to 86. The results showed that the people who regularly napped for at least 30 minutes at least three times a week had a 37% lower risk for death from heart disease than the non-nappers.

Taking a nap in the afternoon doesn't usually affect a person's ability to get to sleep at his/her normal bedtime or to sleep for the normal number of hours at night. In fact, many people who start taking daytime naps report that they fall asleep more easily at bedtime and feel more refreshed in the morning.

Exception: Don't nap within two to three hours of your usual bedtime—it could keep you from getting to sleep on schedule.

Sleep and Age

Older adults often find themselves waking up earlier than they used to and having trouble getting back to sleep. Shifting to an earlier wake-up time—and feeling the need for an earlier bedtime—is a natural part of the changes in body rhythm that come with aging. Rather than fighting your body's normal needs, accept them. A great way to make up for the lost sleep and help yourself stay up later? Take a nap!

Customize Your Nap

To use the Nap Wheel (*saramednick.com/htmls/book/napwheel.htm*) to design your own custom nap, drag the "wake-up time" dial to the hour you woke up. Then follow the hours clockwise until you reach the point in the day when rapid eye movement (REM) sleep and slow-wave sleep (SWS) cross—the point of ultimate balance.

Example: If you woke up at 7 am, that balance point would be 2 pm. Naps taken before the crossing point will have more REM sleep...naps taken after it will have more

SWS. All you have to do is decide what type of nap you want.

Also helpful if you have trouble falling asleep for your nap, try the Apple Sleep Cycle Power Nap app, available on iTunes. It includes three different nap modes, including one that wakes you gently after 20 minutes.

Secrets to Staying "Regular": Common Mistakes That Can Lead to Constipation

Anish Sheth, MD, a gastroenterologist at Princeton Medical Group and an attending physician at the University Medical Center of Princeton at Plainsboro, New Jersey. He is coauthor of *What's Your Poo Telling You?*

With so much attention being focused these days on irritable bowel syndrome, colitis, diverticular disease and other gastrointestinal (GI) problems, many people forget about the granddaddy of them all—constipation.

It's hands down one of the most common GI challenges, and 15% of American adults regularly suffer from the condition. And if you believe TV and magazine advertisements, more fiber (often from a supplement) is the solution.

What you're not being told: While fiber is helpful, it's not always the answer. In fact, constipation isn't as straightforward as most people imagine. There are many common mistakes that prevent some people from getting relief from constipation—and cause others to worry unnecessarily.

Among the most common...

MISTAKE #1: **Assuming that "normal" means daily.** Constipation is usually defined as having fewer than three bowel movements a week. But there's a wide range of "normal"—some people routinely have three bowel movements a week...others go three times every day.

Doctors usually do not worry about a few missed bowel movements. There is almost always a simple explanation—travel, a new medication (see below), changes in diet or simply a busy schedule that causes people to delay using the toilet.

When to be concerned: When constipation is persistent—especially when it occurs along with other symptoms, such as lumpy, hard stools, straining to have a bowel movement and/or feeling as though you can't completely empty the stool from your rectum. It's also cause for concern when someone's normal bowel habits suddenly change for no obvious reason. This could indicate irritable bowel syndrome, a thyroid condition or even colon cancer.

MISTAKE #2: **Not taking medication into account.** Many prescription and over-the-counter drugs as well as supplements can cause constipation as a side effect. People who aren't aware of this may resort to treatments, such as enemas, that they don't really need—or book unnecessary visits with their doctors.

Psychiatric medications, including tricyclic antidepressants, such as *imipramine* (Tofranil) and *amitriptyline* (Elavil), are notorious for causing constipation.

Other offenders: Blood pressure drugs, including calcium channel blockers and beta-blockers…narcotic painkillers…antihistamines such as Benadryl…and iron supplements.

My advice: If a new medication is causing constipation, ask your doctor if you can get by with a lower dose—or switch to a different drug. If that's not possible, you might need to be more aggressive with lifestyle changes—such as drinking more water and getting more exercise—both help keep stools soft and intestinal muscles active.

MISTAKE #3: **Depending only on fiber.** Getting more fiber from plant foods (especially pears, apples and sweet potatoes—all with skins on—and cooked greens) will usually increase the frequency and comfort of bowel movements…but not for everyone.

A form of constipation known as slow-transit constipation (STC) occurs when the intestinal muscles contract less often and with less force than normal. Some patients with STC improve when they get more fiber, but others will still need laxatives or other treatments.

My advice: If you have constipation that hasn't responded to dietary changes, ask your doctor whether you might have STC. You may need a colonic transit study, which involves swallowing a capsule containing a small amount of material that can be traced with X-rays to show its movement over a period of several days. This test will help your radiologist and gastroenterologist determine how quickly stool moves through your colon.

MISTAKE #4: **Rejecting laxatives.** Many people have the mistaken notion that laxatives should always be avoided. Admittedly, some of the laxatives used in the past were harsh—people who took them were nervous about being more than a few steps away from a bathroom. But newer laxatives are much gentler.

I usually recommend one of the osmotic laxatives, such as polyethylene glycol 3350 (MiraLAX) or good old Milk of Magnesia. They help stool retain fluid, which softens stools and stimulates bowel movements. It's obviously preferable to have "natural" bowel movements, but these laxatives are gentle enough for long-term use (under a doctor's supervision) and can be a good choice for those with health problems (such as Parkinson's) that often cause constipation.

Note: People with heart or kidney failure should avoid these laxatives—they can cause dehydration and/or a mineral imbalance.

MISTAKE #5: **Not checking the bowel.** Some people would rather not see what comes out (others closely examine their stools). I advise patients to take at least a quick look before they flush. The appearance of stools can provide important information about your GI health.

Color is a big one. Stools that are extremely dark could be a sign of intestinal bleeding. Bright red can indicate a recent meal of beets, a bleeding hemorrhoid or even colon cancer. Gray can mean that something's obstructing the flow of bile to the intestine.

Texture/shape is also important. Stools that are hard and pelletlike can indicate more severe constipation, which could have many underlying causes, including chronic conditions such as thyroid problems, diabetes or Parkinson's disease. "Floaters" are usually normal (they're caused by gas in the stools) but can also be a sign of conditions that impair fat absorption, such as pancreatitis.

MISTAKE #6: Avoiding enemas. Simple fixes might not help when you haven't had a bowel movement for a week or two. Stools that stay that long in the intestine can become almost rocklike and painful to pass. Enemas are also the best treatment for fecal impaction, a hard-stool blockage that's usually caused by lengthy constipation.

An enema, available as an over-the-counter saline laxative, increases the flow of water into the intestine. It softens hard stools and usually promotes a bowel movement within a few minutes. Follow package instructions. Fecal impaction that is not relieved by an enema may require a health-care provider to manually remove stool.

MISTAKE #7: Not eating enough prunes. Your grandparents were right—prunes (and prune juice) are an effective treatment for constipation. Prunes are high in fiber, but the main benefit comes from sorbitol, a sugar that draws water into the intestine. Two servings of prunes (about 10 fruits) contain 12 g of sorbitol...and eight ounces of juice has about 15 g.

Note: Drinking warm prune juice seems to be more effective at relieving constipation in some people. If you don't like prunes, consider trying rhubarb, artichokes and/or peaches—all of which promote regular bowel movements.

Important: If you're prone to constipation, limit your intake of processed foods, cheese and meat—these foods can slow down your digestive system.

You Don't Have to Give Up Those Car Keys

Patrick Baker, an occupational therapist, certified low-vision therapist and certified driver-rehabilitation specialist at the Cleveland Clinic in Cleveland, Ohio.

Driving may be the most hazardous thing that most of us do each day, but simply growing older—or having a chronic medical condition, no matter what your age, that affects your vision, thought process or physical abilities—doesn't mean that you can't continue to be independent.

To drive safely as long as possible: It's crucial to proactively avoid problems that can limit your car-handling competence. *Here's how...*

Preempt Problems

Beyond commonsense imperatives such as getting regular medical, vision and hearing checkups, a few simple steps will help ensure that your driving abilities are intact.

At your checkup with your primary care doctor, have a candid talk to discuss any medical conditions you may have that could affect your driving now or in the future.

For example, a stroke may result in lingering visual or movement problems...diabetes might be causing neuropathy in your feet, making it difficult to feel the gas or brake pedals...and cataracts, macular degeneration or glaucoma may limit vision if it's not carefully treated. A conversation with your doctor can help you minimize these issues and prevent them from becoming a bigger problem down the road. *Also...*

Manage Your Meds

Some prescription or over-the-counter medications can impair your ability to drive by triggering drowsiness, cutting concentration, inducing shakiness or uncoordinated movements, or increasing your reaction time. Taking multiple drugs—a common practice among older adults and those coping with chronic medical problems—can make matters even worse by amplifying medication side effects. Certain dietary supplements, such as *melatonin* or *valerian*, may also have an effect.

What to find out: Show your doctor or pharmacist a list of all the medications (prescription and over-the-counter) and dietary supplements you take and ask how they interact and may affect your driving abilities.

Also: Ask if the timing of when you take any drugs or supplements that may affect cognition or coordination can be altered—for example, taken before bedtime instead of in the morning.

Important: If you are on painkillers or narcotics, also ask your spouse or a trusted friend if the medication makes you "loopy"—an effect that you may not notice but is perhaps obvious to another person.

Customize Your Car

Age can compromise your eyesight and bring physical changes that make it more difficult to see the road while driving—for example, many people lose one to three inches of height due to bone loss and spinal compression. Or a stroke or eye condition (such as cataracts) may affect your peripheral vision, interfering with your ability to spot traffic alongside your car. To address these changes, it helps to customize your car. *Here's how…*

• **Set power seats at the highest level.** Also, consider adding a firm cushion (such as the durable type used for outdoor furniture) to the driver's seat so that your chin is at least three inches higher than the top of the steering wheel.

• **Use extra (or bigger) mirrors inside and/or outside your car to increase your field of vision.** For example, you can get a mirror that attaches to your rearview mirror to expand your view to the rear. Or you can get bigger mirrors or extra mirrors that can be bolted onto existing side mirrors or the side of the car itself. Check with your car dealer for details for your make and model.

• **Keep your headlights clean.** Also, consider replacing the bulbs—even before they burn out. The bulbs get dimmer before they've completely burned out.

• **Opt for automatic.** If you're buying a new car, be sure to get one with automatic transmission, power steering and power brakes, which don't require as much strength to operate. Also, consider a car with backup alert sensors, which detect objects in your blind spots.

Spruce Up Your Skills

A driving refresher course (ideally taken every three to five years) will keep you up to date on the newest traffic rules and can reduce road mishaps.

Good news: Some car insurance companies even lower premium rates if you take one of these courses, which usually lasts four to eight hours.

Good choice: A course such as those offered by AAA or AARP is likely to have an instructor who is well versed in issues facing older adults—as well as classmates who are true peers. If you are interested in taking a driver course because of a medical condition, consult The Association for Driver Rehabilitation Specialists (*ADED.net* and search "CDRS provider") to find a program near you.

Don't Cut Back on Water Intake When You Drive!

Limiting water intake to avoid bathroom breaks while driving can be dangerous.

Recent finding: Drivers who were mildly dehydrated made twice as many errors as drivers who were adequately hydrated. These errors included lane drifting, late braking and crossing the rumble strip.

Self-defense: Drink plenty of fluids.

Phillip Watson, PhD, a visiting professor in the department of human physiology at Vrije Universiteit Brussel in Brussels, Belgium. He led a recent study at Loughborough University, Leicestershire, UK, published in *Physiology & Behavior*.

Focus on Footwear

When it comes to hitting the gas and brake, what's on our feet can be just as important as our ability to see and react. Consider these important footwear-related issues...

• **Choose the right sneaker.** Running-style sneakers with soles that are thick, chunky and/or beveled can catch on pedals as you move your foot, so opt for a flat sole, such as a tennis-style or walking sneaker.

• **Go for thin soles.** People with diabetic neuropathy or limited foot sensation should wear thinner-soled shoes while driving. Thin soles, which don't have much padding between the bottom of the feet and the car pedals, give you a better sense of how hard you are pushing the brake and accelerator.

Important: Be sure to choose a car that "fits" you well—with good sight lines to the sides and rear...controls that are easy to reach...and a model that is easy for you to get in and out of.

Save Your Sight: Natural Ways to Fight Common Eye Problems

Jeffrey R. Anshel, OD, founder of the Ocular Nutrition Society and president of Corporate Vision Consulting, based in Encinitas, California, where he also has the private optometry practice E Street Eyes. He is author of *What You Must Know About Food and Supplements for Optimal Vision Care: Ocular Nutrition Handbook.* SmartMedicineForYourEyes.com

Vision problems in the US have increased at alarming rates, including a 19% increase in cataracts and a 25% increase in macular degeneration since 2000.

Why the increase? Americans are living longer, and eyes with a lot of mileage are more likely to break down. But not getting the right nutrients plays a big role, too—and the right foods and supplements can make a big difference.

Of course, people with eye symptoms or a diagnosed eye disease should work closely with their doctors. I also recommend medical supervision for people who are taking multiple supplements.

But here are common eye problems and the foods and supplements that can fight them...

Dry Eyes

The eyes naturally get drier with age, but dry-eye syndrome—a chronic problem with the quantity and quality of tears—often is due to nutritional deficiencies. Poor nutrition can permit damaging free radicals to accumulate in the glands that produce tears.

What to do: Take one-half teaspoon of cod liver oil twice a week. It's an excellent source of DHA (docosahexaenoic acid, an omega-3 fatty acid) and vitamins A and D, nutrients that improve the quality of tears and help them lubricate more effectively.

Also helpful: BioTears, an oral supplement that includes *curcumin* and other eye-protecting ingredients. (I am on the scientific advisory board of BioSyntrx, which makes BioTears and Eye & Body Complete, see next page, but I have no financial interest in the company.) I have found improvement in about 80% of patients who take BioTears. Follow the directions on the label.

Cataracts

Cataracts typically are caused by the age-related clumping of proteins in the crystalline lens of the eyes. More than half of Americans will have cataracts by the time they're 80.

What to do: Eat spinach, kale and other dark leafy greens every day. They contain *lutein*, an antioxidant that reduces the free-radical damage that increases cataract risk. (Lutein and *zeaxanthin*, another antioxidant, are the only carotenoids that concentrate in the lenses of the eyes.)

Important: Cook kale or other leafy greens with a little bit of oil...or eat them with a meal that contains olive oil or other fats. The carotenoids are fat-soluble, so they require a little fat for maximal absorption.

I also advise patients to take 500 milligrams (mg) of vitamin C three or four times a day (cut back if you get diarrhea). One study found that those who took vitamin C supplements for 10 years were 64% less likely to have cataracts.

The supplement Eye & Body Complete contains a mix of eye-protecting compounds, including bioflavonoids, bilberry and vitamins A and D. Follow instructions on the label.

Computer Vision Syndrome

The National Institute of Occupational Safety and Health reports that 88% of people who work at a computer for more than three hours a day complain of computer-related problems, including blurred vision, headaches, neck pain and eye dryness.

What to do: Take a supplement that contains about 6 mg of astaxanthin, a carotenoid. It reduces eyestrain by improving the stamina of eye muscles.

Also helpful: The 20/20/20 rule. After every 20 minutes on a computer, take 20 seconds and look 20 feet away.

Reduced Night Vision

True night blindness (nyctalopia) is rare in the US, but many older adults find that they struggle to see at night, which can make night driving difficult.

What to do: Take a daily supplement that includes one-half mg of copper and 25 mg of zinc. Zinc deficiencies have been associated with poor night vision—and you'll need the extra copper to "balance" the zinc. Zinc helps the body produce vitamin A, which is required by the retina to detect light.

Also helpful: The foods for AMD (see next article).

The Best Nutritional Defense Against Macular Degeneration

Robert Abel, Jr., MD, ophthalmologist and eye surgeon based in Wilmington, Delaware, and author of *The Eye Care Revolution*.

Andrew Rubman, ND, medical director, Southbury Clinic for Traditional Medicines, Southbury, Connecticut. SouthburyClinic.com.

Nutrition is a widely accepted ally in the fight against macular degeneration, the leading cause of vision loss in the US. But you can do more to protect your eyes than follow the standard recommendations, according to Robert Abel, Jr., MD, author of *The Eye Care Revolution*.

Current recommendations emphasize a few key nutrients once you have the disease. According to the National Eye Institute, a specific daily nutritional formula called AREDS—500 mg of vitamin C, 400 IU of vitamin E, 10 mg of *lutein*, 2 mg of *zeaxanthin*, 80 mg of zinc and 2 mg of copper—can slow the progression of existing macular degeneration from early stage to its advanced stage.

But Dr. Abel argues that certain foods and supplements are not only effective at slowing the progression of the eye disease but can prevent the disease as well. To be sure, there is no large-scale study proving that any one nutrition formula definitively prevents this sometimes devastating eye disease. But there is a substantial body of evidence that a variety of nutrients, including many that are not currently in the AREDS formulation, are important for prevention, according to Dr. Abel. We also spoke with naturopath Andrew Rubman, ND, for his recommendations on nutrient dosages that can protect your vision.

Here's the plan...

Starvation of the Retina: The Cause of Macular Degeneration

Age-related macular degeneration (AMD) is a condition that causes progressive damage to the delicate center of the retina called the macula. The macula is composed of light-sensing cells that allow us to see objects clearly. If you have AMD, over time you develop a blurry, distorted or dark area near the center of vision that interferes with the ability to see. People with advanced macular degeneration lose the ability to drive, read and recognize faces and, in some cases, they go blind.

The nutrition connection: Because the macula is so sensitive to light, it needs protection against the oxidation caused by exposure to UV radiation as well as environmental toxins and smoking. Many antioxidant nutrients work together to protect the eye and, in particular, the macula from this damage. When the eye isn't properly "fed," metabolic waste accumulates in tiny deposits called drusen, leading to AMD.

In short, according to Dr. Abel, AMD develops because our eyes are starved of the nutrients they need to protect themselves.

Feed Your Eyes With These Nutrients

• Docosahexaenoic Acid (DHA)

Why you need it: DHA is an omega-3 fatty acid found in high levels in algae and cold-water fish. Even though the AREDS 2 study didn't find that omega-3 supplementation slowed progression of AMD, Dr. Abel believes it is key for prevention. DHA is a major component of retina receptors and cell membranes.

Benefit by: Including cold-water fish such as tuna, salmon and mackerel in your diet two to three times a week. Supplement with DHA (500 mg) twice a day. It doesn't matter whether it's derived from fish oil or microalgae. Consult your doctor if you are taking a blood thinner such as *coumadin* (Warfarin)—even aspirin—since DHA also has blood-thinning effects. Dr. Rubman points out that because tuna is likely to contain high levels of mercury, it's best to limit consumption to no more than twice a week for people who are age 18 and older...and to no more than once a week for people who are younger.

• Lutein and Zeaxanthin

Why you need them: The cone cells in the macula have a very high density of yellow pigments, derived primarily from two carotenoids—*lutein* and *zeaxanthin*—that neutralize ultraviolet light damage to the retina, filter dangerous wave-lengths of blue light (from TVs, computers, tablets and smartphones) and stabilize the pigment layer beneath the retina.

Benefit by: Eating green leafy vegetables such as spinach, kale, mustard and turnip greens. Supplement with *lutein* (10 mg) and *zeaxanthin* (2 mg) daily. According to Dr. Rubman, even higher amounts of these two nutrients might be more beneficial. Check with a doctor who is knowledgeable about supplements for what would be best for you.

• Vitamin D

Why you need it: Vitamin D reduces inflammation in the retina by clearing amyloid beta, a waste product that can impair vision. Many studies have found that people who have a normal blood level of vitamin D (30 mg/dL to 60 mg/dL) are much less likely to develop AMD.

Benefit by: Getting your doctor to test your vitamin D level and, depending on the results, taking 2,000 IU to 5,000 IU daily of vitamin D-3.

• B-12 and Folic Acid

Why you need them: These B vitamins protect the macula and the optic nerve. A 10-year study published in *American Journal of Clinical Nutrition* (2013) showed that deficiencies of folic acid and B-12 substantially increased the risk for macular degeneration.

Benefit by: Eating plenty of leafy green vegetables for folic acid. Animal foods (seafood, red meat, poultry) are good sources of vitamin B-12. Supplement with sublingual (under-the-tongue) B-12 (100 micrograms to 500 mcg) and take a folic acid pill or capsule (500 mcg to 1,000 mcg) daily. Dr. Rubman also recommends periodic testing to make sure blood levels of B-12 are adequate.

• **Vitamin C**

Why you need it: Vitamin C protects against free-radical damage from exposure to UV light.

Benefit by: Eating fruits (oranges, grapefruit, strawberries, kiwi, mango, pineapple) and vegetables (broccoli, kale, peppers). Supplement with vitamin C (at least 1,000 mg) daily in a split dose twice a day between meals.

• **Vitamin E**

Why you need it: Highly concentrated in the retina, vitamin E prevents lipid per-oxidation (deterioration of fats) and protects against free-radical damage from UV light.

Benefit by: Taking 400 IU daily with DHA to support the cell membrane function.

• **Flavonoids**

Why you need them: Flavonoids are powerful antioxidants found in a wide variety of plants (especially blueberries and grapes) that improve the eye's adaptation to darkness (night vision) and improve or retard progression of macular degeneration. Studies find that moderate consumption of wine, which contains not only flavonoids but also other antioxidants, is associated with a lower risk of developing macular degeneration.

Benefit by: Drinking wine in moderation—one glass a day for women and up to two glasses a day for men—if you can drink alcohol safely. Flavonoids, such as bilberry, are widely available in supplement form as well. Dr. Rubman recommends 750 mcg to 1,000 mcg daily of a mixed flavonoid formula.

• **Taurine**

Why you need it: This amino acid, found in high levels in the retina, is thought to protect against both ultraviolet light and toxic substances.

Benefit by: Taking 500 mg daily.

• **Glutathione**

Why you need it: A super antioxidant, glutathione squashes free radicals that can damage vision. If you have macular degeneration, it's likely that you already have a significantly diminished level of glutathione.

Benefit by: Eating avocados, asparagus, eggs and garlic. And supplement with 500 mg daily, taken between meals with a small amount of fruit.

• **Garlic**

Why you need it: In food or as a supplement, garlic improves circulation, including in the eye. Improved blood flow through the tiny capillaries in the eyes brings in needed nutrients and helps eliminate waste products.

Benefit by: Including garlic in your meals and taking one odorless capsule (100 mg to 1,000 mg, depending on tolerance) daily. You may want to choose an "odorless" garlic supplement, such as Kyolic aged garlic extract.

• **Magnesium**

Why you need it: Magnesium helps improve the function of the small blood vessels such as those found in the eye, which helps to bring in nutrients and eliminate waste products.

Benefit by: Taking 500 mg daily.

• **Selenium**

Why you need it: Selenium, present in very high levels in the eye, protects against free-radical damage from UV light and is needed for the body to take full advantage of both vitamin E and glutathione.

Benefit by: Taking 50 mcg to 200 mcg daily.

• **Zinc**

Why you need it: Zinc, found in high concentrations in the eye (especially in the retina and its underlying tissues), helps bind the protective pigment layer of the retina to the underlying tissue. Zinc also helps to form connections between nerve cells.

Benefit by: Taking 80 mg zinc as zinc oxide daily.

Got Glaucoma? Skip Downward Dog

Study titled "Intraocular Pressure Rise in Subjects With and Without Glaucoma During Four Common Yoga Positions" New York Ear and Eye Infirmary of Mount Sinai, New York City, et al., published in *PLoS ONE*.

If you're one of more than three million Americans with glaucoma, certain yoga poses could put your vision at risk. In a recent study of older yoga practitioners (average age 62), including some with glaucoma, four yoga moves significantly increased pressure inside the eye, known as intraocular pressure. *The moves are…*

- **Downward-Facing Dog**
- **Standard Forward Bend**
- **Plow Pose**
- **Legs-Up-the-Wall Pose**

It's normal for eye pressure to increase in these positions even if you don't have glaucoma, and pressure did quickly return to baseline for both groups after they completed the moves. If you have glaucoma, which is more common over age 65, you may want to avoid head-down yoga positions.

Fortunately, you can find many other energizing and healing poses in the practice of yoga. If you have a teacher, ask him or her to guide you in developing a routine that doesn't put extra pressure on your eyes.

Better Vision in 6 Weeks or Less: Without New Glasses or Surgery

Larry Jebrock, OD, founder and director of Natural Vision Correction, Orthokeratology & Vision Therapy, in Novato, California. EyeExercises.com

If you're over 40, it's likely that you're not seeing as well as when you were younger—and if you're over 60, it's nearly certain that your eyesight has declined.

Breakthrough approach: Behavioral optometry—using eye exercises to improve vision—is an effective but usually overlooked method for stopping, slowing and even reversing the age-related decline of eyesight.

Vision Problems

If your eyesight has declined, you probably have presbyopia, a decrease in your ability to focus and see clearly at close distances, such as when you're reading or looking at the computer.

You also might have diminished contrast sensitivity—less light is reaching the retina, the lining at the back of the inner eye that transforms light into electrical impulses that are sent to the visual cortex in the brain. As a result, vision is "washed out" and the contrast between objects becomes less distinct. It may be difficult to see the difference between the sidewalk curb and the street, for example. Lessened contrast sensitivity also worsens glare from headlights at night or sun reflecting off windshields during the day.

The danger: Poor contrast sensitivity increases the risk for falls and car accidents.

Aging also decreases overall visual acuity, or sharpness of vision. And visual reaction time is diminished. It takes longer for the brain to register what has been seen.

The typical solutions to declining vision are corrective lenses (eyeglasses or contacts) and Lasik laser surgery, in which the cornea is reshaped. But for many people, stronger corrective lenses are needed every six to 18 months, as vision continues to worsen…and Lasik surgery often is not covered by insurance, doesn't always restore perfect vision and can cause dry eyes, glare and hazy vision.

Exercises Work

New scientific evidence: Researchers from University of California, Riverside and Brown University used eye exercises to improve the eyesight of 16 younger people (average age 22) and 16 older people (average age 71), and published their results in *Psychological Science*.

After just seven days, diminished contrast sensitivity was eliminated in the older group—in other words, their contrast sensitivity reversed, becoming the same as that of the younger group. And both younger and older adults had improved visual acuity in the problem areas common to their age—older people saw near objects more clearly, and younger people saw far objects more clearly.

Here are three vision-restoring exercises you can do at home. Results can be immediate or take up to six weeks. Once your eyes have improved, keep up the exercises, but you can do them less often. Your eyeglass/contact prescription may change, so see your eye-care professional.

● **Improve near vision and far vision.** Practice this simple eye exercise for three or four minutes a few days a week.

Instructions: Look at a calendar on a wall about 10 feet away. In your hand, have another object with numbers or letters, such as a small calendar or an open book. Cover the left eye with your hand. Look back and forth from the far object to the near object, focusing on and calling out a letter or number from each.

Example: The "J" in June from the far calendar and the "12" in June 12 from the near calendar. Do this five to 10 times, calling out a different letter or number each time. Cover the right eye, and repeat the exercise. (You also can use an eye patch to cover one eye and then the other.)

Bonus benefit: It's common after a car accident for the person who is at fault to say that he "never saw" the other vehicle. I call this inattentional blindness—your eyes are on the road, but your vision system is not fully activated, because you're thinking or moving or otherwise preoccupied. The near-far exercise also improves visual attention.

● **Improve peripheral vision**—the "other" visual system. Corrective lenses correct only central vision, when the eyes focus straight ahead, so that you can read, drive and see details sharply. But there are two key parts to the visual system—central and peripheral vision. And improving peripheral vision improves every aspect of seeing, from visual acuity to contrast sensitivity.

Everyday enemy of peripheral vision: Stress. Under stress, people see less, remember less and typically the visual field constricts. But there's a simple exercise called "palming" that relieves stress and eases eyestrain.

Instructions: Sit at a table with your elbows on the table. (Put a pillow under your elbows if that's more comfortable.) Breathe easily and deeply, relaxing your body. Close your eyes, and notice what you're seeing—it's likely there will be visual "chatter," such as spots and flashes of light. Now cup your palms over your closed eyes, and visualize (create mental imagery of) blackness.

Example: Visualize yourself out on the ocean on a moonless night on a black ship on a black sea. The goal of the exercise is to see complete blackness.

Relaxing, breathing deeply, blocking out light and "visual chatter"—and even the warmth of your palms—relaxes the visual system and helps to open up peripheral vision.

Do the exercise for as long as you like, from 30 seconds to 30 minutes.

● **Improve "binocularity"**—seeing out of both eyes. A common but little-recognized vision problem in older adults is a lack of binocularity—one eye is not processing visual detail, which decreases visual acuity and depth perception (crucial for stepping off a curb or walking up stairs without stumbling or falling). This exercise can help you see with both eyes.

For this exercise you'll need a Brock String, named after its inventor, the optometrist Frederick Brock. It's a simple device—a 10- or 12-foot string with several colored beads on it. (The Brock String is widely available online for around $10 or less.)

Instructions: Attach one end of the string securely to a wall with a nail, tack or tape. Sit 10 feet away from the wall, holding the string so that there is no slack. The closest bead should be about four feet from your eyes.

Hold the string to the side of your nose and look directly at the closest bead, using both eyes—you should see two strings going toward the bead and crossing either in front of or behind the bead. You're "seeing double" because the device is engineered to generate a double-image, similar to what you might see when your eyes are relaxed and unfocused. This experience helps you become aware that you're seeing out of both eyes. If you see only one string, you're not seeing fully out of both eyes. And if the strings cross in front of or behind the bead, your eyes aren't aimed right at the bead. The goals of the exercise...

• **Keep both strings "turned on" (your eyes will get a "feel" for how to do this).**

• **The strings should cross at the bead—if the string crosses ahead of the bead, look a few inches beyond the bead...if the string crosses behind the bead, look in front of the bead.**

Do the exercise for three or four minutes, two or three times a week.

The Critical Test Most Doctors Don't Do

Katherine Bouton, author of *Living Better with Hearing Loss: A Guide to Health, Happiness, Love, Sex, Work, Friends...and Hearing Aids* as well as *Shouting Won't Help*. She is a member of the board of trustees of the Hearing Loss Association of America, Hearing-Loss.org, and has had progressive bilateral hearing loss since she was 30.

If you get an annual checkup, you probably assume that you're doing everything you need to do to take good care of your health. But chances are your physicals have not included a test that's crucial to your physical and mental well-being.

Shocking fact: Only about 30% of primary care physicians do a basic screening of their patients' hearing. In fact, most adults haven't had their hearing tested since they were in grade school! For most people with hearing loss, this means their problem (or the severity of their deficiency) goes undetected.

And don't assume that only the oldest adults are affected. More than half of the 48 million Americans who have trouble hearing are under age 55, and most of them aren't getting treatment.

Ignoring hearing loss is dangerous: In addition to the social isolation and depression that sometimes occur when people have trouble hearing, the condition has been linked to an increased risk for dementia. While there is more research to be done, many neuroscientists believe that if you are working hard to comprehend what's being said, you are using up the brain's stores of "cognitive reserve," which would instead be devoted to analytical thinking or memory.

That's not all. Because most age-related hearing loss occurs in the inner ear, which regulates balance, ignoring the problem increases one's risk of falling by three-fold. Hearing loss also makes driving and walking on the streets less safe because you don't hear car horns and other traffic noises.

My story: My hearing loss began suddenly when I was 30. Like many people, I resisted getting help and didn't get hearing aids for 20 years. That was a mistake!

Keeping It Simple

Testing for hearing loss is painless and easy. *My advice...*

• **Start now!** No matter what your age, ask your primary care physician to do a hearing screening during your annual physical. Professional guidelines vary on the frequency for such testing, but I believe that it's important enough to get screened every year—subtle changes can easily go unnoticed if you wait too long between testing.

As an initial screening, your primary care doctor will likely ask you a series of questions such as: "Does your spouse complain that the TV is too loud?" and "Do you find that people often say, 'Oh, never mind. It's not important.'?" The doctor may also snap his/her fingers behind your head or rub his fingers together next to your ear. If you seem to be having trouble hearing, he'll refer you to an audiologist for diagnostic testing. (An otolaryngologist, or ear, nose and throat specialist, may also employ an audiologist who gives hearing tests.)

•**Go to a true professional.** Try to stick to your doctor's referral. Lots of hearing-aid shops employ people who may not have adequate training to accurately diagnose hearing loss. You want to be sure to see an audiologist. They're trained to diagnose, manage and treat hearing and/or balance problems. An audiologist can also fit you with hearing aids.

The Best Testing

When you go to an audiologist, you'll be asked about your general health history, work history, exposure to noise and use of certain medications—drugs such as nonsteroidal anti-inflammatory drugs (NSAIDs), certain antibiotics and loop diuretics (commonly used to treat heart failure) can cause temporary hearing loss...and repeated doses of other drugs, including the cancer drug *cisplatin* (Platinol), can cause permanent hearing loss. The audiologist will then take you to a soundproof room for the following tests...

•**Pure-tone test.** This test provides a baseline of the softest level at which you can hear sounds.

What happens: You put on headphones, and the audiologist activates tones at different pitches and loudness. You respond by raising a finger or pressing a button when the tone is heard. The test is given in one ear at a time. If the test is normal, the audiologist will probably send you home. If not, other tests follow.

•**Bone-conduction test.** This test helps identify whether hearing loss originates from the inner, middle or outer ear.

What happens: You will be fit with a headset that has a vibrator placed on the bone behind the ear. This bypasses the ear canal (outer and middle ear) and sends vibrations directly to the cochlea (inner ear).

Again, the audiologist will activate tones at different intervals.

If the result is normal or better than the pure-tone test, it suggests the problem is in the middle or outer ear—sound is not getting through to the cochlea. If the result is worse than the pure-tone test, it points to a problem in the cochlea.

•**Speech perception test.**

What happens: While hiding his mouth (so there's no cheating by lipreading), the audiologist reads a list of common two-syllable words (or a recording is played) to determine the lowest level at which you can correctly identify 50% of the words spoken. If you cannot hear 50% of the sounds, the volume is turned up until you can. The test is given in quiet or with noisy background sounds. It helps to determine the extent of hearing loss and the need for a hearing aid.

•**Tympanometry test.** This test helps detect problems in the middle ear. It can reveal tumors, fluid buildup, impacted earwax or a perforated eardrum—all of which can lead to hearing loss.

What happens: The audiologist uses a probe that changes the air pressure in the

Calcium Is Linked to Vision Loss

Taking more than 800 mg/day of calcium was associated with nearly twice the risk of being diagnosed with age-related macular degeneration (AMD), which can cause severe vision loss.

Important: Calcium has important benefits for many medical conditions, including osteoporosis and high blood pressure. Do not reduce or discontinue use of calcium supplements without speaking to your doctor.

Caitlin Kakigi, BA, a medical student in the department of ophthalmology, University of California, San Francisco, and coauthor of a study of 3,191 national health survey participants, age 40 or older, published in JAMA Ophthalmology.

ear canal and causes a healthy eardrum to easily move back and forth.

Important: While you're being tested, stay still and do not speak or swallow to make sure your results are accurate.

What's Next?

If your audiologist recommends hearing aids, don't panic. Unlike the bulky devices you may have seen in the past, today's hearing aids are comfortable, highly effective—and most are small enough to not be seen when looking at the wearer's face. But they are also expensive—up to $4,000 per aid—and are not covered by insurance.

For people with mild-to-moderate hearing loss, personal sound amplification products (PSAPs) are a less expensive option (up to $700 a pair). They help in specific situations, such as a noisy restaurant, crowded airport or large lecture hall.

This Supplement Protects Against Hearing Loss

Andrew Rubman, ND, medical director, Southbury Clinic for Traditional Medicines, Southbury, Connecticut. SouthburyClinic.com.

Study titled "Activation of SIRT3 by the NAD+ Precursor Nicotinamide Riboside Protects from Noise-Induced Hearing Loss," by researchers at Weill Cornell Medical College and the Gladstone Institutes, published in *Cell Metabolism*.

A natural, noninvasive remedy that prevents hearing loss would be a big health boon. After all, 38 million Americans have hearing loss, including 14% of people between ages 45 and 65 and 30% to 40% of those over age 65. Hearing aids are a great help, but even the best are a poor substitute for the miraculous miniature machinery of the inner ear.

Now researchers seem to have a strong candidate—a building block of niacin (vitamin B-3) that's already found in tiny amounts in

milk and that has protected hearing in studies. It's called nicotinamide riboside, or NR for short. Even better, NR may have cardiovascular and brain benefits and for that reason is being added to antiaging supplements.

So, for people who want to protect or improve their hearing, is this vitamin-related supplement safe and ready for prime time?

The Big Bang Hypothesis

The most common type of hearing loss is called "noise-induced" and results from exposure to loud and/or high-pitched sounds. This damages the sensitive hair cells of the cochlea, the part of the ear that transmits sound to the spinal ganglion, which sends the information on to the brain. Significant noise exposure also damages the synapses connecting the nerves of the inner ear and the hair cells.

At Weill Cornell Medical College, researchers gave mice NR and then exposed them to noises loud enough to damage the cochlea.

Results: Mice that were given NR five days before the noise exposure and for 14 days afterward had less damage to the synapses of the inner ear than mice that weren't given NR. In separate experiments, similar benefits were found with NR given only before the noise (for five days) or only after the noise (for 14 days).

This evidence of NR's ability to protect the inner ear from noise damage is promising because it follows previous studies showing that a coenzyme that is in all body cells, nicotinamide adenine dinucleotide (NAD+), is a key factor in age-related hearing loss. NR helps the body make NAD+. Digging deeper, the researchers demonstrated that NR and NAD+ both protect cells from hearing damage because they increase the activity of a protein known as sirtuin3 (SIRT3).

SIRT3, it turns out, is a famous molecule. It's been known for decades that feeding animals a nutritious yet very low-calorie diet lengthens life. So does exercise. Both boost SIRT3, which helps keep mitochondria, the cells' energy engines, healthy. SIRT3 protects neurons. Because levels of SIRT3 naturally decline with age, researchers think that lowered levels of the protein might be at the heart of age-related hearing loss…and other age-related diseases including Alzheimer's disease.

So it should come as no surprise that NR, which boosts SIRT3, is hot right now on the supplement market. One company, Niagen, markets 250-mg capsules of NR. Another, called Elysium Health, guided by Nobel Prize winners in molecular biology and related fields, sells Basis, an antiaging supplement that includes 250 mg of NR and 50 mg of pterostilbene, a neuroprotective compound found in blueberries.

Should You Take NR to Protect Your Hearing?

The promise of this new research realm is truly exciting, but let's walk back this particular study. Remember, this is early research. The mice got about 455 mg of NR for each pound of body weight by injection. The human equivalent would be about 50,000 mg of NR for a 110-pound person. How taking 250 mg in an oral supplement (the amount in the products mentioned above) relates to receiving 50,000 mg by injection (the equivalent used in the study) is, well, unclear. On the plus side, NR is found naturally in food—there are tiny amounts in milk and, possibly, in beer—and it appears to have a good safety profile. It's not likely to cause flushing, like large doses of niacin (vitamin B-3) do.

To put all this in perspective, we checked in with naturopathic physician Andrew L. Rubman, ND. He's not quite ready to jump on the NR bandwagon for everyone: "I don't believe that supplementation will be either advisable or productive as a generalized intervention to slow aging or produce other supported claims generated by mouse studies," Dr. Rubman said.

However, if you have hearing loss, Dr. Rubman said, it's a different story—you may want to check with your doctor about your body's level of NAD+. (Yes, some labs can test for this, as part of testing for a B-3 deficiency.)

Reason: "For a limited segment of the population that have pathologies related to NAD+ biosynthesis, some supplementation with NR (which helps the body make NAD+) may be helpful." (In case you're wondering, NAD+ itself is not a stable compound and can't be taken as a supplement.)

Dr. Rubman is comfortable with doses as high as 2,200 mg a day, preferably as a part of a plan that you and your doctor work out. Because of possible interactions with other B vitamins such as thiamin and riboflavin, Dr. Rubman recommends that NR supplements be taken along with a multi-B vitamin supplement. He often prescribes two doses a day to his patients for better absorption.

Sounding "Old" Is Not About Age

Study titled "Voice Changes in Elderly Adults: Prevalence and the Effect of Social, Behavioral, and Health Status on Voice Quality" by researchers at Research Institute and Hospital, National Cancer Center, Gyeonggi, and University of Ulsan, Seoul, both in South Korea, published in *Journal of the American Geriatric Society.*

I f you read "Little Red Riding Hood" aloud to a child, you probably make Grandma's voice weak and quavering to sound "old." But the truth is you can have a strong voice at any age—unless you have a specific health problem…one that affects your whole health, not just your vocal chords.

In a recent study of 420 seniors (average age 72) with *dysphonia,* the medical term for decreased ability to produce a normal voice, South Korean researchers found that, compared to statistical averages, they were 300% more likely to have a particular medical condition—low thyroid function.

The condition, called hypothyroidism, is easy to overlook because many of the symptoms—constipation, fatigue and sensitivity to cold—are also symptoms associated with aging. While the new study doesn't prove causation, it does suggest that in an otherwise apparently healthy 60-plus person, a weakening voice could be a clue—perhaps the only clue—to this health-compromising condition.

So if you have a "grandmotherly" voice or know someone who does, speak up—to a doctor. Ask him or her to test your thyroid function.

Headstand for Health?

A headstand, or the sirsasana pose as it is known in yoga, can provide many health benefits, such as improved muscle strength, circulation and balance. Performing a headstand requires upper-body and abdominal strength, so maintaining overall physical fitness to achieve this position will help keep you mentally sharp and youthful.

If you're not up for a headstand, older adults can get the same benefits by taking brisk walks, swimming or doing other forms of exercise every day. Even working out as little as one hour a week can cut dementia risk, recent research has found. If you want to do headstands, check with your doctor first. They should not be done by anyone with neck or back problems, osteoporosis, high blood pressure or glaucoma (see also page 334).

Rammohan Rao, PhD, associate research professor, Buck Institute for Research on Aging, Novato, California.

Anxiety Disorders Speed Aging

People with untreated anxiety disorders—including social phobia, agoraphobia and panic disorder—had shorter telomeres (the DNA at the end of chromosomes) than people without such disorders. Telomeres get shorter with age. People with untreated anxiety were found to have three to five years more cellular aging than those without anxiety disorders.

But: Treatment of the disorders may reverse the shortening of telomeres. People whose symptoms had improved for 10 years or more had longer telomeres than those whose symptoms had improved for a shorter time.

Study of more than 2,300 people by researchers at VU University Medical Center, Amsterdam, the Netherlands, published in *The British Journal of Psychiatry*.

Eat More Protein, But Do It Right to Avoid Muscle Loss

Douglas Paddon-Jones, PhD, professor, department of nutrition and metabolism, The University of Texas Medical Branch, Galveston.

A re you young at heart? What about "young at body"? We go crazy trying to maintain that goal, but the truth of the matter is that most of us lose 0.5% to 1% of muscle mass per year starting at age 40. So by the time we hit 60, this gradual loss has really added up. Age-related muscle loss increases the risk of falling. It also can cause you to gain or lose too much weight either because of muscle wasting or because you don't have the energy to stay in shape. And not only will you feel old, you'll likely look old. There's an easy way, through diet, to help prevent loss of muscle mass, but there is some controversy about how to do it right.

The Truth About Protein

As we age, we experience anabolic resistance. This means that the body does not turn the protein we consume into muscle as efficiently as it once did. Researchers at the University of Arkansas for Medical Sciences have come up with a solution. They say to eat a lot of protein*—much more than the USDA recommended daily allowance (RDA) of 0.8 grams per two pounds of body weight, which amounts to about 48 grams per day for a 120-pound woman and 68 grams for a 170-pound

*Check with your doctor before increasing your protein intake especially if you are at risk for chronic kidney disease.

man. They recommend doubling that amount. These researchers found that it was OK to protein-load at dinner, as most adults do, as opposed to worrying about getting equal amounts of protein at every meal. You'll still reap the benefits of increased protein intake, they said.

They conducted a study in which they divided 20 adults, ages 52 to 75, into four groups. Two groups were assigned a diet that matched the USDA RDA standard, with one group consuming protein in equal portions throughout the day and the other consuming the majority of it at dinner. The other two groups consumed twice the USDA RDA standard, following the same even and uneven protein-distribution patterns.

The results: After just four days, regardless of the distribution of protein, those who consumed the higher amount of it had higher whole-body net protein gains with higher rates of protein synthesis—the ability to turn protein into muscle—compared with those who ate less of it.

Eat Protein Right

But hold off on packing in the protein at dinner. Douglas Paddon-Jones, PhD, professor of nutrition and metabolism at The University of Texas Medical Branch, Galveston, challenges the study findings and says that we should think in terms of maximum protein consumption per meal and not focus on the total protein consumption per day.

Like most researchers, Dr. Paddon-Jones agrees that increasing protein consumption over the RDA is important when it comes to building and maintaining muscle mass and function, especially for older adults. But protein-loading at dinner or at any meal will not produce the same protein synthesis as eating adequate amounts of protein throughout the day.

Through his research efforts, Dr. Paddon-Jones found that somewhere around 30 grams of protein, which equals about four ounces of lean meat, is close to the maximum amount of protein our bodies can use at one time to build and repair muscle. Although there is no harm and potentially some benefits to consuming additional protein at each meal if your energy demands are high, excess consumption of any macronutrient is increasingly likely to be turned into glucose and eventually fat. Our bodies don't have the temporary storage capacity for excess protein to be used later or the next day in the same way carbohydrates and fat are used.

Between 25 grams and 30 grams of protein is all most of us need per meal.

Treat Meals Right

Breakfast is the low hanging fruit when it comes to improving your protein intake per meal because it's the meal that people most often skip or the one that is usually virtually devoid of any protein. Getting at least 25 grams of protein at breakfast might seem daunting to many. Adults should forgo bagels, croissants and sugary cereals and consider eggs (two scrambled equals 14 grams of protein), yogurt (20 grams per seven-ounce container of 2% fat Greek yogurt) and oatmeal (6 grams per one-cup serving of regular cooked, not instant). Add nuts (6 grams per ounce of almonds), whole-wheat toast (7 grams per two slices) and a latte (8 grams per cup of milk) and you'll be up to

25 grams of protein quicker than you can say mocha cappuccino.

On the flip side, while many people skip breakfast, they overeat protein at dinner, often eating a steak the length of their forearm or a chicken breast the size of their face. OK, maybe we are exaggerating just a bit—but you get the picture. Most lean meats have about 30 grams of protein per four-ounce serving. Anything over that amount is probably not doing you a lot of good even if it's the only protein you've eaten all day.

For vegetarians or vegans, soy, legumes, quinoa, nuts and mushrooms are protein-rich foods and all vegetables have some sort of protein in them. Spinach, for example, has five grams per cup.

If you're too busy to get your protein from food at any given meal, protein powders or bars can be an alternative—but read labels carefully. The 20 to 30 grams of protein that come in a serving of whey protein powder, for example, won't do you as much good if the product is laden with sugar and fat.

Build Muscle Through Diet

As we all know, diet and exercise are both important when it comes to health, regardless of age. But focus first on nutrition in preparation for exercise, because diet is the fundamental to getting the most benefit from fitness routines. Consuming the optimal amount of protein per meal will maximize your body's ability to use that protein efficiently.

Swings for Grown-Ups: Multigenerational Fitness Parks Are the Latest Trend

Chhanda Dutta, PhD, chief, clinical gerontology branch, division of geriatrics and clinical gerontology, National Institutes of Health, Bethesda, Maryland.

Colin Milner, founder and CEO, International Council on Active Aging (ICAA), Vancouver, British Columbia, Canada.

Do you ever get the impression that outdoor fitness spaces are only for the young? Kids get playgrounds, while adults get…walking paths…and park benches. Even if you're lucky and your park has outdoor fitness trails dotted with exercise equipment, they're likely geared toward the young and fit…the Ironman-triathletes-in-training.

What about the rest of us who, no matter what our age, want to stay fit and agile, flexible and strong, and have some fun doing it out in the fresh air? Now there's a movement to create a new kind of outdoor activity space. Call them fitness parks, outdoor gyms or playgrounds for seniors, they're popping up in local and national parks, town recreation centers, retirement communities and senior centers. "I've been to 33 countries now, and almost every single country I've been to has them," says Colin Milner, founder and CEO of the International Council on Active Aging (ICAA) in Vancouver, British Columbia, Canada. "The popularity is really picking up."

Why the sudden interest? Outdoors is where we are. As we age, we're less likely to do strength training in an indoor gym, but we still walk outdoors. "If the older people aren't into fitness centers, take the fitness

---

Strong Arm Yourself

Toned arm muscles can help you look younger. Consider working with a trainer to learn the best exercises for you. Sagging biceps and triceps in the upper arm can make women look old. Exercising with dumbbells is the best way to tone these. Start with very light dumbbells if necessary—even two-pound weights can make a difference. Do bicep curls, hammer curls and tricep exercises several times a week.

Lauren Rothman, style and trend expert. She is a style consultant for individuals and corporations in the greater Washington, DC, area and author of *Style Bible: What to Wear to Work.* StyleAuteur.com

center to them!" says Milner. A related trend: Many parks are replacing outdoor trails and exercise areas designed for a younger fit population with equipment that is more accessible to everyone.

Read on to find out how this new kind of fitness equipment works (spoiler alert—it's fun!) and how you can take advantage of the new fitness movement in your own community.

A Seesaw You Won't Fall Off

Some of these fitness parks are multigenerational, so that, say, grandparents can easily play with their grandchildren. (And that means actually play—not just stand there and watch the urchins go down the slide.) The equipment is easy to use, low impact and designed to prevent falls. It works almost every muscle group, yet can be used by people with limited agility, balance and flexibility. Some equipment allows people in wheelchairs to roll up and participate. *You might see…*

•**A swing that is strong and has wide seats so adults,** and not just kids, can use it.

•**A slide that's adult-sized and has a gentle slope so it's safe for all ages.**

•**A roomy, comfortable outdoor recumbent bike that's easy to get onto and off of—and inviting to use.**

•**A two-person cross-country ski machine that's easy to use** and fun for people of any age from teens to octogenarians—truly multigenerational.

•**An elliptical machine in which you stand and simply swing your legs to and fro**—a great way to improve range of motion.

•**A "Tai Chi Spinner"**—two wheels, one for the right hand and one for the left, that you can rotate this way and that way together or separately to improve flexibility in your arms, shoulders and wrists. (It's also good as a warm-up for golf.)

•**A two-person "rotator"**—think of it as a really safe seesaw—that stretches the backs and hips while strengthening the abs.

•**Stand-alone "activity panels."** One panel has a bar that you lean against to do push-ups (without getting down to the ground), another a bar that you lift over your head to strengthen your shoulder muscles, a third instructs you on how to do easy mini squats, while a fourth has handles that you turn for upper body cycling.

Fitness Benefits—and Beyond

Most multigenerational outdoor fitness parks cover the four key elements of fitness—aerobic activity, strength training, balance and flexibility. Strength training is particularly important as we age, says Chhanda Dutta, PhD, chief of the clinical gerontology branch in the National Institutes of Health's division of geriatrics and clinical gerontology. As we age, it's common to lose muscle mass, but strengthening muscles is key to enjoying our favorite activities and hobbies…and having a good quality of life. Balance is often overlooked, too—by both young and older adults. "It isn't until we run into balance problems that we realize we need to work on it," says Dr. Dutta.

While there isn't much academic research on fitness parks per se, one Finnish study of people aged 65 to 81 found that those who spent time at a fitness park experienced significant improvements in balance, speed and coordination after just three months. There are benefits beyond fitness, too. One is social, creating ways to get older people, who are often socially isolated, together. The other is motivational—having a buddy to exercise with is a proven way to stick with your exercise program.

If that sounds good, check with your local park administration, senior center or, if you're considering it, retirement community. If no multigenerational fitness parks are available near you, you may want to advocate that one gets built in your neighborhood. Try contacting your local parks and recreation department. Also check out these companies that sell senior-friendly playground equipment—LifeTrail, Triactive America and Greenfields. And if a senior playground pops up nearby, swing by and give it a whirl. Don't let the young have all the fun!

Appendix 4
VERY PERSONAL

How Women Can Feel Sexier Again (Without Popping a Pill)

Kathryn Hall, PhD, a licensed psychologist and sex therapist in private practice, Princeton, New Jersey. She is president-elect of the Society for Sex Therapy and Research, and author of *Reclaiming Your Sexual Self: How You Can Bring Desire Back into Your Life.* DrKathrynHall.com

If you're a woman, everyone wants to help you with your sex drive.

The medical profession may classify you as having hypoactive sexual desire disorder (HSDD)…aka, low libido. The drug industry wants to sell you its latest pill.

The good news: If low sex drive bothers you, there are better ways than popping a pill to rekindle the flames of desire.

Beyond the Little Pink Pill

The pharmaceutical industry is excited about *flibanserin* (Addyi), the first-ever drug approved for low libido in women, but many doctors and mental health professionals aren't so jazzed about it. It doesn't move the desire needle much, and there are worrisome side effects. And did you know that you're supposed to take it every day…but can't take it if you drink alcohol?

Even the HSDD diagnosis itself is controversial. "There is no evidence that hypoactive sexual desire disorder is a medical condition," according a report in *Journal of Medical Ethics.* The author documents the extensive marketing campaign that the pharmaceutical industry sponsored to convince physicians that HSDD is, in fact, real—and thus needs to be treated with a drug.

Still, there's no question that many women do struggle with a lack of desire, and that it can have real, sometimes painful, effects on their sense of well-being, as well as on their relationships. If you're dealing with lagging libido—and you can't or don't want to try the new "little pink pill"—what can you do about it?

To find out, we spoke with noted sex therapist Kathryn Hall, PhD, a psychologist in Princeton, New Jersey.

Low Libido Is Very Common and Very Normal

There are many, many reasons why women lose desire for sex—relationship problems, stress, fatigue, body image issues, hormonal changes in menopause, medications such as antidepressants, as well as depression itself. But you don't have to have a reason. *Many women don't. Here's why…*

It's very common for women to lose sexual desire as a relationship progresses over time from lust to love.

We know from a lot of studies that for many women, desire—their spontaneous lust—seems to wane in midlife. It's a normal pattern to lose that sort of lustful feeling, and it doesn't mean there's something wrong with you. The truth is, there's no "normal" when it comes to desire and how it plays out. If you don't want to have sex very often, or at all, and that doesn't bother you or your partner (if you have one), that's fine. Your desire, or lack thereof, is only a concern if it's distressing for you or problematic for your relationship.

If it does bother you, on the other hand, here are some suggestions that have worked for many couples…

Rekindling Desire

For women, what often replaces lust is "responsive desire"—getting in the mood after things have already gotten going because her partner has taken the initiative. That's perfectly fine for many couples. But some partners may resent always having to initiate sex. And many women miss the excitement of lust and eventually start to feel like sex is an obligatory chore, something they have to do so their significant others don't get angry. Fortunately, many couples work with these challenges to improve their sex lives, although it's not necessarily an easy road. *Here are some helpful strategies...*

• **Be realistic about sex, but don't give up on it.** Now that you know that a lot of women struggle with a low sex drive, you can work on bringing desire back into your life. You've made a decision that you need sex in your life and in your relationship and that you're going to put some energy and effort into it. It's not going to happen naturally. And that's OK.

• **Have maintenance sex.** A lot of couples who stay sexual throughout their life span have what is called "maintenance sex." They think, "OK, it has been a while and I don't really feel like it but, you know what? I'm going to put some effort into it because we need sex in our life and in our relationship. These couples understand that bad sex happens and boring sex happens, but they still make lovemaking a priority because most of the time sex is satisfying.

• **Set yourself up for success.** The first step is to get out of the rut of feeling that sex is a chore. Start by challenging the belief that you never want to have sex with your partner. Think about the occasions when you enjoy it more, such as when you've just shared a nice time doing something together, and choose those kinds of situations for initiating sex—rather than if it's late and you have to get up early and go to work the next morning, or when you've been fighting.

• **Reengage with your own desire.** You may feel like you want to get sex over as quickly as possible. For many women, that means focusing only on satisfying their partners to get the deed done. Try slowing down and paying attention to what you need and want sexually. Put on some clothing that makes you feel sexy. Watch some erotica or, if you've ever used one, get your vibrator out. Have a glass of wine if that helps. Do these things not because you think it's going to turn your partner on, but because it's going to turn you on. And don't forget to clue your partner

into what you like. He or she is probably dying to know!

• **Make an effort to initiate sex. This is probably the furthest thing from your mind,** but it may be a big deal to your partner. Often, the man feels, "Look, I'm always the one that initiates this, and I don't like doing that. I want to be desired." Of course he does, right? Men in their midlife want to feel like, "Hey, I'm still vital and attractive and desirable," and, if his partner never wants to initiate sex with him, it doesn't feel great. Being more mindful about initiating sex from time to time can go a long way toward making your partner feel physically cherished—and that can only reap benefits for you.

---

12 Things You Should Know About the New "Female Viagra"

Article titled "Evaluation of Flibanserin: Science and Advocacy at the FDA," by researchers at University of Pittsburgh, Medical College of Wisconsin, Milwaukee, and Johns Hopkins Bloomberg School of Public Health, Baltimore, published in *Journal of the American Medical Association.*

The "little pink pill" called Addyi (pronounced "ADD-ee"—aka "female Viagra") has been approved by the FDA—five long and contested years after it was first submitted. It's the first US prescription medication for female low-sex drive. If you're a woman and low libido is taking a toll on your intimate relationship, you're likely intrigued by a new drug designed to boost desire and improve your sex life.

"Addyi" is kind of a cuddly name, but we think there are a few things you should know about this new drug, whose generic chemical name is *flibanserin*, before you ask your doctor for a prescription. We'll let you know about the slick media campaign sponsored in part by the drug's manufacturer that put enormous political pressure on the FDA to approve a drug that it had previously been very wary of approving. In short, Addyi is hugely controversial and comes with many caveats and warnings…not to mention heated debate among mental health and sexual-health professionals—and women.

Here's what you need to know…

1. It's not really "female Viagra." That drug (and similar ones) works on performance, specifically increasing blood flow to the penis in men who are already aroused. Flibanserin is supposed to act on the step before that—the desire stage. It was originally developed as an antidepressant, and while it didn't work well for boosting mood, researchers noticed an influence on sex drive. Likely mechanism—promoting the release of dopamine, a "feel good" chemical in the brain.

2. It's only for low libido that causes distress. The mental health condition called "female sexual interest/arousal disorder" (formerly "hypoactive sexual desire disorder") is marked by an ongoing lack of fantasies and desire for sexual activity that causes you distress or severely strains your relationship with your partner…and isn't caused by another disorder, another medication or a relationship problem. In short, low libido itself isn't a disorder. If your sex drive, or lack thereof, isn't causing you distress, you don't need Addyi.

3. Not everyone thinks this disorder is… real. No one's contesting that some women experience distressing low libido, but some clinicians say female sexual desire is often over-medicalized—and that it's doubtful that low desire can be effectively treated with a drug. There's debate about this in the medical and psychological health communities.

4. It's not very effective. Women on the drug report small improvements in libido at best. Only about 8% to 13% of women said they were "much improved" or better in terms of desire or sexually satisfying events. Supporters of the drug argue that these improvements, while seemingly small, are meaningful to the women who have them.

5. It has to be taken every day. Unlike Viagra, Addyi is not an "on-demand," fast-acting aid to sex. It's a pill that you take every day, so you have to commit to it—and its side effects—for months, if not years.

6. It's expensive. Addyi is about as expensive on a monthly basis as Viagra, which can cost as much as $400 for 10 pills—typically, a month's supply.

7. It was rejected twice before. The FDA voted against approving flibanserin in 2009 because it wasn't effective enough. In 2013, new trials found it to be effective based on a different parameter, but it was rejected again. This time the agency cited safety concerns, including a risk for low blood pressure, fainting and drowsiness. Research shows that 28.6% of those taking the drug experienced "adverse events" related to sedation or low blood pressure, versus 9.4% of those taking a placebo. The drug can also cause nausea, which, while not a safety issue, isn't exactly an aphrodisiac either.

8. Side effects are still a concern. Those side effects are still there, but now it's recommended to be taken only at night, so drowsiness is less of an issue. New data did reassure the FDA panel that women who took the pill at night were OK to drive the next day. How that works if you're, say, a shift worker who needs to drive at night isn't clear.

9. You can't drink alcohol if you take it. Alcohol makes side effects such as drowsiness and low blood pressure worse. Critics argue that it's unreasonable to expect women who do drink alcohol to stop entirely for the duration of the time they take this drug…and the combination can be dangerous. We'll know how bad the alcohol/Addyi combo is only after women start combining the two in the real world, however. Why? The only study about how alcohol interacts with flibanserin presented to the FDA had just 25 subjects… and 23 of them were men! Many other medications also interact with flibanserin and can make its side effects worse—anxiety medications, sleep aids, oral contraceptives, drugs for yeast infections and more.

10. The FDA was under extraordinary public pressure to approve the drug. After the unfavorable 2013 ruling, an advocacy group called Even the Score was formed to campaign for "gender equality" in treatments for sexual dysfunction. The group—which gets funding from Sprout Pharmaceuticals, the makers of Addyi—claims there are 26 sexual dysfunction drugs for men and none for women. In reality, there are zero low-sexual-desire drugs for men (again, there's a difference between a libido drug and a performance drug). Even the Score has been accused of unfairly politicizing the FDA's rulings on flibanserin.

11. It wasn't a unanimous decision. When the FDA advisory committee voted to recommend approving the drug in 2015, 18 members voted yay, but six voted nay. That shows there are still significant questions about the medication's risks versus its benefits.

12. It's approved only for premenopausal women. That's the only group for whom the FDA has approved this drug. Sprout is now doing studies on postmenopausal women…and may study men in the future, too. But it's not approved for those groups, and it isn't known whether it will work or be safe for them.

Figuring Out What's Right for You

If you do decide to get a prescription, you and your doctor will need to be aware of the many contraindications of this new drug… and that you're sure you're fine with a no-alcohol lifestyle.

If you're postmenopausal and considering trying to get flibanserin as an off-label medication, you may be better off with another medicine that has been shown to help women with low libido—low-dose testosterone. It's not approved by the FDA for this purpose, but many ob/gyns prescribe it to older women for this issue.

Of course, there are also many nondrug ways for woman to enhance libido, including food, flowers, herbal love potions, natural aphrodisiacs…plus a libido-boosting mindset and keener sexual intelligence.

Natural Alternative to "Viagra" for Women

The new "female Viagra" boosts libido only moderately. Unlike Viagra for men, which increases penile blood flow, flibanserin affects the brain and changes levels of serotonin, norepinephrine and dopamine to enhance sexual mood. Side effects include dizziness, fatigue, anxiety, dry mouth, insomnia and nausea.

Natural alternative: ArginMax, which has been shown in clinical studies to boost women's sexual response. It contains L-arginine (an amino acid), herbs, vitamins and minerals. Side effects include headache and nausea.

Laurie Steelsmith, ND, LAc, medical director of Steelsmith Natural Health Center, Honolulu, and author of *Great Sex, Naturally.*

6 Libido Busters for Women—Solved!

The North American Menopause Society, The University of Texas at Austin, Hackensack University Medical Center in New Jersey, University of Guelph in Ontario, Canada.

Laurie Steelsmith, ND, LAc, licensed naturopathic physician and acupuncturist in private practice in Honolulu and coauthor of *Great Sex, Naturally: Every Woman's Guide to Enhancing Her Sexuality Through the Secrets of Natural Medicine.* DrLaurieSteelsmith.com

Marsha Lucas, PhD, licensed psychologist and neuropsychologist in private practice in Washington, DC, and author of *Rewire Your Brain for Love: Creating Vibrant Relationships Using the Science of Mindfulness.* RewireYourBrainForLove.com

Ladies, what's holding your libido back? Let's fix that.

If sex has lost its thrill, if it feels more like a chore than ever, you're not alone. Starting in the 30s, lack of desire is the biggest sexual problem women report.

Maybe your sex drive is just fine, thank you very much—or it is low but you're OK with that. Great. But if low sexual desire bothers you, if it's taking a toll on your romantic relationship and your quality of life, you want solutions.

Sure, the pharmaceutical industry wants to sell you its little pink pill, but Addyi (*flibanserin*) doesn't work very well and has plenty of side effects and drawbacks.

The good news is that there are many reasons why libido may flag—and thus, many ways to bring it back. The key is to identify what's holding you back and find solutions.

Here are some of the most common reasons their patients give for a lack of desire—and targeted solutions.

If sex hurts now…

Consider: A lubricant, a moisturizer or low-dose estrogen.

Vaginal dryness and thinning becomes a huge sexual obstacle for many women as they get older. But you don't have to just accept it as the new normal. There are over-the-counter products that can help. Start with a lubricant that's used during sex to make things go…more smoothly. If that doesn't quite do the trick, add in a moisturizer such as Replens. Moisturizers are used regularly (not just before sex) and have a longer-lasting effect than lubricants. Many women use both lubricants and moisturizers. If those aren't enough, some perimenopausal and postmenopausal women find relief with a prescription for low-dose estrogen. You can get this in the form of a tablet (a vaginal suppository), a cream or even a vaginal ring. According to The North American Menopause Society, these products aren't absorbed much beyond the vagina, so they don't carry the same health risks as hormone-replacement therapy. They make vaginal tissue thicker and more flexible so that sex is more comfortable.

If hot flashes keep you from getting in the mood…

Consider: The Peruvian herb maca.

This is one of naturopathic physician Laurie Steelsmith's favorite natural remedies for a lagging libido. Maca balances the entire hormonal system, helps to reduce stress hormones (which can sap energy), increases sex drive and alleviates desire-dampening symptoms of menopause such as hot flashes, night sweats and insomnia. (It can also help men improve sperm quality.) The recommended dose for women is 1,000 milligrams twice a day. As with any supplement, talk with your doctor first, especially if you have high blood pressure, since maca may increase blood pressure.

If your mood meds are dampening your desire…

Consider: A non-SSRI antidepressant—or exercise.

SSRIs, which are prescribed for depression or anxiety, can have the unfortunate side effect of killing desire, arousal and orgasms. Not all antidepressants work this way, though, so talk to your doctor about an SSRI alternative such as *bupropion* (Wellbutrin) or *duloxetine* (Cymbalta). If switching meds isn't an option for you, being more physically active could help. A 2013 study from The University of Texas at Austin found that 30 minutes of exercise just before sex improves libido and sexual functioning for women on antidepressants.

A possible explanation: Aerobic activity brings blood flow to the genitals. In case you're wondering, the same sexy effect has also been shown in other studies on depressed women who aren't taking mood medications…and in healthy nondepressed women. Of course, exercise is a great mood lifter in general and can help treat depression, so it's a win not only in the bedroom—but in your life.

If you can't stop thinking about your body…

Consider: Being more "mindful."

Many women lack awareness of sensation and arousal during sex because we're too busy thinking about the grocery list or knocking around self-doubts like, Do I look fat right now? If this sounds like you, try practicing mindfulness in the bedroom, suggests neuropsychologist Marsha Lucas, PhD, author of *Rewire Your Brain for Love: Creating Vibrant Relationships Using the Science of Mindfulness.*

The key: Being attuned to the present moment, without judgment. The famous sex researchers Masters and Johnson coined a technique called sensate focus that can help with awareness during sex. To practice sensate focus, you and your partner take turns experiencing what it's like to touch and be touched—when he or she runs his fingers up and down your back, for example—in both nonsexual and sexual ways. This exercise helps you pay attention to the experience so you can enjoy it more.

If you're just never in the mood...

Consider: Low-dose testosterone.

You may think of testosterone as a male hormone, but women have it in their bodies, too, and some doctors think it's actually important for female desire. This hormone gradually declines in women after peaking in their 20s. Some ob-gyns swear by it for their postmenopausal patients dealing with desire issues. Testosterone products aren't FDA-approved for women, but your ob-gyn can still prescribe them off-label to you if you're in menopause. To limit side effects, you need a special low-dose preparation—often 1/10th the amount used for men—which your health-care provider can order at a compounding pharmacy.

Warning: Never use a testosterone product designed for men.

If it's not like what you remember...

Consider: Adjusting your expectations.

That may sound like settling, but here's the thing—experts say that many of us have unrealistic expectations about what sex should be like in our long-term relationships. Very often, we want it to be just as thrilling as it was in the early days. Research has also found that, for every month a woman is in a relationship, her desire lessens a bit. Simply knowing this might help you—and your partner—stress about it less. And knowing that sex usually changes over time (even with the same partner), and that this doesn't necessarily mean anything is wrong with the relationship, can keep us motivated to keep the spark alive. For more tips, see *How Women Can Feel Sexier Again (Without Popping a Pill)* on page 344.

Suppository Eases Vaginal Dryness

Elizabeth Kavaler, MD, urology specialist, Lenox Hill Hospital, New York City.
Menopause, news release.

For postmenopausal women, suppositories containing the hormone DHEA may reduce vaginal dryness, discomfort and pain during sex without raising overall estrogen levels, researchers report.

DHEA is an anti-aging hormone produced by both women and men. In supplement form, it is used to improve thinking skills in older people. But DHEA is also a hormonal precursor of estrogen and testosterone, so some women who have low levels of certain hormones take it to improve well-being and sexuality, according to the U.S. National Library of Medicine.

"Although this medication is considered 'hormonal,' the mechanism appears to be primarily local with minimal side effects beyond vaginal discharge from the suppository," said Dr. JoAnn Pinkerton, executive director of the North American Menopause Society (NAMS).

Generally, without hormonal treatment after menopause, vaginal tissues shrink and produce less moisture, leading to discomfort during sex, and vaginal and urinary problems, according to background information in the study.

In this phase 3 clinical trial, 325 women who used the DHEA suppository daily saw significant improvements in vaginal dryness after 12 weeks, compared to 157 women using a placebo.

"Its action seems to be entirely within [vaginal] cells, and no significant amount of sex hormone gets released into the circulation," Pinkerton said in a society news release.

"That means that intravaginal DHEA avoids the raised hormone levels that might stimulate breast tissue or the lining of the uterus, which are concerns for women at risk of estrogen-sensitive cancers, or cancer recurrence, in these organs," she said.

The findings were published online in the journal *Menopause*, a NAMS publication.

One woman's health expert noted that DHEA may be a better option than estrogen treatments for some women.

"Intravaginal DHEA is a good alternative to estrogen creams in postmenopausal women with vaginal atrophy that manifests as vaginal dryness and pain with intercourse," said Elizabeth Kavaler, MD, an urology specialist at Lenox Hill Hospital in New York City.

"Intravaginal DHEA does not increase a woman's exposure to the effects of estrogen that concern many women, like endometrial hyperplasia [thickening of the lining of the uterus that can raise the risk for cancer] and breast cancer risk," Dr. Kavaler added.

Help for Clitoral Pain

Women with clitoral pain, itching or burning may have a fungal problem. Flare-ups of the yeast Candida, a common fungus, can be triggered by antibiotics or certain other drugs, alcoholic drinks or a diet with too much sugar or gluten.

Self-defense: Reduce consumption of sugar, starch and alcohol. Eat plenty of garlic. Treat the affected area with coconut oil (three or four times daily) or drink three drops of oil of oregano daily in a glass of water.

Also helpful: Swallow one olive leaf capsule twice daily after meals. Insert a gauze-wrapped garlic clove in the vagina for 30 minutes a day.

If the problem persists for more than a week, consult a physician, who may suggest using nystatin, tioconazole or another pharmaceutical.

Barbara Bartlik, MD, sex therapist in private practice and clinical assistant professor of psychiatry and obstetrics, Weill Cornell Medical College, New York City. She is past president of the Women's Medical Association.

Good-Bye, Thigh Hairs

Karen Burke, MD, PhD, associate clinical professor of dermatology, Mount Sinai Hospital, and research scientist and dermatologist in private practice, both in New York City. She has written numerous articles and books, including *Great Skin for Life*.

Some women don't mind those coarse hairs that creep down past the panty line and onto the inner thighs—but some do mind. A lot. *Options...*

•**Shaving.** This is the cheapest, fastest, safest way for most women to get rid of pubic hair on the thighs. The problem is that running a razor over this sensitive area may irritate the skin.

Secret to preventing irritation: Be sure to wait three minutes after applying shaving cream before you use the razor, so hair has time to soften. You can use soap instead of shaving cream if you prefer—but don't skimp on the amount of soap or neglect to wait the three minutes. For the closest shave, it's best to shave against the grain of the hair (for instance, shave upward if your hair grows downward).

To prevent breakouts caused by clogged hair follicles, apply *benzoyl peroxide* (a topical antibacterial and anti-inflammatory medication often used for acne) to the area once or twice daily. Benzoyl peroxide is sold over-the-counter at pharmacies and comes in gel and lotion form. There are even shaving creams that contain benzoyl peroxide—check labels. If your breakouts are not cured with topical benzoyl peroxide, you should see an American Board of Dermatology–certified dermatologist who can prescribe medication or recommend permanent hair removal by laser treatment.

•**Depilatory.** This is a cream that breaks down hair's chemical bonds. Because hair is removed right down to the bottom of the follicle (not just cut off at the skin's surface, as with shaving), a depilatory leaves skin smooth for several weeks. To reduce the risk for skin irritation, use a product made specifically for the pubic area, such as Nair Bikini Cream. Always test it on a small patch of skin before using on the whole area.

Beware: Some women develop a sensitivity to depilatories over time. So, even if you've used a product several times before with no problem, be prepared to stop if any signs of irritation appear.

• **Laser.** The laser's pulsed light is absorbed by the pigment in the hair, heating up the strands and permanently destroying the hair follicles.

But: Laser works only on dark hair—blonde, light brown or light red hair does not have enough melanin to absorb the light. Three to four treatments six to eight weeks apart typically eliminate upper thigh hair for good.

Caution: To minimize the risk for scarring or unintended lightening of the skin, have laser treatments done by a doctor or nurse, not by nonmedical salon personnel.

Cost: $250 or more per treatment.

• **Electrolysis.** For light-colored hair, this is the best permanent solution. It delivers an electrical current that destroys follicles one at a time, so it takes longer and is more uncomfortable than laser treatments. A topical numbing cream applied 30 minutes in advance minimizes discomfort. The number of sessions needed depends on how many hairs you want to eliminate.

To reduce the risk for scarring or pigmentary spotting of the skin, always use a professional electrologist who is accredited by the American Electrology Association.

Cost: $50 to $175 per session. Never use a home electrolysis unit, which can cause burns or leave scars.

Treat Cystic Acne from the Inside Out

Andrew Rubman, ND, medical director, Southbury Clinic for Traditional Medicines, Southbury, Connecticut. SouthburyClinic.com.

Acne—it's not just for kids anymore. Actually, it never was. Whether or not you were plagued by pimples in high school, you can have acne as an adult...after age 50, 15% of women (and 7% of men have acne). Cystic acne is the most severe form—not just pimples but embedded larger cysts that often are red and inflamed and cause scars.

Dermatologists have many interventions for cystic acne. Ointments that contain *benzoyl peroxide*, for example, can dry out oils that clog pores and inhibit acne-causing bacteria. Topical antibiotics and retinoids (vitamin A derivatives) can also work. If they don't, systemic medications may be prescribed, ranging from low-dose antibiotics to hormones to oral retinoids. These treatments often are effective, but like all medications, they have risks and side effects, some serious.

If you're concerned about going too far down that path, you can improve your acne by taking a natural approach. The trigger for acne is often the gastrointestinal system—specifically, the liver. Improve digestion and liver function, and cystic acne often resolves on its own.

The Digestion Connection

It might sound far-fetched to think that something going on in your belly can cause pimples on your cheeks. But there's a strong connection. How can the liver affect the skin? Both organs—yes, your skin is an organ—are involved in ridding your body of toxins. Sebaceous glands act as backup organs of elimination for the liver for certain fat-soluble compounds. When digestion and liver function aren't good, oily toxins flow to the skin in excess, clogging pores and trapping dead skin cells that skin bacteria feed on. The result can be cystic acne.

To improve your acne from the inside out, the first thing you need to do is get your stomach digesting food properly. To do that, it needs to produce enough acid. When acid is too low, food may remain partially digested and fat-soluble compounds will not exit the liver sufficiently...so they get shuttled to the skin. Poor diet, stress and age all can prevent the stomach from producing enough acid.

So do drugs called *proton pump inhibitors,* such as Prilosec and Nexium, which have other health risks, too. Acne patients with chronic heartburn should take DuoZyme, a supplement that provides digestive enzymes such as pepsin along with betaine HCL...which mimics stomach acid. (See a health-care professional before taking this supplement, however, especially if you have an ulcer, which it can make worse.) And for everyone, chew food thoroughly, limiting fluid with meals to about one-half cup and entirely avoiding caffeine-containing beverages with meals (including that cup of coffee after a meal—wait at least an hour). These actions can help stomach acid remain at the proper level.

Improving Liver Function Through Nutrition

The next step: Support the liver. To do this, eat plenty of sulfur- and nitrogen-containing foods such as dark green, leafy vegetables and eggs. That promotes the production of bile, which is key to helping move fat-soluble compounds out of the liver efficiently. Dietary cholesterol (also in eggs) and B vitamins also promote bile production. Talk to your health-care provider about the proper dose of a B vitamin complex for you.

Why a Certain Fiber Helps Acne, Too

Changing your diet isn't always easy, and many people are impatient for results. Take the fiber supplement glucomannan, made from the root of the konjac plant, as well. It's a capsule that you take a half an hour before each meal, with plenty of water, and it can improve cystic acne within seven to 10 days. Glucomannan is often used as an appetite suppressant, but what makes it helpful for acne is that it gets down into the small intestines where it binds to bile acids. That helps move toxins out of the body more efficiently.

Getting Better...and Healthier

Improving diet and taking glucomannan capsules can improve at least 50% of cystic acne cases, with patients often seeing some progress within a few days and significant results in less than two weeks.

In the meantime, you can continue to use topical treatments recommended by your dermatologist or other health-care provider. A particularly good treatment is a face mask made from the Aveeno colloidal oatmeal bar soap. First, work up a stiff lather, then apply to your face, let it dry, and wash it off—morning and night. Also, squalene, a particularly effective moisturizer found in many cosmetics, can be applied to the skin without fear of clogging pores. It helps to reduce inflammation while also moisturizing. Mayumi is a good brand.

The best part of treating acne primarily from the inside out, through digestion and nutrition, says Dr. Rubman, is that it benefits not just the skin, but the functioning of the entire body. It's helpful for less severe forms of acne, too.

Antibiotic That Makes Birth Control Less Effective

Richard O'Brien, MD, associate professor of emergency medicine at The Commonwealth Medical College of Pennsylvania in Scranton. Dr. O'Brien, who died in 2015, was also a spokesperson for the American College of Emergency Physicians, ACEP.org, and a recipient of the group's Communications Lifetime Achievement Award.

Not all doctors agree that all antibiotics have an effect on oral contraceptives, but rifampin has been clearly shown to make the Pill less effective. To be safe, I tell women who are taking a course of antibiotics that is 15 days or less to continue taking their contraceptives to avoid irregular periods—but to not trust the contraceptives for birth control for 28 days, which is one full menstrual cycle. This will virtually eliminate the chance of any obstetrical surprises!

The use of antibiotics can be tricky. There are more significant side effects and interactions with these drugs than perhaps with any other medication. Diarrhea is a risk for anyone taking virtually any antibiotic. But other surprises include violent vomiting if you mix the antibiotic Flagyl with alcohol, and people using ciprofloxacin can suffer ruptured tendons.

Benefits of Sleeping in the Buff...

Michael Breus, PhD, sleep specialist in private practice in Los Angeles, and author of *Good Night: The Sleep Doctor's 4-Week Program to Better Sleep and Better Health.* TheSleepDoctor.com

There are many health benefits to sleeping naked (but it is inadvisable with small children around or pets in the bed). New research has found that sleeping in a chilly room (or staying cool by sleeping naked) increases brown fat, a healthy type of fat that burns calories to make heat. For the best night's sleep, aim for a bedroom temperature of about 65°F and keep your hands and feet warm.

Women (and men) who sleep in their underwear or tight pajamas are more likely to get genital infections due to trapped heat and moisture. But the best benefit of sleeping in the nude may be skin-to-skin contact between bed partners, which triggers the release of the feel-good hormone oxytocin. Studies have shown that oxytocin increases a feeling of connection between partners, relieves stress and lowers blood pressure. So it most certainly won't hurt to shed your winter PJs for a night or two to see if you like it.

Breakthrough Therapies for Women's Hair Loss

Shari R. Lipner, MD, PhD, an assistant professor of dermatology and assistant attending physician at the New York-Presbyterian Hospital/Weill Cornell Medical Center in New York City. Dr. Lipner is board-certified in dermatology, lectures nationally and has authored numerous research articles and book chapters.

If you were a woman suffering from hair loss 25 years ago, your only option was to cover your head with a wig.

Now: Female hair loss is highly treatable—most cases improve within a matter of months—using a variety of breakthrough therapies.

When Hair Loss Strikes

More than half of all women will experience significant hair loss (more than 100 hairs per day) in their lifetimes. Any woman who has this amount of hair loss should see a dermatologist right away to determine the cause.

Some forms of hair loss can be temporary (see next page), while others are typically permanent unless treated within a year of the start of symptoms. If the follicles remain dormant for too long or if there is scarring, stimulating hair regrowth may be impossible. Treatment works best when started at the first sign of hair loss.

Men who have hair loss tend to get a "receding hairline," while women get an expanding center part. This condition, known as female pattern hair loss (FPHL), is the most common type of hair loss in women.

Self-test: Part your hair in the center. With FPHL, the center part is no longer a thin, crisp line. It is wider—and in later stages, it takes on a Christmas tree appearance with balding "branches" extending out from the center.

FPHL is a chronic, progressive hereditary condition often caused by changes in levels of male hormones as women age. It gets worse over time, and the hair won't regrow on its own. That's why you need treatment.

The Best Medication

The only FDA-approved medication for women's hair loss is minoxidil. It has been available as 2% liquid for many years.

Newer treatment option: In 2014, the FDA approved extra-strength 5% *minoxidil* foam for women.

The 5% foam version has a higher concentration of medication and also causes fewer side effects than the liquid version, which contains *propylene glycol*—a trigger for allergic reactions in some women. Both versions, however, can cause hypertrichosis, a form of excess hair growth, particularly along the sides of the face.

Caveats: When using either form of minoxidil, it takes at least six months to see hair growth. Also, you must use the product indefinitely—discontinuing it will cause your new hair growth to fall out again. It costs about $40 a bottle and is not typically covered by insurance.

Even though minoxidil is available over the counter, it's wise to consult a dermatologist before using it. The cause of your particular hair loss may require a different treatment. For example, topical steroids or steroid injections are given for hair loss caused by the autoimmune condition alopecia areata. Finasteride, which is FDA approved for hair loss in men, is sometimes prescribed off-label for women who have elevated levels of male hormones.

When You Need More Help

While 80% of women in clinical studies can regrow hair with minoxidil, for the unlucky few who can't, there are some new treatments that may be worth considering...*

•**Platelet-rich plasma (PRP).** This procedure is thought to jump-start dormant hair follicles. With PRP, some of your own blood is spun down in a centrifuge to separate platelet-rich plasma. Nutrients are added to the plasma, and the mixture is injected into the scalp with small needles.

*To find a hair-loss specialist, go to the website of the International Society of Hair Restoration Surgery, ISHRS.org.

PRP is available in some clinics, but it has not been approved by the FDA. While early findings are moderately positive, most practitioners believe the best results are for PRP combined with minoxidil treatment or hair follicle transplants. PRP is not covered by insurance and costs more than $1,000 for a single treatment, which may need to be repeated every three to six months.

•**Laser phototherapy.** With laser treatments, the idea is that light can stimulate hair growth at the level of the follicle. A few small studies have shown good results with no reported side effects, but there are no long-term studies. Two laser therapies that have been cleared by the FDA...

•**Theradome,** which looks like a bike helmet with 80 tiny lasers inside. It is available online for $895 and should be used for 20 minutes at least twice a week for 12 to 24 weeks.

•**HairMax LaserComb,** which looks like a cordless phone with light-emitting bristles. You turn it on and hold it over one spot on your head until a beep signals you to move it to another location. It is used three times a week. The base model costs $295 and is available online.

•**Hair loss camouflage.** Scalp micropigmentation is a permanent tattoo applied by a trained physician in a stippling pattern on the scalp to fill in areas of hair loss. It effectively disguises areas of hair loss and scars. Cost generally runs from $1,000 to $5,000.

Temporary Hair Loss

For about 20% of women who suffer from hair loss, the condition is temporary.

Here's why: Hair can function as the proverbial canary in the coal mine—follicles react to unhealthy body changes before we know anything might be wrong. Fix the problem, and hair grows back.

Consult a dermatologist to see if one of these conditions could be causing your hair loss...

•**Extreme stress.** A death in the family, hospitalization, moving to a new house or other life-altering change can cause hair follicles to go dormant, and hair falls out several months later. Typically, hair will regrow within a few months, once stress levels are reduced.

•**Weight loss/poor nutrition.** For healthy hair, you need to eat a well-balanced diet. Rapid weight loss, eating disorders and crash diets low in protein can cause hair to fall out. Your doctor may recommend a multivitamin or other supplement if you have any deficiencies and will likely check your iron levels. Healthful eating is all you need to regrow hair, usually within several months.

•**Medical conditions.** Thyroid conditions, scalp infections and anemia can also cause hair loss. Treating these diseases can stop the hair from falling out.

•**Hairstyling practices.** Bleaching, straightening, relaxing or perming can temporarily (or sometimes permanently) damage the scalp and hair follicles.

What's Really Causing Your Gas and Bloating?

Douglas A. Drossman, MD, codirector emeritus at the University of North Carolina Center for Functional GI and Motility Disorders and professor emeritus of medicine and psychiatry at the University of North Carolina School of Medicine in Chapel Hill.

Ugh! Here comes another gas attack. Or maybe it's bloating that's got you feeling so out of sorts. If you're lucky, you can avoid gas and/or bloating by forgoing the usual triggers—carbonated drinks… some high-fiber foods such as beans…chewing gum…and artificial sweeteners and the fruit sugar fructose.

But sometimes the source of this all-too-common gastrointestinal (GI) discomfort isn't so obvious. If your symptoms don't ease within a few weeks…or they have no apparent reason and tend to come and go, you and your doctor may need to do some investigating. The following health problems can cause gas and/or bloating but often go undetected—especially in the early stages…

•**Aerophagia (air swallowing).** Swallowing too much air can stretch the stomach and cause bloating. This often occurs when people are experiencing anxiety or can even become an unconscious habit. It can also happen when chewing gum, using a straw or drinking carbonated beverages.

What to do: Consider stress-reducing activities like deep breathing, meditation or yoga. If symptoms are severe, see a counselor for stress-management techniques.

•**Irritable bowel syndrome (IBS).** As many as one in five adults experiences the chronic symptoms of IBS—abdominal pain, bloating, gas, diarrhea and/or constipation—to some degree. IBS can have many causes, but typically nerves in the GI tract are extremely sensitive to food and gas passing through the bowel, triggering discomfort.

What to do: An IBS diagnosis includes regular abdominal pain that is relieved by a bowel movement, along with symptoms of bloating, diarrhea and/or constipation.

If you have IBS, your doctor may prescribe antispasmodics, such as *dicyclomine* (Bentyl) and *hyoscyamine* (Levsin), that may help relieve your symptoms. Since stress can trigger IBS symptoms, try to manage it with yoga, massage, meditation and counseling, if needed.

•**Functional dyspepsia.** After eating, the stomach in a healthy adult can expand in volume up to four times its normal size. But with functional dyspepsia, the muscles don't relax properly and the stomach remains small, leaving you feeling full and bloated after just a few bites.

What to do: If symptoms are stress-related, relaxation techniques, such as deep breathing or biofeedback, may be effective. An antianxiety drug, such as *buspirone* (BuSpar), can also help because it helps to relax the stomach.

•**Celiac disease.** People with celiac disease are sensitive to gluten, a protein in wheat, barley and rye that can produce inflammation in the bowel, resulting in bloating, gas, abdominal cramps and diarrhea.

What to do: If you suffer from the digestive symptoms described above—especially if you also have any nutritional deficiencies and/or experience frequent fatigue—see your doctor. Celiac disease is diagnosed with a blood test followed by an endoscopic biopsy. By avoiding foods and products that contain gluten, most sufferers can eliminate symptoms. For a list of hidden sources of gluten, go to *Celiac.org*.

More serious but less common causes of gas and/or bloating...

•**Diverticulitis.** This condition occurs when small pouches in the walls of the colon become inflamed and/or infected—often due to small tears caused by stool trapped in the pouches. It not only causes gas and bloating but also pain in the lower left side of the pelvis, where pouches get infected.

What to do: If you're having severe abdominal pain with fever and vomiting, see your doctor right away—you could have a serious infection that requires antibiotics and possibly emergency surgery. Sometimes, however, diverticulitis is mild, and symptoms may improve if you apply heat to the painful area...go on a liquid diet—including clear broth, clear fruit juice (such as apple), gelatin and plain tea—for a few days to "rest" your digestive system...and/or take antibiotics if needed to treat an infection.

•**Gallstones.** They often cause no symptoms, but if gallstones block the duct where the gallbladder empties, the gallbladder stretches, resulting in distension and pain, as well as bloating and gas.

What to do: If you suffer bloating and gas, pain in the upper-right abdomen (where the gallbladder is located), nausea and fever, see your doctor. He/she will perform an ultrasound to check for gallstones. Gallstone removal, which is routinely performed via laparoscopic surgery or, in some cases, endoscopy, is often recommended.

•**Certain cancers.** With advanced colorectal cancer, the bowel can become blocked, which leads to gas, bloating and blood in the stool. Ovarian cancer often causes subtle symptoms that may include bloating and feeling full quickly.

What to do: With colorectal cancer, regular colonoscopies after age 50 (or after age 40 if a close family member has had the disease) will catch suspicious polyps before a malig-

nancy develops. Women who experience the symptoms described above for more than two or three weeks—especially if they are accompanied by pelvic pain and/or an urgent or frequent need to urinate—should see a gynecologist.

Quick Relief

If your gas and/or bloating is only occasional, consider trying...

•**Probiotics,** which promote the growth of "good" bacteria in the bowel. One study found that *Lactobacillus acidophilus* and *Bifidobacterium lactis* helped bloating by replacing the bad (gas-causing) bacteria with good (gas-relieving) bacteria in people with bowel disorders, such as IBS or functional dyspepsia. In another study, probiotics were found to relieve intestinal gas.

What to do: Try a daily probiotic in supplement form or via probiotic-rich fermented foods and beverages such as kefir, miso or kimchi.

Good News for IBS Sufferers

Mark Pimentel, MD, director of the GI Motility Program and Laboratory at Cedars-Sinai Medical Center in Los Angeles, where he specializes in irritable bowel syndrome. He is the creator of the IBS blood tests described in this article. (Disclosure: Dr. Pimentel receives consulting fees from Commonwealth Laboratories, which produces the tests.)

If you're unlucky enough to get hit by a day or two of diarrhea, you can write it off as a short-lived bit of unpleasantness. But for those with irritable bowel syndrome (IBS), diarrhea—as well as constipation and/or other digestive problems—can be a way of life.

Imagine that you are afraid to leave the house because you might get caught without a bathroom. You suffer from gut-wrenching abdominal pain...daily bloating...and/or frequent (and unpredictable) bouts of diarrhea or constipation—or both. That is what it's like to live with IBS.

A Challenge to Diagnose

IBS is the most common gastrointestinal problem in the US. Studies estimate that 10% to 15% of adults—as many as 37 million Americans—are affected to some degree. But without a definitive test, the approaches to diagnosis and treatment have been scattershot.

Problem: The same symptoms that occur with IBS can also be caused by other, more serious conditions (such as inflammatory bowel disease, ulcerative colitis and diverticulitis). As a result, IBS patients often undergo a multitude of tests (including stool analyses, blood tests and imaging tests) as well as doctor visits to rule out what's not causing their problems.

Because IBS has traditionally been so difficult to diagnose, many doctors have not fully understood the disorder and blamed their patient's IBS symptoms on stress, anxiety and/or depression…or told them that their symptoms are "all in your head" and recommended psychological counseling.

Now that's all about to change.

Latest development: Rather than spending months—or even years—going from doctor to doctor seeking help for this condition, new blood tests allow IBS patients to learn within a matter of days what's causing their symptoms so they can begin treatment much sooner.

Uncovering the Cause of IBS

The underlying cause of IBS was not known until pioneering research at Cedars-Sinai Medical Center in Los Angeles recently found that the majority of IBS patients were at some point infected with Salmonella, Escherichia coli or other harmful (and often food-borne) bacteria.

The bacteria secrete toxins that damage the intestinal nerves that control motility, the synchronized contractions that move digested food through the intestine. The nerve damage, which persists long after the infection is gone (and perhaps indefinitely), explains all of the typical IBS symptoms.

The blood tests that researchers have developed identify evidence of past infections that can cause IBS. This means that patients can describe their symptoms to a doctor, receive the new blood tests and get an accurate diagnosis after a single visit to a doctor.

Doctors send the patient's blood samples to a laboratory (Commonwealth Laboratories, *IBSchek.com*) to be analyzed. The results are generally available within 24 hours.

Typical cost: $500, which is usually covered by insurance.

How Your Diet Can Help

If you get a diagnosis of IBS, what you eat can affect how well you manage your symptoms. (If you simply suspect that you have IBS but have not been diagnosed with it, it's also worth trying the dietary changes below.) *What helps…*

• **Avoid "FODMAP" foods.** Scientists have identified a class of hard-to-digest carbohydrates that ferment in the small intestine and increase IBS symptoms. These so-called FODMAP (shorthand for fermentable oligosaccharides, disaccharides, monosaccharides and polyols) foods include wheat, dairy, onions, apples, high-fructose corn syrup, beans, stone fruits (such as apricots, nectarines and cherries) and artificial sweeteners (such as sorbitol and mannitol).

There's some evidence that people who feel better when they give up gluten are actually responding to the reduction in FODMAPs that occurs when they go on a gluten-free diet. No one loves restrictive diets—and a low-FODMAP diet is restrictive. But it can help if you stick with it. For a comprehensive list of FODMAP foods, go to *IBSDiets.org*.

• **Get less fiber.** In the past, doctors advised IBS patients to eat a lot of fiber to firm up stools and reduce diarrhea as well as constipation. We now know that too much fiber can increase bacterial overgrowth in the small intestine.

My advice: Limit your daily fiber intake to no more than 20 g to 35 g. For example, eat white bread (such as Italian) instead of whole wheat…avoid super-high-fiber cereals (more than 8 g of fiber per serving)...and limit beans, whole grains and other high-fiber foods.

Medication That Helps

While many IBS sufferers get relief from the dietary changes described in the main article, medication is usually also necessary. Until recently, there were only two drugs specifically approved for IBS—*alosetron* (Lotronex) for diarrhea-predominant IBS, or IBS-D...and *lubiprostone* (Amitiza) for constipation-predominant IBS, or IBS-C.

New options: In May, the FDA approved two new drugs, which may benefit a greater number of IBS patients...

• **Rifaximin (Xifaxan).** This drug is an antibiotic, but it isn't used to treat the infections that cause IBS (those infections are usually long gone by the time patients develop symptoms). Instead, it curtails the bacterial overgrowth in the small intestine that results from months or years of impaired motility that typically accompanies IBS symptoms. Rifaximin is taken orally three times a day, for 14 days. It is expected to become the first-line therapy for IBS-D, since it has far fewer side effects than Lotronex.

• **Eluxadoline (Viberzi).** This medication is an antidiarrheal. It targets opioid receptors in the intestine, while having little effect on similar receptors in the brain. This means that it's less likely to cause drowsiness or other side effects than other medications used to treat diarrhea. It improves stool consistency and reduces abdominal pain/cramping.

Natural Ways to Quiet Tremors

Monique Giroux, MD, a neurologist and medical director and cofounder of the Movement & Neuroperformance Center of Colorado in Englewood, CenterforMovement.org. She is the author of *Optimizing Health with Parkinson's Disease.*

Most people think of tremors—rhythmic trembling in your hands, voice, head or other parts of your body—as a red flag for neurological disorders such as Parkinson's disease and multiple sclerosis (MS).

That can be true. But this constant shakiness can also accompany a wide range of other conditions, including so-called essential tremor (ET), a chronic but harmless disorder that often is inherited and affects an estimated seven million Americans—a greater number than those affected by MS and Parkinson's disease. In some people, tremors also can occur as a side effect of common prescription drugs such as certain antidepressants, asthma inhalers, seizure medicines and immune-suppressing drugs. Even pain and anxiety can cause mild shaking or worsen tremors that are due to disease or medication.

If you suffer from tremors, there's no question how disruptive the problem can be to everyday life. Simple movements most of us take for granted—such as putting on make-up, eating or simply writing a check—can turn into a shaky endurance test.

But quieting tremors is no small feat. Medications such as antiseizure drugs and mild tranquilizers are effective only about half of the time and can have troubling side effects, including drowsiness and confusion. Injections of *botulinum toxin* (Botox) can help head and voice tremors but are less effective for hand tremors because weakness can result as a side effect. An invasive procedure called deep brain stimulation (DBS) is reserved for the worst cases. This treatment, which can be quite effective, involves surgically implanting electrodes in the brain that are connected to a pacemaker placed under the skin near the collarbone. Electrical pulses are continuously delivered to block the impulses that cause tremors.

Good news: If drugs or surgery aren't for you or leave you with lingering symptoms, several natural therapies can help calm tremors by easing the stress and altering the brain chemicals and emotional responses that exacerbate the condition.

Important: Before trying natural remedies, be sure to avoid caffeine, smoking and/or excess alcohol—all of which can worsen tremors. Also, make regular exercise (especially strength training) a priority—tremors are more common when muscles become fatigued. *Natural treatments to tame any type of tremor…**

Aromatherapy

Breathing in the aroma of certain flowers and herbs can reduce tremors by enhancing brain levels of gamma-aminobutyric acid (GABA), a widely circulated neurotransmitter with proven stress-fighting effects. Raising GABA levels helps calm the overexcited neurons that can worsen tremors. *What to try for tremors…*

• **Lavender.** This fragrant blue-violet flower has been shown in a number of small studies to produce calming, soothing and sedative effects when its scent is inhaled. Lavender essential oil is widely available and can be inhaled in the bath (add five to eight drops to bath water for a long soak) or by dabbing a drop on your neck or temples.

Supplements

Certain supplements can ease tremors by enhancing muscle relaxation and/or reducing the body's overall stress levels or load of inflammatory chemicals, which can play a role in tremors caused by neurodegenerative diseases. Check with your doctor to make sure these supplements don't interact with any medication you may be taking and won't affect any chronic condition you may have…**

• **Magnesium.** This mineral helps to regulate nerve impulses and muscle contraction. Magnesium-rich foods include sesame seeds, beans, nuts, avocados and leafy greens. To ensure that you're getting enough magnesium, consider taking a supplement.

*Consult your doctor before trying these therapies to determine the cause of your tremors and for advice on the approaches best suited to your situation.

**Because supplements aren't regulated by the FDA for purity, I advise looking for products that bear the "USP-verified" stamp on the label—this means they have met rigorous testing standards to ensure quality by the scientific nonprofit US Pharmacopeial Convention.

Typical dose to ease tremors: 200 mg to 400 mg daily.

• **Fish oil.** The omega-3 fatty acids in fish oil offer proven anti-inflammatory effects—systemic inflammation is implicated in neurodegenerative diseases such as MS and Parkinson's disease. Fish oil is abundant in fatty fish such as salmon, albacore tuna, mackerel and herring. Aim for two servings per week. If you don't like fish, consider trying a supplement.

Typical dose to ease tremors: 1,000 mg to 1,500 mg daily.

• **Valerian, skullcap and passionflower.** These calming herbs have been successfully used as part of a regimen to ease tremors. The supplements can be found in combination products, including capsules, teas and tinctures. Follow instructions on the label.

Beat Tremors with Your Mind

If you suffer from tremors, it's common to think—Oh no…my arm (or other body part) is shaking again…this is so embarrassing! I hate this! While such thoughts are perfectly natural when tremors emerge, they are potentially destructive when trying to calm your condition.

What helps: Mindfulness can reset this negative thought pattern so that you stop viewing tremors as a problem, which only leads to distress that often worsens the condition.

Mindfulness is more than just relaxation. Often done in conjunction with deep-breathing exercises, mindfulness helps you simply observe your thoughts, feelings and sensations and let them pass without judging them, labeling them or trying to control them. By reducing the distress you feel about the tremors, you are no longer fueling the condition.

You can learn mindfulness from CDs or books.

My recommendations: Consult your local hospital to see if it offers mindfulness-based stress-reduction classes. Also consider trying other mind-body therapies that may help, such as hypnosis, biofeedback and breath work.

Non-Surgical Fibroid Treatment Can Boost Your Sex Life

Marc Sapoval, MD, PhD, professor, clinical radiology, Hopital Europeen Georges-Pompidou, Paris, and Robert Vogelzang, MD, chief of vascular and interventional radiology, Northwestern Memorial Hospital, Chicago.

Scott Chudnoff, MD, director of gynecology, Montefiore Health System, New York City.

Society of Interventional Radiology annual scientific meeting and news release, Vancouver, Canada.

Women with bothersome uterine fibroids saw improvements in their sex lives and significant symptom relief a year after undergoing a type of non-surgical treatment called uterine fibroid embolization, a French study finds.

Nearly eight in 10 women who completed surveys a year after treatment reported improved sexual function, a measure that reflects pain, desire, arousal and satisfaction.

About nine in 10 had better overall quality of life, researchers said.

"UFE [uterine fibroid embolization] is not a new intervention," said Marc Sapoval, MD, PhD, one of the study coauthors. Dr. Sapoval is a professor of clinical radiology at Hopital Europeen Georges Pompidou in Paris.

"What's new in this data is the fact that we focused on sexual function," he said.

About Uterine Fibroids

Uterine fibroids are a type of solid tumor. They are usually non-cancerous. Fibroids can form in and around the uterus and within the uterine walls, according to the U.S. Office on Women's Health.

Women with fibroids often experience significant symptoms and discomfort, Dr. Sapoval said. These symptoms may include heavy menstrual bleeding, pain during sexual intercourse, and pelvic, back and leg pain.

Hysterectomy—removal of the uterus—is the only treatment that can guarantee fibroids won't return. But it's not the only treatment option available, the Office on Women's Health says.

Uterine Artery Embolization Explained

UFE, also known as uterine artery embolization, is one alternative to surgery.

For the procedure, an interventional radiologist makes a tiny snip in the skin of the groin. A thin tube is inserted in the artery at the top of the leg. Using real-time imaging, the tube is snaked into the uterine artery, which supplies blood to the uterus, the researchers explained.

Then, sand-sized particles are released, blocking blood flow to the tiny arteries that feed the fibroid. With the blood supply choked off, the tumor shrinks and dies, the study authors said.

Study Details

The study included more than 260 women from 25 centers throughout France who had the embolization procedure. The women completed assessments on their sexual function and quality of life before and one year after the procedure.

Initially, 189 women reported abnormally heavy menstrual bleeding. Just over 170 experienced pain due to fibroids, the study revealed. But a year after treatment, only 39 patients reported abnormal bleeding. And, only 42 still had pelvic pain, the study found.

After a year, the procedure was associated with significant improvement in all aspects of sexual function, the investigators found.

The study results were presented at the Society of Interventional Radiology's annual scientific meeting in Vancouver, Canada.

Implications

"Not only is UFE an effective treatment for uterine fibroids, but it allows women to return to a more normal life, increase their sexual desire, and enjoy an overall improved quality of life," Dr. Sapoval said.

One caveat: it's not recommended for women who want to get pregnant because there are still some unknowns about fertility after the procedure, he said.

Despite the positives, UFE is not widely used in the United States, noted Robert Vogelzang, MD. He's chief of vascular and interventional radiology at Northwestern Memorial Hospital in Chicago and a past president of the Society of Interventional Radiology.

"Sadly, the patients who have fibroids are often not being told about embolization," Dr. Vogelzang said.

Asked why doctors aren't talking about it, Dr. Vogelzang said he believes "it's largely an economic issue," implying that obstetrician/gynecologists have no financial incentive to recommend a treatment they don't perform.

Expert Commentary

Not everyone agrees, however. Scott Chudnoff, MD, said that most obstetricians and gynecologists are forthright in discussing all of the surgical and medical options for treating fibroids, including embolization. He's director of gynecology at the Montefiore Health System Moses Campus in the Bronx, New York.

If surgery would be risk for a woman, Dr. Chudnoff said he often highly recommends embolization. But there are a lot of factors that go into the final decision, he said. One is the tumor's location. Another is a woman's personal history with fibroids and whether she wants to get pregnant, he noted.

Better answers about which uterine fibroid treatments work best are likely on the horizon. The U.S. Agency for Healthcare Research and Quality is building a nationwide registry of women undergoing fibroid treatment at centers across the country through 2019. This data will allow researchers to compare the effectiveness of various approaches.

Learn what's being done to help women make informed decisions about fibroid treatment options through COMPARE-UF (Comparing Options for Management: Patient-centered Results for Uterine Fibroids), *compare-uf.org*.

Lack of Stem Cells May Be Key to Repeat Miscarriages

University of Warwick, news release.

A lack of stem cells in the lining of the uterus may cause recurrent miscarriages, a new study suggests.

"We have discovered that the lining of the womb in the recurrent miscarriage patients we studied is already defective before pregnancy," said research team leader Jan Brosens, a professor of obstetrics and gynecology at the University of Warwick in England.

Brosens said the researchers will use the findings to begin seeking solutions to the problem.

"I can envisage that we will be able to correct these defects before the patient tries to achieve another pregnancy. In fact, this may be the only way to really prevent miscarriages in these cases," Brosens said in a university news release.

Between 15% and 25% of pregnancies end in miscarriage. And one in 100 women trying to have children suffers recurrent miscarriages, defined as the loss of three or more consecutive pregnancies, the researchers noted.

Stem cells, meanwhile, have the potential to develop into many different cell types in the body, scientists say.

For the current study, the research team analyzed uterine lining samples from 183 women. They found that those who miscarried repeatedly had a lack of stem cells in the tissue.

The researchers noted that the lining has to renew itself after each menstrual cycle, miscarriage and birth. This shortage likely accelerates aging of the uterine lining, increasing the risk of miscarriage, they said.

"Cultured cells from women who had had three or more consecutive miscarriages showed that aging cells in the lining of the womb don't have the ability to prepare adequately for pregnancy," Brosens said.

The study was published in the journal *Stem Cells*.

"The real challenge now is to develop strategies to increase the function of stem cells in the womb lining," study coauthor Siobhan Quenby, a professor of obstetrics, said in the news release.

Quenby's research team began piloting new interventions to improve the lining of the womb in spring 2016.

The researchers' focus has been twofold, Quenby said. First, they want to develop new tests of the uterine lining, or endometrium, to improve the screening of women at risk of repeat miscarriages.

"Second, there are a number of drugs and other interventions, such as endometrial 'scratch,' a procedure used to help embryos implant more successfully, that have the potential to increase the stem cell populations in the womb lining," Quenby said.

The March of Dimes has more about miscarriage at *marchofdimes.org/complications/ miscarriage.aspx.*

INDEX